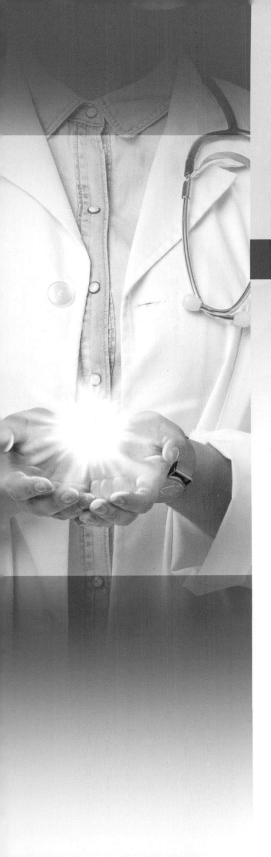

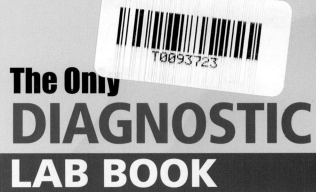

T0093723

The Only
DIAGNOSTIC
LAB BOOK
You'll Ever Need

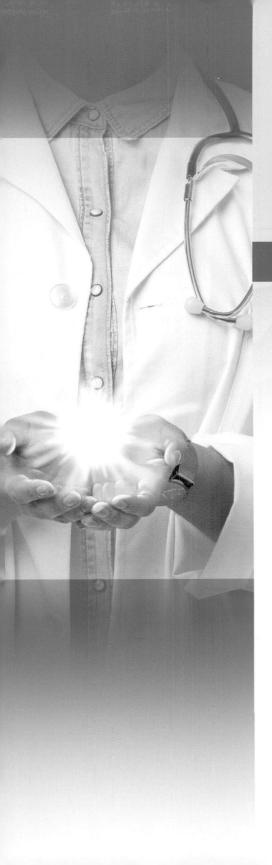

The Only
DIAGNOSTIC
LAB BOOK
You'll Ever Need

JONATHAN E. THALER, MD

MALCOLM S. THALER, MD

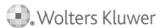
Wolters Kluwer

Philadelphia • Baltimore • New York • London
Buenos Aires • Hong Kong • Sydney • Tokyo

Acquisitions Editor: Matt Hauber
Development Editor: Amy Millholen
Editorial Coordinator: Venugopal Loganathan
Editorial Assistant: Parisa Saranj
Marketing Manager: Danielle Klahr
Production Project Manager: Frances Gunning
Manager, Graphic Arts & Design: Stephen Druding
Manufacturing Coordinator: Margie Orzech
Prepress Vendor: S4Carlisle Publishing Services

9 8 7 6 5 4 3 2 1

Printed in Mexico

Library of Congress Cataloging-in-Publication Data
ISBN-13: 978-1-975194-70-3
ISBN-10: 1-975194-70-5
Cataloging in Publication data available on request from publisher.

shop.lww.com

QUADM0324

Dedication

This is the easy part. To Tracey, Miles, Nancy, Ali, Ben, Eliana, and Maia. You inspire us and bring so much meaning and joy to our lives. We love you all very much.

Preface

There are, by our count, a gazillion lab tests out there. How do you know which ones to order when, which ones to avoid, and what they all mean? If you plow ahead without the tools to choose and interpret your patient's lab tests, things can get messy very quickly. Our intent with this book is to help you clear a path through the muddle so that you can find and understand the best tests for your patient.

This book is not intended to be encyclopedic. There are other excellent—and very large!—sources that can provide you with all the details of every lab test under the sun. That being said, we have packed a lot of information into these pages. And—we think most critically—our emphasis is always on how you can apply each test in clinical practice. We will explore the most common, most important, and most useful lab tests. We will point out those tests that fail to make the grade, and we will tell you why. This book is a practical guide. It is meant to be used.

We have tried our best to keep the text short and conversational. We will share the facts you need to know, the opinions of experts, and our own perspectives as well. Don't worry—we will let you know when we are offering you our own advice.

One quick word of caution: when it comes to the interpretation of lab results—for example, what is normal or abnormal in a given clinical context—there are many instances in which various experts and organizations disagree. In order not to be over-burdensome, we have selected those normal ranges and interpretations that we have found to be used most frequently. We point out when a test or its interpretation is particularly controversial. Don't hesitate to check with experts at your own institution whenever such a situation arises.

And now we need to pause and thank all the extraordinary clinicians—drawn from so many different backgrounds and clinical professions—who read, edited, and critiqued this book as we were creating it. We couldn't have done it without you: Shreya Chablaney, MD; Karmela Chan, MD; Matthew Copeland, DO; Doruk Erkan, MD, MPH; David Lam, MD; Erin Love, PA; James Malatack, MD; Virginia Malatack, MD; Amanda Reyes, MD; Anthony Rowe, MD; Jonathan Salik, MD; Varun Sharma, MD; Molly Shay; Ritu Shrotriya, MD; Lindsay Stagg, PA; and Alison Thaler, MD. We also want to thank all our friends at Wolters Kluwer, especially Joe Cho, Amy Millholen, Tom Conville, Venugopal Loganathan, Frances Gunning, and Bhuvaneswari Rajendran.

Now, welcome to *The Only Diagnostic Lab Book You'll Ever Need*. We are so pleased to have you on board!

Jonathan E. Thaler, MD
Malcolm S. Thaler, MD

Contents

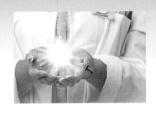

An Introduction, Because Every Book Should Have One

The average human body contains, by most estimates, more than 37 trillion (37×10^{12}) cells. Each cell carries out approximately one billion (1×10^9) chemical reactions every second. So it takes no great feat of mathematical wizardry to calculate that our bodies carry out 37×10^{21} chemical reactions every second. That is an insanely large number, way more than, for example, the number of stars in our Milky Way galaxy (a paltry 100-400 billion).

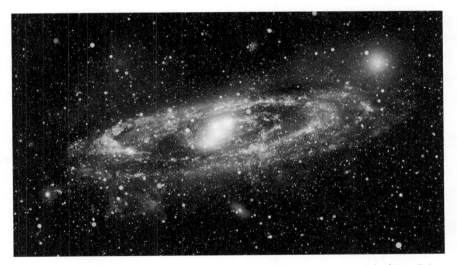

Figure I.1 Our Milky Way galaxy, 100,000 light years across, is a model of simplicity when you compare it to what is going on in our bodies every second. (Courtesy of NASA/Zakharchuk/Shutterstock.)

So when it comes to the practice of medicine, it is remarkable that we can ever figure out how things work and—perhaps more importantly—how they don't work when things go wrong. How extraordinary is it that we can draw a small tube of blood, often no more than a single milliliter's worth, and use it to diagnose so many disorders ranging from the barely consequential to the profound and life-altering?

That's what this book is about: lab tests—what they can tell us, what they can't tell us, which ones to order (and when), which ones *not* to order, and how to interpret them.

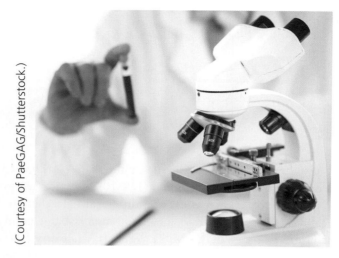

(Courtesy of PaeGAG/Shutterstock.)

We have divided the book into three major sections:

1. **Finding the Sweet Spot:** Here we get a chance to philosophize a bit, but don't worry—you won't be subjected to categorical imperatives or Cartesian dualism. This is where you will be introduced to the best ideas out there about:

   - what labs really tell you,
   - how to interpret normal and abnormal values (it's not as simple as you may think, but not outrageously difficult either), and
   - how to integrate the laboratory into the overall context of your patient in order to arrive—to the best of your ability—at an accurate diagnosis and help your patient achieve the best possible outcome.

   You will be introduced to Bayesian reasoning, the best way to figure out how to think about a particular test result, and how much confidence you should put in it. You will also become familiar with—and (we hope) really understand—terms such as sensitivity, specificity, predictive values, and likelihood ratios (no worries; with a few important exceptions the only math you will encounter in this book will be the page numbers).

2. **Profiles and Panels: Common Lab Tests That Come in Families:** Labs are rarely looked at in isolation, but are grouped into profiles that are used (and, alas, overused) frequently. Why certain profiles and not others? What are the pluses and minuses of ordering a particular profile for a particular patient? We'll answer these and many other questions besides.

   Because profiles are so widely used, you should not be surprised to learn that they include many of the most common lab tests available. You will be introduced to them here. In many ways, this section is the heart of the book.

3. **Other Tests You Need to Know:** There are a ton* of lab tests out there, way beyond those you will find in the most common profiles and panels. We can't cover them all, so we've picked out

---

*Not technically a ton; we don't actually know what they weigh (or even what that means), but there are a whole lot of them for sure

the most important and useful among them to help you work up everything from abdominal pain to arthritis to altered mental status to anemia (and we are still just in the A's!).

So let's get going. We are delighted to have you along for the ride. We have tried to make your journey both fun and rewarding. And because we like inspiring quotes, let's close this very brief introduction with this one from the great Nobel laureate, physicist, and teacher, Richard Feynman: *Nobody ever figures out what life is all about, and it doesn't matter. Explore the world. Nearly everything is really interesting if you go into it deeply enough.*

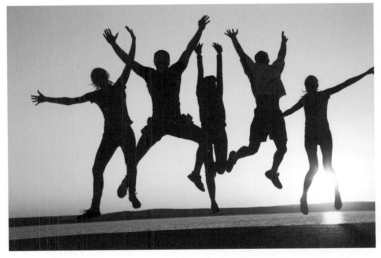

Figure I.2 By the time you have finished this book, we can't promise you will jump for joy, but your patients may! (Courtesy of YanLev Alexey/Shutterstock.)

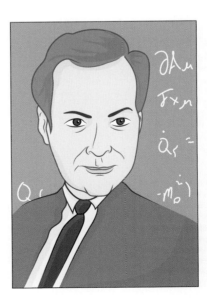

Figure I.3 Richard Feynman, who also knew a thing or two about the Milky Way galaxy.

Section 1
Finding the Sweet Spot

 What This Section Is All About

In this section, you will learn:

- How to think like a Bayesian: in other words, how to combine new lab results with what you already know about your patient in order to determine the likelihood of a particular diagnosis

- How to incorporate sensitivity, specificity, predictive values, and likelihood ratios—each a valuable shortcut for understanding how effective a particular lab test is in ruling in or out a diagnosis—into your analysis

- How "normal" and "abnormal" lab results are defined

- The key clinical factors that help you decide when and when not to order a particular lab test

It's easy to order a lab test. Anyone can do it. Just one click of the mouse or touchpad and you're done. Then you can sit back, turn off your brain, and wait for the numbers to come cascading in. And after all, who doesn't love numbers? Whereas so much of clinical medicine is subjective ("what does my patient really mean when she says she has chest *discomfort*?"), numbers seem so absolute and reliable.

Of course, it's not really so simple. Whereas a glucose of 150 mg/dL is always and inarguably 150 mg/dL, that number, precise as it is, has no meaning outside its clinical context. In a hospitalized patient with diabetes, a blood sugar of 150 mg/dL is typically considered normal (or at least good enough). In an otherwise healthy outpatient, the very same blood sugar could represent a new and concerning diagnosis of diabetes. In both cases, the number is the same, but the meaning and management are very different.

In this section, we are going to help you make sense of the numbers you will see. This will involve a little math (just a little, we promise), but much more importantly it will involve thinking (more than a little, but—after all—that's why you're here!).

The basic concepts underlying everything that follows are these:

- Order and interpret lab results only within their appropriate clinical context and only when they will affect your management; and

- Understand that a lab result (especially a single result in isolation) is almost never the same thing as an absolute, unequivocal answer, although it can help point you in the right direction.

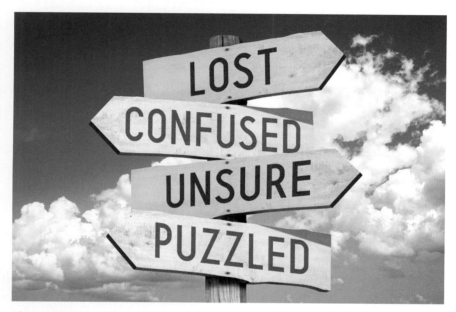

Figure S1.1 The differential diagnosis of many conditions can be long and complicated, filled with dead ends and wrong turns. The lab—when used appropriately—can help you find your way. (Courtesy of PX Media/Shutterstock.)

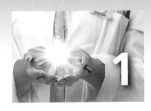

1 Bayesian Thinking

Thomas Bayes was a mathematician and theologian who devised a simple formula to describe the probability that a given hypothesis (in our case, a diagnosis) is true. But we care less about the formula (for those of you who are interested, we spell it out in the box below) than in the concept that underlies it: *Bayesian thinking.*

Bayes' Formula

$$P(A|B) = \frac{P(B|A)P(A)}{P(B)}$$

where

- $P(A|B)$—the probability of event A occurring, given event B has occurred
- $P(B|A)$—the probability of event B occurring, given event A has occurred
- $P(A)$—the probability of event A
- $P(B)$—the probability of event B

Know this formula exists. Don't memorize it.

According to Bayes, when deciding how likely a hypothesis (diagnosis) is, there are two things we care about:

1. Our prior knowledge, that is, what we already know

2. New (in our case, lab) results that alter that knowledge base

On the face of it this seems obvious and, in a way, it is. It turns out we use Bayesian thinking all the time in our daily lives.

Imagine sitting on the beach and looking out at the ocean extending out to the horizon in front of you. Your new results—what's in front of you right now—would suggest that the earth is flat. What prevents you from taking that piece of data to mean the earth really is flat?

Here's where your prior knowledge comes in. An overwhelming preponderance of previous evidence (eg, photos of the Earth from space) makes the concept of a flat Earth so unlikely that your observation today is very unlikely to shift your overall "diagnosis." In this case, the new data do not alter your conclusion at all.

Now let's consider another example. Suppose that you live on a beach near the ocean and—in a state of prelapsarian bliss—you have had no exposure to books, computers, radio, or TV. You look out at the horizon every day and think, "the earth is flat," a perfectly reasonable assumption. That's your baseline, your prior knowledge. Now along comes someone who happens to have a laptop with her. She shows you pictures of the Earth

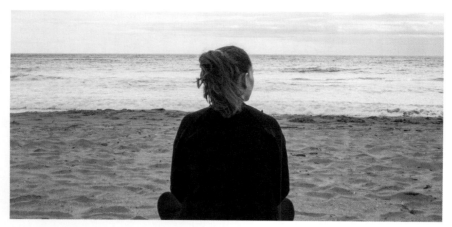

Figure 1.1 Sure looks flat to me! (Courtesy of Daniel VG/Shutterstock.)

taken from space. These new data will—at least should—have a profound impact on your hypothesis that the Earth is flat. Presumably, if you think like a Bayesian, your faith in your baseline belief will be substantially altered.

We can think of our prior knowledge as a baseline. In medicine, this baseline is what we use to establish the likelihood of a given diagnosis *before* ordering a new lab test. We call this likelihood the *pretest probability*.

This pretest probability is something you arrive at through taking a careful history, performing an appropriate physical exam, your knowledge of medicine (previous academic studies, the informed expertise of those around you, etc.), and looking at any other diagnostic tests that you already have on hand. Assigning a precise probability is less important than estimating how likely you think it is that a patient has a particular diagnosis (eg, "I think it is somewhat unlikely that this patient has a pulmonary embolism." You might go further and consult a medical calculator, feed in the information you have, and get an actual estimate: "The chance of a pulmonary embolism is 15%.").

Any new lab results will nudge that pretest probability up or down, sometimes to a large extent and sometimes—as in the first example of the "flat earth" earlier—not at all. The end result is a *posttest probability*. ("Now that the D-dimer test has come back and is negative, I think it is far less likely that this patient has a pulmonary embolism—closer to 1%.")

Used in this way, Bayesian thinking simply refers to the process of constantly weighing what we already know against new results as they come in.

The Quality of Your Prior Knowledge Matters

Using prior knowledge is helpful only when that knowledge is reliable. Making blind assumptions or careless leaps of judgment is not helpful. You should arrive carefully at a pretest probability through data such as your accumulated medical knowledge and the patient's history and physical examination. Coming up with a pretest probability can be challenging—it's a big part of "the art of medicine"—but it is very important in guiding which tests you will or will not order.

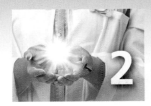

2 Moving the Needle: Sensitivity, Specificity, Predictive Values, and Likelihood Ratios

How do we know how good a given lab test is at shifting the likelihood of a particular diagnosis up or down? We'll call this process "moving the needle."

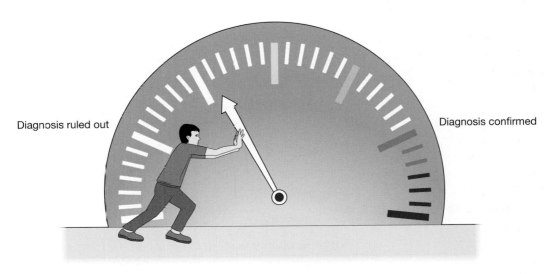

Diagnosis ruled out

Diagnosis confirmed

Figure 2.1 Moving the needle to the left makes the diagnosis less likely. Moving it right makes it more likely.

The concepts of *sensitivity, specificity, predictive value,* and *likelihood ratio* (LR) serve as shortcuts to help us understand how much a given test result will move the needle one way or the other. Don't let these terms intimidate you—although they have very specific mathematical definitions, they actually mean the same things that they mean in real life. We've included the respective formulas for each in Table 2.1, but in actual clinical practice it's much more important to understand the concepts than the formulas. Follow along with this scenario and you'll get the idea:

Table 2.1 Sensitivity, Specificity, Predictive Values, and Likelihood Ratios. These can all be expressed in terms of true positives, false positives, true negatives, and false negatives. If you're a math person, it may be worthwhile to spend a few minutes playing with these formulas and plugging in examples to understand how the math lines up with the concepts

	Disease/Diagnosis Positive	*Disease/Diagnosis Negative*	
Test Positive	True Positive (TP)	False Positive (FP)	Positive Predictive Value $\dfrac{TP}{TP+FP}$
Test Negative	False Negative (FN)	True Negative (TN)	Negative Predictive Value $\dfrac{TN}{TN+FN}$

$$\text{Sensitivity}\quad \frac{TP}{TP+FN} \qquad \text{Specificity}\quad \frac{TN}{TN+FP}$$

$$\text{Positive Likelihood Ratio (PLR)} = \frac{\text{Sensitivity}}{1-\text{Specificity}}$$

$$\text{Negative Likelihood Ratio (NLR)} = \frac{1-\text{Sensitivity}}{\text{Specificity}}$$

Imagine going through an airport security checkpoint (if this example doesn't get you excited, we don't know what will). Just like in medical lab testing, the goal of airport security screening is to make a "diagnosis" of sorts—in this case, to accurately determine the presence or absence of a dangerous item.

 ## The Sensitive Test: Scanning Your Bag

The airport security scanner is designed not to miss any items that might be dangerous. It is, literally, very *sensitive*—it has a low threshold for being set off (a positive test result). If no alarms go off, security can trust the negative result and no further testing is required. There are very few false negatives. *This is what we mean by a sensitive test: it can reliably rule out a diagnosis.*

Because we like mnemonics, try thinking "Snout" to link the terms *sensitive* ("Sn") and *rule out* ("out").

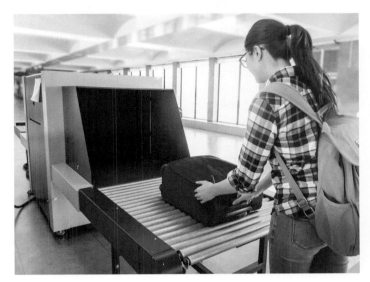

Figure 2.2 The sensitive airport security scanner won't miss a thing. Very few false negatives! (Courtesy of PR Image Factory/ Shutterstock.)

A scanner that won't miss any dangerous items sounds great. Unfortunately, many of us are all too familiar with the downside of such a sensitive scanner: perfectly benign items set it off. In other words, there are many false positives. Many tests in medicine work the same way. As we make them more sensitive, more people *without* disease tend to test positive (more false positives).

 ## The Specific Test: Searching Your Bag by Hand

The follow-up test we all know and love—the bag search by hand—is great for confirming that whatever set off the scanner really is, *specifically*, a dangerous item.

Just as the scanner can reliably rule out a dangerous item, the manual search can reliably rule it *in*. TSA agents who quickly go through your bag can't possibly catch every detail picked up by the scanner (the scanner is more sensitive), but they can identify a dangerous item when they find one. With this test, there are very few false positives. Security can trust a positive result. *This is what we mean by a specific test: it reliably rules in a diagnosis.*

Think "Spin" to link *specific* ("Sp") and *rule in* ("in").

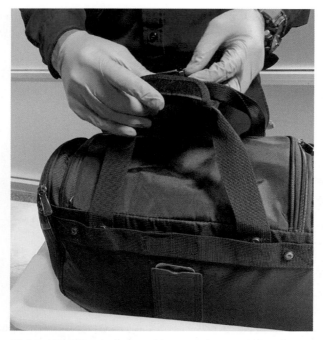

Figure 2.3 TSA agents searching your bag can identify a specific item when they come across one. Very few false positives! (Courtesy of Rosamar/Shutterstock.)

Notice how these two tests work together to avoid false negatives (scanner) and false positives (manual search). Combining a sensitive screening test and a specific confirmatory test is a theme that comes up repeatedly in clinical medicine.

Can We Design the Perfect Test That Will Do It All?

The "perfect" lab test would have 100% sensitivity and 100% specificity. Do such tests exist? No, although some do come surprisingly close, and we will point them out as they come up.

 ## Positive and Negative Predictive Values

The predictive value of a test is very closely related to its sensitivity and specificity. The predictive value answers the question: *How likely is it that the result in front of me is accurate?*

Positive predictive value (PPV): This term refers to the likelihood that the patient has the diagnosis in question given a positive test result. Think of this as similar (but not quite identical) to specificity.

Negative predictive value (NPV): This term refers to the likelihood that the patient does *not* have the diagnosis in question given a negative test result. Think of this as similar (but not quite identical) to sensitivity.

PPV and NPV are straightforward ways of telling us whether a result is likely to be a true positive/negative (as opposed to a false positive/negative). Here's the catch:

> *Unlike sensitivity and specificity, PPV and NPV are not constant or inherent characteristics of a given lab test. They change depending on the disease prevalence, that is, how common the disease is in the relevant patient population at the time.*

To nail this concept, let's do a short example using fictional "disease Z" and corresponding diagnostic "lab test A":

Suppose that disease Z is more common among people living in large cities than in rural areas. Matteo, a 45-year-old healthy male living in New York City, takes lab test A that comes back positive for disease Z. Andres, also a 45-year-old healthy male but living in rural Montana, gets the same positive lab test result.

The lab test has the same sensitivity and specificity wherever it is run—New York City, Montana, or Timbuktu. But because the *prevalence* of disease at the time is much higher among people living in large cities, the *PPV* of lab test A is significantly higher for Matteo, who lives in New York City, than for Andres, who lives in Montana.

So to repeat: sensitivity and specificity are always the same for a given test, but predictive value varies with the prevalence of disease. For this reason, it is often (including in this book) more useful to discuss the *general* characteristics of tests in terms of their sensitivity and specificity rather than in terms of their predictive values. But for any one individual, predictive value can matter a great deal.

Positive and Negative Likelihood Ratios

How do these test characteristics (sensitivity, specificity, predictive value) tell us how much a new result will move the needle? Remember, à la Bayes, that we need to combine our new result with our prior knowledge. Let's return to the airport. Suppose you put your bag through the scanner and it beeps—a positive result. Compared to before you passed through the scanner, now that the test has come back positive, how much more likely is it that your bag contains a dangerous item (a "true positive")? The answer is the *likelihood ratio*.

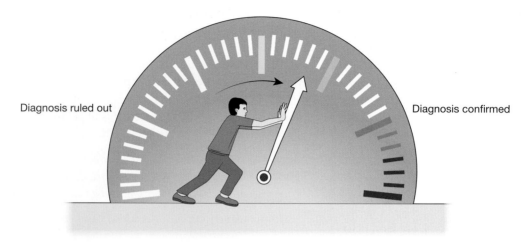

Diagnosis ruled out

Diagnosis confirmed

Figure 2.4 The likelihood ratio tells us how much a test result moves the needle.

We can anticipate your first question: ratio of what? The LR compares the likelihood of a given result (the scanner beeps or doesn't) in someone carrying a dangerous item to the likelihood of the same result in someone who is not. Or, to return to medicine, the LR compares the likelihood of a given result in a patient with a particular diagnosis to the likelihood of the same result in a patient without that diagnosis.

Any given test has a *positive likelihood ratio* for positive results and a *negative likelihood ratio* for negative results. As you might have guessed, these ratios are based on the test's sensitivity and specificity (again, feel free to take a look at the formulas in Table 2.1).

- A very high positive LR (much greater than 1, say around 10) means that a positive test result will make your diagnosis much more likely.

- A very low negative LR (much less than 1, say around 0.1) means that a negative test result will make your diagnosis much less likely.

- The closer the positive or negative LR to 1, the less your positive or negative test result, respectively, will move the needle.

Table 2.2 shows how LRs take us from pretest probability to posttest probability.

Table 2.2 How Likelihood Ratios Affect Diagnosis Probability

Likelihood Ratio (LR)	Approximate Change in Probability (%)
Values Between 0 and 1 *Decrease* the Probability of Disease (−LR)	
0.1	−45
0.2	−30
0.5	−15
1	−0
Values Greater than 1 *Increase* the Probability of Disease (+LR)	
1	+0
2	+15
5	+30
10	+45

 Let's Pause to Review

1. We don't interpret lab results in a vacuum. Instead, we consider what we already know and start with a *pretest probability* of a given diagnosis.

2. Each new test result changes the *likelihood* of that diagnosis and results in a *posttest probability*.

3. How much a given test changes that likelihood depends on its sensitivity and specificity (from which we can derive positive and negative LRs).

Notice the words *probability* and *likelihood*—we are dealing with degrees of uncertainty, not absolutes.

Medicine's ground state is uncertainty. And wisdom—for both the patients and doctors—is defined by how one copes with it.

—Atul Gawande

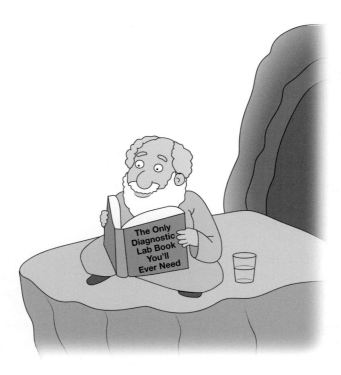

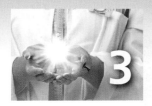

3 Four Things That Matter

There is nothing magic about the number four. It just so happens that we identified four principles of diagnostic lab testing that should serve you well in your clinical career. If they sound obvious to you, good. But sometimes the simple truths are the most important and the most easily forgotten in the hustle and bustle of a busy day (and night) of patient care. And there are some nuances here worth highlighting.

 ## *Understand the Meaning of "Normal" and "Abnormal"*

Suppose you order a comprehensive metabolic panel (see Chapter 5) and the sodium comes back at 143 mEq/L. You hover over the result and the electronic medical record (EMR) tells you that the "reference range" or "normal range" is 136 to 145 mEq/L. You breathe a sigh of relief. Your patient's sodium is normal. Interesting, though, isn't it, that normal is not a single number but a range. Even though you may have learned that a normal sodium is 140 mEq/L, small fluctuations—apparently 4 to 5 mEq/L in either direction—are "allowed." Why?

There is normal variation in lab values among perfectly healthy people (sodium is just one example out of thousands), just as there is normal variation in basic traits like height and weight. This variation can be modeled as a bell-shaped (or "normal distribution") curve, where most people fall fairly close to the center (140 mEq/L for sodium). The curve drops off as it moves out in either direction from the center, indicating fewer and fewer healthy people with increasingly more extreme results.

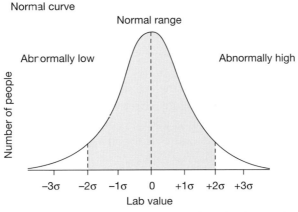

Figure 3.1 A typical bell-shaped ("normal distribution") curve. The σ stands for standard deviation.

We usually define "normal" as falling within the middle 95% of all values ("within two standard deviations from the mean" for those of you who are statistics enthusiasts; the actual standard deviation will vary from curve to curve depending on how dispersed the data are from the mean—that is, a curve that is narrow and pointy [the standard deviation will be small] versus wide and flat [the standard deviation will be large]).

Any lab result not falling within that middle 95% is labeled as "abnormal."

Why are we telling you all of this? *Because, for any given test, 5% of perfectly healthy people—1 out of 20—will have an "abnormal" result.*

So when you are interpreting lab results, remember these two key points:

1. "Abnormal" or "outside the reference range" does not always mean the same thing as *clinically* abnormal. The patient may be perfectly healthy but is just an outlier.

2. Don't get too hung up on whether the lab report or your EMR flags the number as abnormal or not (we know that that little exclamation point, warning flag, or red number can be scary). *How* abnormal is often more important, and the clinical context is most important of all.

An Important Note About Reference Ranges

When you see that a lab's reference range differs from one patient to another, it is usually because of demographic factors such as age or birth sex (eg, testosterone levels for men and women). These different reference ranges are meant to account for physiologic differences among populations. However, there have been instances where reference ranges have been adjusted inappropriately. For example, the "normal" range of a critical measure of kidney function, the GFR (glomerular filtration rate), was historically defined differently for self-identifying African American patients. This separate "African American GFR" was based more on racial bias than evidence-based science and has now been eliminated at most institutions.

 ## *Order Only Tests That Will Change or Guide Your Management*

No matter how well a test performs on its own (think sensitivity and specificity), it will be useless to you if the result won't meaningfully affect your clinical management.

Before ordering a lab, get in the habit of asking yourself, "What will I do with a positive result? What will I do with a negative result?" If the answers to those two questions are the same, you probably shouldn't order the test.

But remember that "clinical management" can mean more than just concrete changes such as starting or stopping medications or ordering additional testing. Thus, for example, an abnormal lipid panel may help provide extra perspective and motivation to a patient who is on the fence about making changes to diet and lifestyle, even if starting a medication isn't

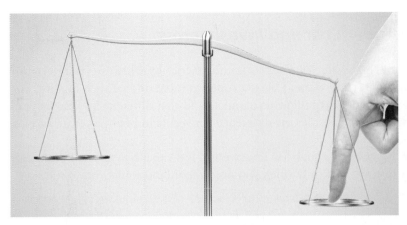

Figure 3.2 Order tests that are likely to tip the scales. (Courtesy of Golden Dayz/Shutterstock.)

indicated. In these kinds of situations—where the lab result *might* change management—it is essential to engage your patient in shared decision-making.

An extra blood draw or urine sample is easy enough to order, but for the patient it can mean another trip to the lab, another uncomfortable stick in the arm, another bill, and another source of psychological stress. Think twice before ordering tests only to reassure your patient. Although there are instances when this can be helpful, you may not get the "normal" result you are looking for. A false-positive result in these cases can be extremely stressful, costly, and even dangerous to the patient if it leads to an invasive procedure.

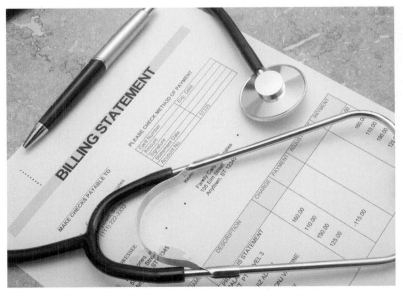

Figure 3.3 Overtesting isn't fun for anyone and can lead to unpleasant and even disastrous outcomes. (Courtesy of aastock/Shutterstock.)

Consider Cost and Invasiveness

The concept of "high-value care" refers to the practice by which we aim to improve health while avoiding harm and waste. This is a complex topic riddled with nuance. For the purposes of this book, it is sufficient to understand that different tests vary significantly in cost and invasiveness (consider the difference between a lumbar puncture and a simple blood draw).

All other things being equal, less invasive and less expensive tests are preferred. Order expensive or invasive tests only when you need them (and sometimes you do).

Don't Miss the Big Picture: How Sick Is Your Patient?

Consider clinical urgency and disease severity when deciding what labs to order. Sicker patients often warrant a more aggressive approach.

Suppose an immunocompromised cancer patient in the hospital develops a new fever. She likely needs blood cultures. The same fever in an otherwise healthy outpatient most often doesn't necessitate any lab work at all. Why? Although our suspicion for bacteremia is low in both patients, the potential consequences of missing a bloodstream infection in the sicker cancer patient are far more serious.

You are now ready to start exploring the specific lab tests that will be a part of your clinical armamentarium.

Section 2

Profiles and Panels: Common Lab Tests That Come in Families

 What This Section Is All About

In this section, you will learn:

- Why so many tests are grouped together in panels
- When (and when not) to order and how to interpret these diagnostic panels:
    - Complete blood count (CBC)
    - Comprehensive metabolic panel (CMP)
    - Lipid panel
    - Thyroid function tests (TFTs)
    - Urinalysis (UA)
    - Blood gases: arterial blood gas (ABG) and venous blood gas (VBG)
    - Cerebrospinal fluid (CSF)
    - Pleural fluid
    - Peritoneal (ascitic) fluid
    - Synovial fluid

Why Are We Starting Here?

The most common lab orders are not for single, isolated lab tests but rather for standard collections of tests—some small in number, some quite large—that we refer to as *profiles* or *panels*. After all, if you are going to the trouble of drawing blood (or performing a spinal tap or even just obtaining a urine specimen), procedures that are never any fun for your patient and that can in some cases be quite difficult and traumatizing, why settle for getting only one result out of your sample when you can get many? Plus, the automated machines that run the tests are already designed to run a whole battery of tests at the same time with little additional cost.*

The are several upsides to ordering a preset panel of lab tests:

- You spare your patient repeated procedures.
- You may discover something important you were previously unaware of.
- Most importantly, you get context. You aren't just looking at one result in isolation, but rather a collection of related tests that—often synergistically—tell you much more about what may or may not be going on with your patient.

There is, of course, a downside:

- More information can sometimes turn into too much information, and you may run into the problem of what to do with an abnormal result you weren't counting on for a test you really didn't need in the first place.

Whatever you may think of them, these panels are here to stay. They include many of the lab tests you need to understand, so they are a good place to begin.

---

*Although most tests can be run at a cost to the lab of just pennies, your patients will almost certainly find themselves with a bill for much more.

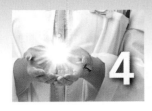

4 The Complete Blood Count

 ## A Quick Overview

Most blood tests measure relatively simple substances found in the blood—electrolytes, proteins, gases, products of the body's metabolism, and so on. The one big exception is the complete blood count (CBC), which measures cells. This not only adds complexity to the test but also makes it a uniquely powerful tool.

All the cellular elements of the blood originate in the bone marrow from a common pluripotent cell. This pluripotent cell, also called a "hematopoietic stem cell," may differentiate into distinct cell lineages, each of which ultimately yields the various cells we see in the circulation. The CBC is a snapshot in time of the cellular elements that are present in the blood.

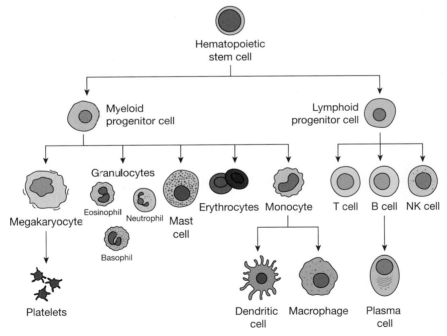

Figure 4.1 A simplified view of hematopoiesis, that is, the pathways by which red blood cells, white blood cells, and platelets evolve from a population of pluripotent hematopoietic stem cells.

The CBC looks at all the major cellular elements of the blood: the red blood cells (erythrocytes), white blood cells (leukocytes), and platelets. It also comes in a more expanded form, the *CBC with differential*, which also provides a breakdown of the different types of white blood cells.

There are many reasons for ordering a CBC, but among the most common reasons are concern for possible:

- anemia (eg, in a patient with unexplained fatigue or lightheadedness)

- infection or inflammation (eg, in a patient with unexplained fever)

- malignancy (eg, in a patient with unexplained weight loss)

- bleeding disorder (eg, a patient with spontaneous bruising)

In each of these situations, the CBC will rarely give you the definitive answer as to what is going on, but it is usually one of the first steps in identifying the problem and guiding you toward what to do next.

Figure 4.2 shows what the results from a CBC with differential can look like.

A CBC is drawn in a lavender top tube (Figure 4.3) that contains EDTA. EDTA is a chemical that prevents the blood sample from clotting, which would make it impossible to count and examine the cells. (Clotted cells are just that: a thick, amorphous clot or thrombus. Good luck trying to count anything in that mess!)

The Red Blood Cells

The CBC provides a lot of information about the number and appearance of a person's red blood cells. The most fundamental measures are the hemoglobin and hematocrit. These are the tests that will tell you if your patient is anemic or, less often, polycythemic (too many red blood cells). It also allows you to classify the anemia into one of several categories, in this way helping you begin to narrow down the list of possible reasons your patient is likely to be anemic, although you will need additional testing to arrive at a precise diagnosis (see Chapter 20).

Hematocrit

The hematocrit is a measure of the *percentage of the total volume of blood that is made up of red blood cells.* It is measured by spinning a tube of blood in a centrifuge (or just waiting awhile and letting the cells settle out), watching the red blood cells drop to the bottom, and seeing how tall their column is compared to that of the entire sample (see Figure 4.4). Thus, the hematocrit is reported as a percentage.

A normal hematocrit is typically 41% to 51% in men and 36% to 47% in women.

YourLab

Patient Report

Specimen ID: **020-992-9212-0**   Acct #: **90000999**   Phone: Rte: **00**
Control ID:

SAMPLE REPORT, 005009

|||₁₁||¹·ᵘ·ₗ|₁ₚ|₁ ₘₚ|·ₗ₁ₗₗ||||||¹°||¹₁·ₚ||·º||¹º·¹¹·|·¹||¹ₗₗₚ·||¹º·¹

Patient Details	Specimen Details	Physician Details
DOB: **01/02/1960**	Date collected: **01/20/2023**	Ordering:
Age(y/m/d): **060/00/18**	Date received: **01/20/2023**	Referring:
Gender: **F** SSN:	Date entered: **01/20/2023**	ID:
Patient ID:	Date reported: **01/27/2023 0000 ET**	NPI:

General Comments & Additional Information
Clinical Info: ABNORMAL REPORT

Ordered items
CBC With Differential/Platelet

TESTS	RESULT	FLAG	UNITS	REFERENCE INTERVAL	LAB
CBC with Differential/Platelet					
WBC	**11.4**	**High**	×10E3/µL	3.4-10.8	01
RBC	**3.50**	**Low**	×10E6/µL	3.77-5.28	01
Hemoglobin	**10.0**	**Low**	g/dL	11.1-15.9	01
Hematocrit	**31.2**	**Low**	%	34.0-46.6	01
MCV	89		fL	79-97	01
MCH	28.6		pg	26.6-33.0	01
MCHC	32.1		g/dL	31.5-35.7	01
RDW	**18.3**	**High**	%	11.7-15.4	01
Platelets	**109**	**Low**	×10E3/µL	150-450	01
Neutrophils	55		%	Not Estab.	01
Lymphs	22		%	Not Estab.	01
Monocytes	6		%	Not Estab.	01
EOS	2		%	Not Estab.	01
Basos	11		%	Not Estab.	01
Immature Cells	Note				01
Bands	1		%	Not Estab.	01
Metamyelocytes	**2**	**High**	%	0-0	01
Myelocytes	**1**	**High**	%	0-0	01
Neutrophils (Absolute)	6.4		×10E3/µL	1.4-7.0	01
Lymphs (Absolute)	2.5		×10E3/µL	0.7-3.1	01
Monocytes (Absolute)	0.7		×10E3/µL	0.1-0.9	01
Eos (Absolute)	0.2		×10E3/µL	0.0-0.4	01
Baso (Absolute)	**1.3**	**High**	×10E3/µL	0.0-0.2	01
NRBC	**16**	**High**	%	0-0	01
Hematology Comments:					01

Verified by microscopic examination.
Manual differential was performed.

Figure 4.2 Results from a complete blood count with differential. The abnormal values—and there are many—are bolded to catch your eye.

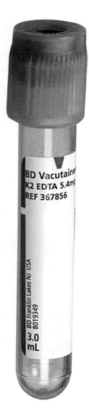

Figure 4.3 A complete blood count tube.

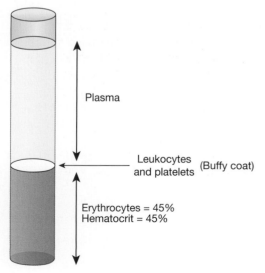

Plasma

Leukocytes and platelets (Buffy coat)

Erythrocytes = 45%
Hematocrit = 45%

Figure 4.4 A spun sample of whole blood showing the column of red blood cells at the bottom of the tube constituting 45% of the total height. Plasma makes up most of the rest. Note that the contribution of white blood cells and platelets to the sample is very small.

Hemoglobin

Although the hematocrit is a useful number to know, we rely more often on the hemoglobin. The hemoglobin, the molecule inside red blood cells that carries both oxygen to the body's tissues and carbon dioxide to the lungs, is measured directly. Why is this the preferred test? The reason is simple: not all red blood cells contain the same amount of hemoglobin. And when we think about red blood cells, what we are primarily concerned about is their oxygen-carrying capacity, not—as the hematocrit tells us—how many there are.

A normal hemoglobin is 14 to 17 g/dL in males and 12 to 16 g/dL in females.

Red Blood Cell Count

What about the red blood cell count itself?

Again, we are usually more interested in the amount of hemoglobin than in the actual number of red blood cells. You would expect that the red cell count would be low in most patients with anemia, and you would be right: fewer red blood cells usually means less hemoglobin. However, this is not always the case—the red blood cell count and the hemoglobin do not always march in tandem (see the box below). Knowing both the red blood cell count and the hemoglobin can help you determine if such a discordance is present, which in turn allows you to narrow your differential diagnosis considerably.

A normal red blood cell count is 4.2 to 5.9 $\times$ 10^6/μL.

> ### Thalassemia: A Mismatch Between the Hemoglobin and the Red Blood Cell Count
>
> The thalassemias are the second most common of the hemoglobinopathies (ie, disorders in the structure or production of hemoglobin). Only sickle cell disease is more common. The thalassemias are a group of inherited blood disorders in which the production of globin chains (constituents of hemoglobin) is defective, creating an imbalance in the number of α- and β-chains. One result of this mismatch is that the hemoglobin level is low. Another result, surprisingly, is that the red blood cell count is usually high, presumably because the body is trying to compensate for the red blood cells' impaired oxygen-carrying capacity by churning out more cells. So with a low hemoglobin and a high red blood cell count, is the patient anemic? Yes, because it is the hemoglobin that defines anemia. We will discuss testing for thalassemia more in Chapter 20.

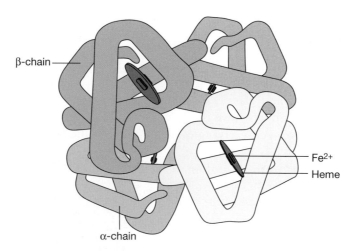

β-chain

Fe²⁺

Heme

α-chain

Figure 4.5 The normal hemoglobin molecule consists of two α-globin chains and two β-globin chains containing the heme components that bind iron.

Red Blood Cell Indices

The hemoglobin tells you if your patient is anemic. The red blood cell indices help you begin to sort through the different causes of anemia and narrow your differential diagnosis. The CBC reports three of these red blood cell indices:

- Mean corpuscular volume (MCV)
- Mean corpuscular hemoglobin (MCH)
- Mean corpuscular hemoglobin concentration (MCHC)

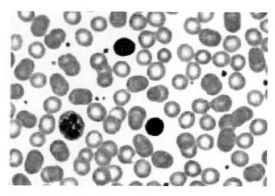

Figure 4.6 A blood smear showing normal, healthy red blood cells. Note their round-to-oval shape, the small clearing in the center (normally <1/3 the diameter of the cell), and the absence of a nucleus. (From Nath JL. *Programmed Learning Approach to Medical Terminology*. 3rd ed. Wolters Kluwer; 2019.)

The Mean Corpuscular Volume: The MCV is a measure of the average size (volume) of a patient's red blood cells. The normal MCV is 80 to 100 fL.* In a patient with anemia, the MCV can be low (small size/volume), in which case we say the patient has a *microcytic anemia*. When it is high, the patient has a *macrocytic anemia*. And, yes, in case you are wondering, there are *normocytic anemias*, too.

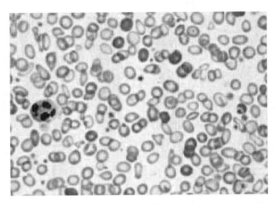

Figure 4.7 Microcytic anemia. The red blood cells are small and in this case also hypochromic (pale). (From Nath JL. *Programmed Learning Approach to Medical Terminology.* 3rd ed. Wolters Kluwer; 2019.)

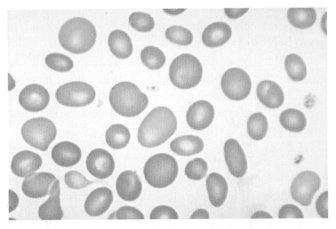

Figure 4.8 Macrocytic anemia. Some of the red cells are large and so packed with hemoglobin that you can't see much of a central clearing. (From Nath JL. *Programmed Learning Approach to Medical Terminology.* 3rd ed. Wolters Kluwer; 2019.)

---

*fL stands for femtoliter, a unit of volume equivalent to 10^{-15} L, that is, very small.

Evaluation of Anemia—First Steps

Once you know if your patient has a microcytic, normocytic, or macrocytic anemia, you are well on your way to pinning down the diagnosis:

- The small, usually pale cells of *microcytic anemia* are most often caused by iron deficiency (see Chapter 20). Other causes include the thalassemias, lead poisoning, and hereditary sideroblastic anemia.

- The most common cause of *normocytic anemia* is what is often called the anemia of chronic disease (or the anemia of chronic inflammation). Many chronic diseases can cause this condition, from infections to inflammatory conditions to chronic conditions such as diabetes, heart failure, and even normal aging. Most likely what is going on here is that red blood cell production decreases as the body tries to hoard its iron stores, preventing any invading pathogen or active disease process from making use of them.

  - While most often normocytic, the anemia of chronic disease can sometimes be microcytic.

- *Macrocytic anemia* is usually due to vitamin B12 or folate deficiency (see Chapter 20), but there are multiple other causes including myelodysplastic syndrome, liver disease, excessive alcohol use, hypothyroidism, copper deficiency, and aplastic anemia.

You can see how distinct the differential diagnosis is for each of these types of anemia and therefore how useful the CBC can be in guiding you toward the correct diagnosis.

The Mean Corpuscular Hemoglobin: This is a measure of the average amount of hemoglobin in each red blood cell. It tends to mirror the trend in the MCV; if one is low, the other is low, and if one is high, the other is high. This makes sense: the larger the cell, the more hemoglobin it can hold.

Because the microcytic cells seen with iron deficiency anemia have a low hemoglobin content, their MCH is low and they appear pale, or *hypochromic*. Macrocytic cells, as seen in B12 and folate deficiency, tend to have a lot of hemoglobin per cell, and thus the MCH is high (*hyperchromic*). It is safe to say that the MCH usually doesn't add much to what we already know from the MCV.

The normal MCH is 28 to 32 pg.*

The Mean Corpuscular Hemoglobin Concentration: This number is calculated by multiplying the hemoglobin by 100 and dividing the result by the hematocrit. This, too, has limited utility, but is the most useful red blood cell index in evaluating patients for hereditary spherocytosis (a condition in which red blood cells appear spherical rather than disk shaped), in whom the MCHC is elevated.

The normal MCHC is 32 to 36 g/dL.**

---

*pg stands for picograms, one of which is 0.000000000001 g.

**g/dL stands for grams per deciliter; you will see this abbreviation a lot; other popular units used elsewhere, not to belabor the point, are mg/dL, μg/mL, ng/mL, and U/L (units per liter).

Red Cell Distribution Width: One healthy red blood cell looks pretty much the same as any other. But when disease kicks in, you may begin to see red blood cells of varying appearance, particularly with regard to size. The red cell distribution width (RDW) is a measure of the variation in the size of the red blood cells. A higher RDW implies a greater variation in size, whereas a lower number implies that the red cells are all largely uniform. For example, you can see a variety of sizes in the picture of macrocytic anemia (Figure 4.8).

The normal RDW is 12.1 to 14 fL.

The RDW was intended to help distinguish between the different causes of anemia, but it has not proven to be as helpful as we would like. A high RDW can be seen in some patients with iron, B12, or folate deficiency, but it can also reflect two totally homogeneous populations of cells that coexist, for example, when a patient has a microcytic or normocytic anemia but is also releasing a lot of immature red cells into the population to compensate. These immature cells are called *reticulocytes*, and they are larger than mature red blood cells. It is therefore generally more useful to examine a blood smear than to rely on the RDW for clues as to what may be causing a patient's anemia.

The Reticulocyte Count

Reticulocytes are immature red blood cells. The reticulocyte count is not traditionally a part of the CBC, but its value is so interwoven with that of the CBC that we feel it is appropriate to discuss it here. You will often order it at the same time as the CBC because it can be extremely helpful in determining the cause of anemia.

In a patient who is not anemic, a normal reticulocyte count is 0.5% to 1.5% of the red blood cells in the circulation; this translates to an absolute count of between 23,000 and 90,000 reticulocytes per microliter.

In a patient with anemia, a *high reticulocyte count* implies a relatively healthy bone marrow churning out lots of red blood cells before they have had time to fully mature as a way to compensate for the low hemoglobin. This is often seen when the bone marrow is trying to make up for the peripheral red blood cell destruction that occurs with hemolysis or when there is massive loss of blood from trauma. This type of anemia is often called *hyperproliferative*.

A *low reticulocyte count* can occur when the bone marrow is not up to the task in a patient with hemolysis or blood loss. Alternatively, and more commonly, it indicates that the bone marrow may be the primary problem—that is, the source of the anemia. This is what happens in iron deficiency, when the bone marrow lacks one critical ingredient (iron) to make enough red blood cells. As you would expect, these anemias are often referred to as *hypoproliferative*.

Because the reticulocyte count should be high in patients with anemia (to compensate for the low hemoglobin), a "normal" count of approximately 1% may not really be normal in this circumstance. There are various formulas for calculating a corrected reticulocyte count. One that is widely used is:

Corrected reticulocyte percentage = reticulocyte percentage $\times$ hemoglobin $\div$ 15

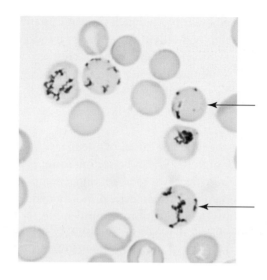

Figure 4.9 A blood smear showing reticulocytes (*arrows*) mixed in with normal red blood cells. Reticulocytes are larger and often more irregular in shape than mature red blood cells. They often contain cytoplasmic densities (excess ribosomal RNA compared to mature cells) that, as here, can be visualized with appropriate stains. (From Cohen BJ. *Medical Terminology: An Illustrated Guide*. 6th ed. Wolters Kluwer Health; 2011.)

Thus, for example, if the hemoglobin is 15 g/dL (normal) and the reticulocyte percentage is 0.5%, the corrected reticulocyte percentage is 0.5%, which is normal. But if the patient is anemic with a hemoglobin of only 10 g/dL and the reticulocyte percentage is 0.5%, the corrected reticulocyte percentage is 0.33%, which is low and points an accusatory finger at a sluggish bone marrow.

Reticulocyte Production Index

The formula on the previous page gives you a decent estimate of the corrected reticulocyte percentage. An even more precise value can be obtained by calculating the *reticulocyte production index* (RPI), which takes into account the reticulocyte life span. The more severe the anemia, the earlier in their development reticulocytes are forced out of the marrow, and the longer their life span in the circulation before they mature into red blood cells. This life span can range from 1 day in mild anemia to 2.5 days in severe anemia. Calculation of the RPI is simple:

RPI = corrected reticulocyte percentage ÷ reticulocyte life span (in days)

You can plug your patient's reticulocyte percentage and hematocrit into an online calculator that will give you both the corrected reticulocyte percentage and the RPI. An RPI less than 2 indicates an inadequate bone marrow response.

In addition to distinguishing hyperproliferative from hypoproliferative anemias, the reticulocyte count can also be monitored to see if a patient with anemia is responding to therapy. A healthy bone marrow response is indicated by an increase in the reticulocyte count—typically before significant improvement in the hemoglobin itself is seen—followed by a gradual decline back to normal.

Red Blood Cell Morphologies

In addition to all the numbers on the CBC, the report will indicate if there are any red blood cells that are unusually shaped or that contain abnormal intracellular inclusion bodies. These interpretations are usually made by the automated machinery (often confirmed by microscopic evaluation by a hematologist) and reflect any red blood cells on a peripheral blood smear that don't resemble ordinary red cells.

Any of five red blood cell alterations will trigger a report:

1. Size

2. Shape

3. Color

4. Arrangement (are the red cells not distributed randomly but are grouped in some discernible pattern?)

5. Inclusions within the cells

Table 4.1 is by no means exhaustive, but reviews some of the morphologies you may encounter, along with an example of a diagnosis each can suggest.

Table 4.1 Abnormal Red Blood Cell Morphologies

Change in Morphology	Description	Most Often Seen With
Acanthocyte (aka spur cell)	Shrunken cells with irregular, sharp projections	Severe liver disease
Echinocyte (aka burr cell)	Regularly spaced rounded projections	Chronic renal disease
Elliptocyte	Oval-shaped cells	Hereditary elliptocytosis
Hypochromia	Central pallor >1/3 diameter of the cell	Iron deficiency anemia
Schistocyte	Angular, fragmented cell, looks like it has been through the mill	Microangiopathic hemolytic anemia
Sickle cell	Looks like a sickle or a narrow boat	Sickle cell crisis
Spherocyte	Small, dark round cell	Autoimmune hemolytic anemia
Stomatocyte	Linear central pallor	Alcoholic liver disease

(continued)

Table 4.1 Abnormal Red Blood Cell Morphologies (*continued*)

Change in Morphology	Description	Most Often Seen With
Target cell	Central red area within the central pallor—that is, looks like a target	Thalassemia
Teardrop cell	Tapered at one end like a tear	Myelofibrosis
Inclusion Bodies		
Basophilic stippling	Dark granular discolorations	Lead poisoning
Heinz body	Small round mass only seen with special stains	Hyposplenism
Howell-Jolly body	Round mass stains purple on usual blood stain	Hyposplenism
Pappenheimer body	Multiple granular inclusions	Hemochromatosis
Unusual Groupings		
RBC agglutination	Cells stuck randomly to each other	Cold agglutinin disease
Rouleaux formation	Linear aggregations	Multiple myeloma

As you can see, the simple red blood cell can be quite a shapeshifter. In fact, it is not unusual to find one or two of these altered red blood cell morphologies on what is otherwise a normal peripheral blood smear in a completely healthy patient. When the clinical significance of one or more abnormal red blood cell morphologies is unclear, or the automated read seems odd in the clinical context, it can be helpful to involve a hematologic pathologist who can review the smear manually.

 ## The White Blood Cells

Unlike the red blood cell population, which in a healthy individual is monotonously uniform, there are many different types of white blood cells. The CBC with differential reports the total white blood cell count as well as the *percentages* and *absolute numbers** of the different types of white blood cells: neutrophils, lymphocytes, monocytes, eosinophils, and basophils.

---

*The absolute number of each cell type is calculated by multiplying the total white blood cell count by the percentage of that particular cell type in the blood.

Total White Blood Cell Count

Look at the total white blood cell count first. Normal values typically range between 4,000 and 10,000/µL.

When the white blood cell count is increased, we call that a *leukocytosis*. A leukocytosis accompanies many infectious and inflammatory disorders. It is an indication—albeit highly nonspecific—that something may be wrong.

When the white blood cell count is decreased, we call that a *leukopenia*. Like leukocytosis, leukopenia can be a sign of underlying disease. However, some individuals have chronic mild leukopenia (around 3,000-4,000/µL) that is perfectly harmless. When you see a patient with leukopenia, pay particular attention to the severity and trend over time (is it new?).

The total white cell count is most useful when you want to assess the following:

- *Infection*—The white blood cell count can give an idea of the likelihood and severity of infection. As a very general rule, an elevated white count is consistent with infection when this is the diagnosis under consideration, and you can often follow the white blood cell count to see if your patient is responding to therapy (it should decline!). However, you should know upfront that the preceding statement is our painting with a very broad brush; not all infections elevate the white blood cell count, and some—including many common viral and tick-borne infections and even severe sepsis—can lower it.

- *Suspected hematologic malignancy*—Elevated white blood cell counts are one of the hallmarks of leukemia and some lymphomas. Whereas extremely high white blood cell counts, over 50,000/µL, are usually indicative of leukemia, they can also be seen with severe infections or widespread tissue damage (eg, burns). In the latter cases, when malignancy is not the cause, we call the high white blood cell count a *leukemoid reaction*.

- *Bone marrow health and immunologic status*—A low white blood cell count can be a sign of bone marrow failure. It is also a hallmark of HIV/AIDS.

More information can be gleaned by looking at the breakdown of the white blood cell count into its component cell types, that is, the differential. We generally divide the different types of white blood cells into two categories:

- *Granulocytes* are (no surprise here) cells with granules in their cytoplasm. These include the neutrophils, eosinophils, and basophils. All granulocytes are able to phagocytose (eat or envelop) bacteria, although neutrophils do it best of all. The response of granulocytes to foreign invaders is not specifically tailored to any one particular pathogen but rather serves as a part of a larger, generalized inflammatory response—more cudgel than scalpel.

- *Non-granulocytes* include the lymphocytes and monocytes. These cells play key roles in the immune response, capable of honing a precise, specific response to an infection that allows for targeted attacks (here is your scalpel), both cell-mediated and antibody-mediated, against invading pathogens.

Roughly, of the total white blood cell population, the normal percentages of these different cell types are:

- Neutrophils 40% to 60%

- Lymphocytes 20% to 40%

- Monocytes 2% to 8%

- Eosinophils 1% to 4%

- Basophils 0.5% to 1%

Granulocytes

Neutrophils: By far the most abundant of the granulocytes, neutrophils are essential for killing and destroying invading bacteria.

Neutrophilia, a high neutrophil count, is typically seen with *bacterial infections;* the total white blood cell count is elevated and the percentage of neutrophils is high. High neutrophil counts can also be seen *early in viral infections* as well as with many *inflammatory conditions* (acute and chronic) and *major stresses* such as surgery, seizures, and even intense exercise, presumably due to the release of cortisol by the body. Cortisol demarginalizes neutrophils, that is, it pops them off of the blood vessel walls where they like to linger, and thrusts them back out into the circulation, thereby increasing the number of neutrophils freely circulating in the blood where they can be counted. Keep in mind that exogenous corticosteroids such as prednisone have the same effect, hence the leukocytosis and neutrophilia seen in patients taking these medications. Other causes of neutrophilia include *myeloproliferative diseases,* such as chronic myelogenous leukemia (CML). *Obesity* and *smoking* can both raise the neutrophil count, probably because of associated low-grade inflammation.

Neutropenia, a low neutrophil count ($<$1,500/µL), can be seen with *bone marrow failure, autoimmune diseases,* many *chemotherapeutic agents,* and with *certain infections,* notably some viruses (eg, Epstein-Barr virus, HIV) and even some bacteria (eg, *Salmonella typhi*). Severe neutropenia ($<$500/µL) is a significant risk factor for infection.

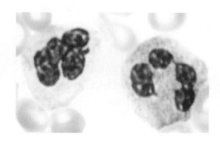

Figure 4.10 Two normal, mature neutrophils. Note the multilobed nuclei and granular cytoplasm, which are their hallmarks. (From Weksler BB, Schechter GP, Ely SA. *Wintrobe's Atlas of Clinical Hematology.* 2nd ed. Wolters Kluwer; 2018.)

Some individuals have an inherited form of mild to moderate neutropenia called Duffy-null-associated neutrophil count (previously called benign ethnic neutropenia), with counts usually between 1,000 and 1,500/μL, and almost always greater than 500/μL. The chronic neutropenia in these patients does not appear to have any clinical repercussions. Consider this diagnosis in a patient with otherwise unexplained chronic, stable, mild to moderate neutropenia *without* an associated history of recurrent infections, particularly if the patient is of African, Arab, Greek, Sephardic Jewish, Yemenite, or West Indian descent.

Eosinophils and Basophils: These cells earned their names because of the way their granules take up stains: eosinophils love acidic stains such as eosin and stain a beautiful pink, whereas basophils love basic stains and typically stain a deep, cerulean blue. Unlike neutrophils, neither eosinophils nor basophils are critical in the fight against most infections, although they do participate each in their own way. Much of the time, however, we don't really know exactly what they are doing (hopefully they do). These cells generally prefer to hang out in the body's tissues rather than in the circulation, and partly for that reason—under normal circumstances—their contribution to the overall white blood cell count is quite small.

Eosinophilia, defined as an absolute eosinophil count ≥500/μL, is most often associated with either *parasitic infections* (eg, *Strongyloides*, *Trichinella*, many others) or—much more often in developed countries—*allergic diseases* (allergic asthma most commonly). The other relatively common causes of a high eosinophil count are various *medications* (eg, nonsteroidal anti-inflammatory drugs [NSAIDs] as well as some antibiotics and antiepileptics). Many *solid tumors*, *hematologic malignancies*, and *autoimmune disorders* (eg, sarcoidosis, inflammatory bowel disease) are also associated with a high eosinophil count. However, if you see a high eosinophil count, most of the time you are looking at a patient with an allergic disorder or with one of the less common—but increasingly diagnosed—eosinophilic disorders, such as *eosinophilic esophagitis*.

Any persistent *hypereosinophilia*, defined as an absolute eosinophil count ≥1,500/μL, usually warrants its own workup unless there is an obvious cause or precipitating factor such as a drug hypersensitivity reaction or known parasitic infection. Particular diagnostic considerations among such patients include parasitic infections, hematologic malignancies (especially if the eosinophil count is ≥20,000/μL), and eosinophilic granulomatosis with polyangiitis (EGPA, a vasculitis of the small blood vessels).

Basophilia, an isolated increase in basophils, is quite rare and is generally limited to *malignant proliferation of mast cells* (the name given to basophils that are residing inside tissues). You will rarely find that the basophil count impacts your patient management.

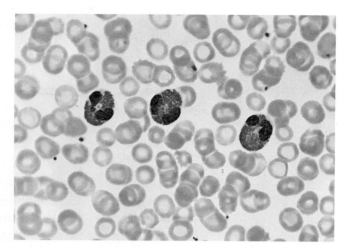

Figure 4.11 An eosinophil. It looks a lot like a neutrophil, only pinker! (Courtesty of SIRIKWAN DOKUTA/Shutterstock.)

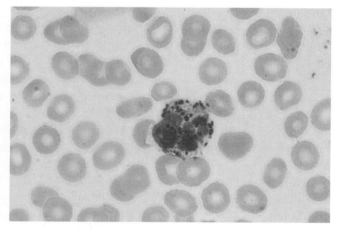

Figure 4.12 A basophil. It looks much like its granular cousins, only it stains a dark blue. (From Anderson SC. *Anderson's Atlas of Hematology*. Wolters Kluwer Health/Lippincott Williams & Wilkins; 2013.)

Because the eosinophil and basophil counts are normally very low, there is never any concern about *eosinophilopenia* or *basophilopenia*.

Non-granulocytes

Lymphocytes: Smaller than the granulocytes, lymphocytes are the heart and soul of the body's immune system. We could spend the rest of this book expounding on their complex role in the immunologic defenses of the body, autoimmune disorders (when things go wrong), transplant medicine, and many other circumstances both good and bad. But that would be a different book.

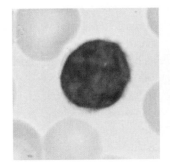

Figure 4.13 A normal mature lymphocyte can be seen mixed among red blood cells. Lymphocytes are approximately the same size as red blood cells. (From Greer JP, Arber DA, List AF, Foerster J. *Wintrobe's Clinical Hematology*. 13th ed. Lippincott Williams & Wilkins; 2014.)

Lymphocytes come in a variety of flavors: some indiscriminately attack foreign invaders, serving as first responders, whereas others are capable of a very directed attack against one specific pathogen, either by producing antibodies or evolving highly regulated, specific cell-mediated mechanisms of attack. Lymphocytes also have a memory—that's why vaccines work.

Lymphocytosis is classically associated with *viral infections*. Almost any viral infection can be implicated—influenza, mumps, measles, rubella, hepatitis A/B/C, etc. *Extreme stress* can also cause a lymphocytosis. There are also primary hematologic causes of lymphocytosis such as chronic lymphocytic leukemia (CLL), acute lymphoblastic leukemia (ALL), and non-Hodgkin lymphoma.

The CBC may report the presence of *atypical lymphocytes*. Although classically associated with infectious mononucleosis, they can also be seen with several other infections including HIV and cytomegalovirus (CMV).

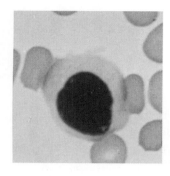

Figure 4.14 Close-up view of an atypical lymphocyte. Note that it is larger than a normal lymphocyte with more cytoplasm and irregularly shaped. (From Greer JP, Arber DA, List AF, Foerster J. *Wintrobe's Clinical Hematology*. 13th ed. Lippincott Williams & Wilkins; 2014.)

Lymphocytopenia (also called *lymphopenia*) is commonly seen with *primary or secondary immunodeficiency syndromes*, especially inadequately treated HIV infection. It is a common feature of many autoimmune diseases (eg, lupus). Like neutropenia, lymphocytopenia can be seen in patients with sepsis. Any medication that causes bone marrow suppression may cause lymphocytopenia, as may corticosteroids (note that corticosteroids tend to have the opposite effect on the neutrophil count).

As mentioned earlier, there are many types of lymphocytes. They are grouped under several rubrics that became common parlance during the COVID-19 pandemic. These include natural killer (NK) cells, T cells, and B cells. T cells are further subdivided into distinct populations based on the presence of unique membrane proteins (eg, CD4 and CD8), each of which serves a specific function. Thus, for example, there are CD8 T killer cells and CD4 T helper cells. However—and this is our main point—*all lymphocytes look alike on a blood smear*. The various subsets will only be reported if you request them via additional testing (see "Flow Cytometry" section in Chapter 20). Knowing the numbers of the different T-cell types is an essential part of the evaluation of HIV/AIDS (see Chapter 14).

While we are on the subject of lymphocytes, recall that when B cells are activated and acquire the ability to release prodigious amounts of antibody, they change their appearance and are then called *plasma cells*. You will generally not see more than the occasional plasma cell on a typical blood smear, but if you do, consider the possibility of a *plasma cell malignancy* (also called a *plasma cell dyscrasia*) such as multiple myeloma.

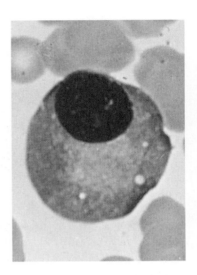

Figure 4.15 A plasma cell. (From Greer JP, Arber DA, List AF, Foerster J. *Wintrobe's Clinical Hematology*. 13th ed. Lippincott Williams & Wilkins; 2014.)

Monocytes: These cells are the other category of non-granulocyte. Monocytes are important producers of interferon, a group of proteins that stimulate the overall inflammatory and immunologic response.

The differential diagnosis of *monocytosis* includes *asplenia, pregnancy, corticosteroid therapy*, and a host of *inflammatory* and *infectious diseases*. However, except in certain types of *leukemia* (eg, acute monocytic or myelomonocytic leukemia), the monocyte count will not need to be foremost in your thinking. And as with the eosinophils and basophils, monocytopenia is not a concern.

One Other (Surprising) Cause of Monocytosis

If you are really into monocytes, then you should know that a monocytosis can develop following an acute myocardial infarction (MI). In that setting, a high monocyte count is associated with a high risk of left ventricular dysfunction and the formation of a ventricular aneurysm. However, monitoring the monocyte count in post-MI patients has not been shown to affect clinical outcomes.

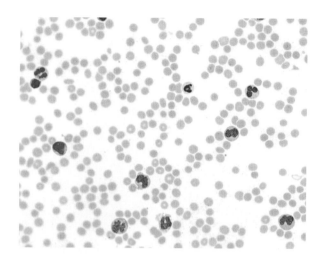

Figure 4.16 A whole lot of monocytes scattered among the red blood cell population. They resemble neutrophils but without the granules. This patient has chronic myelomonocytic leukemia. (From Weksler BB, Schechter GP, Ely SA. *Wintrobe's Atlas of Clinical Hematology*. 2nd ed. Wolters Kluwer; 2018.)

Left Shift

No, this box is not about politics or some obscure athletic maneuver. The term "left shift" refers to *the release of immature blood cells into the circulation*. This is most often seen with neutrophils and their precursors, but can occur with any of the white blood cells as well as with red blood cells (we already saw this in our discussion of reticulocytosis) and even platelets.

Why the term "left" shift? The explanation is simple: years ago when blood cells were counted manually, the least mature cell types were entered on the left side of the ledger, the most mature on the right.

In the case of neutrophils, a left shift is most often the result of diffuse inflammation and/or infection. The release of cytokines prompted by the body's immune response stimulates the bone marrow to release neutrophil precursors into the circulation before they have had time to fully mature. The neutrophil precursor you will most often see is called a *band*, the most mature of the precursor cells; we colloquially refer to the presence of many bands in the circulation as *bandemia*. Sometimes even earlier forms in the neutrophil maturation pathway can be seen—examples include *myelocytes* and *metamyelocytes*. If any of these immature forms are present, the CBC will report their presence.

If you see a large number of one type of immature white blood cell in the peripheral circulation, then you are probably looking at a leukemic clone of malignant cells.

The presence of immature red blood cells (recognizable because they have not yet lost their nuclei) in the blood along with immature white blood cells is called a *leukoerythroblastic reaction*. This can be a normal physiologic response to a dramatic drop in the hemoglobin (the immature white blood cell precursors are incidental accompanists to the nucleated red cells), but it can also reflect a sick bone marrow that has been infiltrated with carcinoma or an expanding clone of leukemic cells.

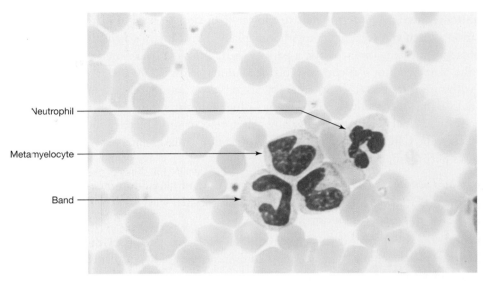

Figure 4.17 One neutrophil, one band, and two metamyelocytes. Note the absence of the nice lobular nucleus in the immature forms. (From Anderson SC. *Anderson's Atlas of Hematology*. Wolters Kluwer Health/Lippincott Williams & Wilkins; 2013.)

 ## Platelets

The last of the cellular elements in the blood that we need to discuss are the *platelets*. Nothing complicated or mysterious here. Platelets are the cellular limb of the body's hemostatic (blood clotting) mechanism. They work hand-in-glove with the coagulation system of proteins (see Chapter 20) and the vascular system to make sure we don't bleed to death every time we suffer a minor injury. However, when there are too many platelets, or when they are activated inappropriately, the result can be serious, even life-threatening thrombosis.

Platelets are tiny and cannot easily be seen on most routine blood smears. The automated CBC machinery, however, can give you a precise account of how many there are.

The platelet count normally lies between 150,000 and 400,000/μL.

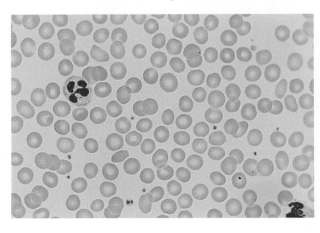

Figure 4.18 On this peripheral blood smear you can see fine little purple dots scattered among the red blood cells and one neutrophil—these are platelets. (From Greer JP, Arber DA, List AF, Foerster J. *Wintrobe's Clinical Hematology*. 13th ed. Lippincott Williams & Wilkins; 2014.)

Thrombocytopenia: This term refers to a lower-than-normal level of platelets in the circulation. When you see a patient with unexplained bruising or small hemorrhages (petechiae) in the skin, or encounter a patient with unusually heavy menstrual bleeding, check the platelet count. Patients with platelet counts below 20,000/μL are prone to bleed with minor trauma (eg, with dental work or with straining to pass urine or stool). Potentially dangerous spontaneous bleeding —for example, an unprovoked cerebral bleed or large gastrointestinal hemorrhage—usually will not occur until platelet counts drop below 10,000/μL. The CBC will flag these results so you don't miss them.

Causes of thrombocytopenia include:

- *Increased peripheral destruction or consumption*: An example is immune thrombocytopenic purpura (ITP), either as a primary disorder or associated with other autoimmune conditions such as systemic lupus erythematosus.

- Because the spleen removes platelets from the circulation, patients with *hypersplenism* may have low platelet counts. The two most common causes of hypersplenism are *cirrhosis* (in which platelet production is also impaired due to decreased levels of thrombopoietin) and *hematologic malignancies.*

- Many *infectious diseases* can cause thrombocytopenia. To name just a few: HIV/AIDS, hepatitis C, infectious mononucleosis (Epstein-Barr virus), measles, mumps, rubella, tuberculosis, malaria, and babesiosis. Any patient with sepsis, regardless of the cause, may have thrombocytopenia.

- Any *heparin* preparation can induce an immune response that destroys platelets, resulting in heparin-induced thrombocytopenia (HIT; see Chapter 20).

- Many *medications* besides heparin, including statins, aspirin, and some antibiotics, can cause a thrombocytopenia that is usually mild to moderate. In a patient with unexplained thrombocytopenia, be sure to check the medication list.

- Excess *alcohol* intake commonly causes mild thrombocytopenia. The mechanism involves both direct bone marrow suppression and liver toxicity.

- *Pregnancy*: usually the low platelet count is not severe and tends to be benign and self-limited, posing no threat to the baby or mother.

- *Primary bone marrow failure* (eg, aplastic anemia): Isolated thrombocytopenia is rare. Usually there will be abnormalities of other cell lines as well.

Watch out for a false decrease in the platelet count called *pseudothrombocytopenia*. This is just a laboratory artifact and occurs most often when the platelets clump in the blood sample, sometimes as a result of interaction of the sample with EDTA (the anticoagulant used to prevent the sample from clotting). Pseudothrombocytopenia is surprisingly common. Most labs

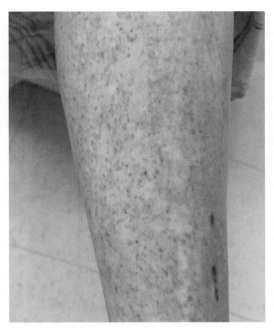

Figure 4.19 Petechiae on the legs of a patient with thrombocytopenia. (From Weksler BB, Schechter GP, Ely SA. *Wintrobe's Atlas of Clinical Hematology*. 2nd ed. Wolters Kluwer; 2018.)

will catch this, but some may not. If you have a patient with an isolated low platelet count and no discernible cause, make sure to repeat the test using a tube with a non-EDTA anticoagulant to rule out pseudothrombocytopenia before embarking on an extensive evaluation.

Bleeding When There Shouldn't Be Bleeding

There are many reasons why a person might bleed excessively or inappropriately with minor trauma or no trauma at all. Thrombocytopenia is just one of the reasons, but not an uncommon one. We felt it was important to remind you here that your work is not done once you have checked a platelet count and found that it is normal. The problem could lie in a defect in the blood vessels themselves or in any of the components of the coagulation pathways (eg, an inherited or acquired coagulation factor deficiency). In addition, there could be a disorder of platelet *function* despite a normal platelet count. Measuring the platelet count is just one piece of what can be a complex—but not complicated—evaluation. That being said, if you find a very low platelet count in the setting of bleeding, you are likely on the right track. See Chapter 20 for more on abnormal bleeding.

Thrombocytosis: The differential diagnosis for a high platelet count is shorter than that for thrombocytopenia.

- By far the most common cause is *reactive thrombocytosis*, a nonspecific response that may accompany infections, acute inflammatory conditions, malignancies, or hemorrhages.

- Most patients who have undergone *removal of the spleen* (splenectomy) develop a thrombocytosis.

- Thrombocytosis, often profound, is the cardinal laboratory feature of *essential thrombocythemia*, a rare myeloproliferative disorder.

- Mild thrombocytosis is a common finding in patients with *iron deficiency anemia*, probably because the iron deficiency leads to stimulation of progenitor cells that impact both the red cell and platelet cell lines.

Giant Platelets

Unusually large platelets are most often seen on a peripheral blood smear when there is profound *destruction of platelets* in the circulation (eg, in ITP), leading the bone marrow to release large, immature platelets or even megakaryocytes, the progenitor cells of platelets. Giant platelets can also be seen in myeloproliferative disorders and myelodysplastic syndromes. Very rare causes include certain inherited disorders of platelet dysfunction such as Bernard-Soulier syndrome.

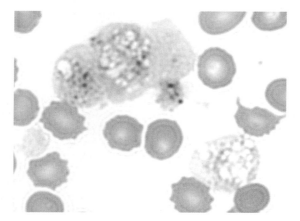

Figure 4.20 The large, irregular, smudgy looking things are giant platelets. This patient has primary myelofibrosis (a type of myeloproliferative disorder). (From Weksler BB, Schechter GP, Ely SA. *Wintrobe's Atlas of Clinical Hematology.* 2nd ed. Wolters Kluwer 2018.)

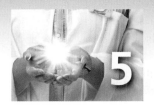

The Comprehensive Metabolic Panel (CMP)

5

The comprehensive metabolic panel (CMP) is just what it sounds like—a general overview of the body's metabolic status. Here is what a report looks like:

Patient Report   ●**YourLab**

Specimen ID: **301-992-9006-0**   Acct #: **90000999**   Phone: Rte: **00**
Control ID:

SAMPLE REPORT, 322000

||₁ᵢₗₗᵢₗᵢₗₗₗ|ₗₗₗₗₗ||||||||ₗₗ||ₗₗ|₁ₗₗₗₗ||ₗₗₗ||ₗₗ||ₗᵢₗ||ₗₗₗ||ₗₗ

Patient Details	**Specimen Details**	**Physician Details**
DOB: **11/13/1960**	Date collected: **10/28/2023 0000 Local**	Ordering:
Age(y/m/d): **062/11/15**	Date received: **10/28/2023**	Referring:
Gender: **M**	Date entered: **10/28/2023**	ID:
Patient ID:	Date reported: **10/31/2023 0000 ET**	NPI:

General Comments & Additional Information
Clinical Info: ABNORMAL REPORT

Ordered items
Comp. Metabolic Panel (14), Litholink CKD Program

TESTS	RESULT	FLAG	UNITS	REFERENCE INTERVAL	LAB
Comp. Metabolic Panel (14)					
Glucose	88		mg/dL	70 – 99	01
BUN	15		mg/dL	8 – 27	01
Creatinine	**1.50**	**High**	mg/dL	0.76 – 1.27	01
eGFR	**52**	**Low**	mL/min/1.73	>59	
BUN/Creatinine Ratio	10			10 – 24	
Sodium	**150**	**High**	mmol/L	134 – 144	01
Potassium	3.8		mmol/L	3.5 – 5.2	01
Chloride	100		mmol/L	96 – 106	01
Carbon Dioxide, Total	25		mmol/L	20 – 29	01
Calcium	9.0		mg/dL	8.6 – 10.2	01
Protein, Total	7.5		g/dL	6.0 – 8.5	01
Albumin	**4.9**	**High**	g/dL	3.8 – 4.8	01
Globulin, Total	2.6		g/dL	1.5 – 4.5	
A/G Ratio	1.9			1.2 – 2.2	
Bilirubin, Total	1.2		mg/dL	0.0 – 1.2	01
Alkaline Phosphatase	66		TU/L	44 – 121	01
AST (SGOT)	25		TU/L	0 – 40	01
ALT (SGOT)	33		TU/L	0 – 44	01

Litholink CKD Program

Figure 5.1 A typical CMP report with a few highlighted abnormalities. CMP, comprehensive metabolic panel.

The CMP is often your first look at the overall body chemistry of your patient. It can be divided into four distinct subsets:

- Several of the tests are so fundamental that they are often ordered alone as a single entity called the *Basic Metabolic Panel** and include:

  - glucose

  - electrolytes: sodium, potassium, chloride, and carbon dioxide (CO_2)

  - two tests of kidney function: blood urea nitrogen (BUN) and creatinine (which allows you to calculate the estimated glomerular filtration rate, or eGFR)

- A potpourri of liver function tests:

  - total bilirubin

  - alkaline phosphatase (ALP)

  - aspartate transaminase (AST; this was previously referred to as the SGOT, or serum glutamic-oxaloacetic transaminase)

  - alanine transaminase (ALT; this was previously referred to as the SGPT, or serum glutamic-pyruvic transaminase)

- The major proteins circulating in the blood:

  - total protein

  - albumin

  - globulins

  - the ratio of albumin to globulins

- The calcium

You can see how, with just this single panel, you can get a pretty good idea of the molecular milieu circulating throughout the body, bathing every organ, tissue, and cell at one moment in time. Reliance on this panel is pervasive in medicine, and clinicians have an understandable tendency to order it almost without a second thought, sometimes repeatedly with no clear idea exactly what they are looking for. But if you paid any attention to what we talked about in the previous section, you know that this modus operandi is rarely a good idea. *A CMP, like all laboratory tests, should be ordered only when the information it provides will affect the management of your patient.* If all you need is one result—say, a calcium—then order a calcium. But you will find that it is often valuable to know more than just a single value in isolation. For example, the serum calcium (specifically its biologically active ionized

---

*A BMP is often all you need when, for example, you are monitoring a patient's electrolytes or renal function. There is no need to order a CMP when a BMP will suffice.

form) is affected by the serum albumin level (see page 77), so it is often important to know both.

Like the complete blood count (CBC), the CMP is a relatively inexpensive test. It requires only a single serum separator tube.

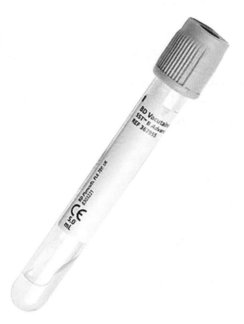

Figure 5.2 A serum separator tube. Note the gel at the bottom that serves as a filter to separate the cellular elements from everything else. The CMP is run on the remaining serum. CMP, comprehensive metabolic panel.

The Comprehensive Metabolic Panel: Why These Particular Tests?

While undeniably useful, the CMP is actually an odd, eclectic collection of items. It includes a test of one of the body's primary sources of energy (glucose), a measure of the body's metabolic capacity (the protein tests), tests of how two organ systems are functioning (kidneys and liver), the charged ions responsible for nerve and muscle function (the electrolytes), and another substance critical for bone and muscle function (calcium). Note what is not included: no hormones, no lipids, no measures of heart or lung function, no screens for infectious or inflammatory diseases. Why, then, this particular grouping?

The truth is, we don't know. We'll confess we didn't look all that hard to find the answer, but it must lie somewhere in the dusty, historical arcana of medicine. Let us know if you find out and we'll add it to the next edition (and thank you as well!). In any event, we are stuck with the CMP for the foreseeable future and should appreciate it for what it does offer us rather than fault it for what it does not.

Glucose, Electrolytes, and Kidney Function

Glucose

Among the many different types of sugars, glucose earns top billing because it is our major source of energy. Measuring the serum glucose is essential in many clinical settings (some would argue, convincingly, in almost all situations). Either an elevated glucose (*hyperglycemia*) or a glucose that is too low (*hypoglycemia*) can have immense health ramifications both acutely and chronically. Normal fasting glucose values are 70 to 100 mg/dL.

The serum glucose can vary tremendously depending on what and when your patient has last eaten. If you are ordering a CMP in the outpatient setting and are concerned about hyper- or hypoglycemia, you may want your patient to come in fasting (generally in the morning having eaten nothing after midnight). All of the other tests in the CMP do not vary so acutely and dramatically with diet, and fasting is not necessary. Recommend fasting before a CMP only if you are concerned about obtaining an accurate reading of the serum glucose.

If sufficiently high, a fasting glucose may be all you need to diagnose diabetes. However, we have other tests that can assess a patient's *long-term* glucose control over the preceding weeks that can provide additional and often more helpful information. The best known of these is the hemoglobin A1c (see Chapter 19). Sometimes, however, you need to know exactly what the glucose is at the very moment you are seeing the patient—for example, in a patient who presents obtunded or comatose, or simply as an easy, initial, on-the-spot screen for diabetes—and that "snapshot" picture is what this test is for.

Hyperglycemia: Definitions

- A *normal* value of the fasting glucose is considered to be less than 100 mg/dL.

- A fasting glucose of 126 mg/dL or more is diagnostic of *diabetes*.

- A fasting glucose between 100 and 126 mg/dL has been called *prediabetes*, a term we do not like because it implies an inevitable progression to frank diabetes, which is simply not the case. Nevertheless, you will see this term over and over again, so we offer it to you with this caveat. A better approach would be to refer to these patients as having *hyperglycemia* or *impaired glucose tolerance* and give the precise number.

There is no uniform glucose concentration above which patients develop symptoms associated with *hyperglycemia*. One patient may develop severe polyuria and polydipsia with a glucose of 300 mg/dL, whereas another patient may remain asymptomatic with a glucose of 400 mg/dL. Most patients with diabetic ketoacidosis (classically associated with type 1 diabetes) have a serum glucose in the 350 to 500 mg/dL range, and most with hyperosmolar hyperglycemic state (classically associated with type 2 diabetes) have a serum glucose closer to 1,000 mg/dL.

Hypoglycemia, defined as a serum glucose less than 70 mg/dL, occurs most often in patients with medication-treated (eg, insulin- or sulfonylurea-treated) diabetes. Those without diabetes may develop hypoglycemia from severe malnourishment, critical illness, adrenal insufficiency, medication or substance toxicity (alcohol is a common offender), or—rarely—endogenous overproduction of insulin (eg, insulinoma). In practice, symptoms associated with hypoglycemia (palpitations, sweating, anxiety, paresthesias) typically do not occur unless the glucose is less than 55 mg/dL, but this varies from patient to patient. Profound hypoglycemia can be life threatening and requires prompt correction (eg, oral administration of sugary juice or candy, or intravenous [IV] dextrose in more severe cases).

Special Note: If your patient is receiving an IV infusion containing dextrose, which is chemically identical to glucose, do not draw the blood sample immediately downstream from the IV; the glucose will be artificially high.

Electrolytes

The electrolytes include the two positive ions, sodium (Na^+) and potassium (K^+), and the two negative ions, chloride (Cl^-) and bicarbonate (HCO_3^-, but confusingly indicated on the CMP as carbon dioxide; we will explain this on page 61).

An electrolyte is any substance that—by virtue of its electric charge—can conduct electricity when dissolved in a solution. These four electrolytes are about as fundamental as it gets when you talk about laboratory tests. The body meticulously maintains their values within very small ranges, because a significant deviation can have severe clinical repercussions. The positive ions get most of the attention, and deservedly so, but it is important to look at all the electrolytes when assessing your patient.

Sodium: Why do we care about the serum sodium concentration? To answer this, we need to talk about osmolality.

Osmolality is defined as the total concentration of solute particles in a solution. Any substance that cannot passively cross a cell membrane—including sodium—contributes to osmolality; it is said to be "osmotically active." Sodium (Na^+) is by far the most ubiquitous extracellular cation and is the largest contributor to plasma osmolality under normal circumstances.* If the sodium increases on one side of a cell membrane, let's say intracellularly, water will move into the cell to restore normal osmolality. In essence, where sodium goes, water follows. Any problem with sodium usually means a problem with osmolality and, consequently, a problem with water. Throw off the osmolality of the blood, and massive fluid shifts can ensue, leading to potentially devastating consequences (eg, cerebral edema).

It makes sense, then, that the body tightly regulates the serum osmolality (and therefore the sodium concentration), largely through two mechanisms: (1) *thirst* and (2) *antidiuretic hormone* (ADH).** Thirst is easy to understand: when serum osmolality is high, you crave water, drink

---

*There is one important exception: when the plasma glucose is very high—for example, in poorly controlled diabetes—it can become the major determinant of the plasma osmolality.
**There are other smaller contributors to sodium regulation. Among these are hormones that respond primarily to volume status rather than osmolality: *aldosterone*, which enhances renal retention of both sodium and water, and the natriuretic hormones, atrial natriuretic peptide (ANP) and brain natriuretic peptide (BNP) (see Chapter 15), which act on the kidneys to decrease reabsorption of sodium from the urine.

water, and dilute out excess sodium. At the same time, ADH is secreted by the posterior pituitary and acts on the kidneys to cause reabsorption of water from the urine. The result is a more concentrated urine and a more dilute serum (lower sodium and osmolality). When plasma osmolality is low, you aren't thirsty. ADH levels decline and more water remains in the urine, resulting in a dilute urine and a more concentrated serum (higher sodium and osmolality).

The serum sodium and serum osmolality are both maintained within a narrow range (136-145 mEq/L and 275-295 mOsm/kg H_2O, respectively). The urine sodium and urine osmolality, on the other hand, can both vary dramatically in a perfectly healthy individual, ranging from less than 10 to more than 40 mEq/L and 50 to 1,200 mOsm/kg H_2O, respectively.

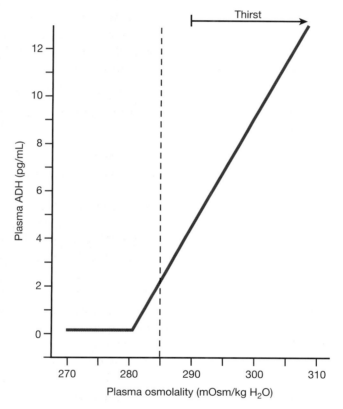

Figure 5.3 ADH and thirst increase as serum osmolality increases. ADH, antidiuretic hormone. (From Rhoades RA, Bell DR. *Medical Physiology: Principles for Clinical Medicine.* 6th ed. Wolters Kluwer; 2023.)

Why is the normal range for both the urine sodium and urine osmolality so much larger than for their serum counterparts? Because the kidneys, with the help of ADH, have to be able to quickly and powerfully adjust the amount of sodium and water that is excreted in the urine and reabsorbed back into the circulation in order to maintain tight control of the serum osmolality. Put another way, the serum osmolality is the key clinical end point; the urine osmolality (along with the urine sodium) reflects the moment-to-moment process of regulating the serum osmolality.

Hyponatremia: Most people can tolerate mild hyponatremia (sodium around 130-135 mEq/L) just fine, with no symptoms at all, particularly if the deviation from normal has occurred gradually or has been persistent for some time. Symptoms of hyponatremia usually begin below 125 mEq/L. A sudden drop in the serum sodium can lead to cerebral edema with headache, seizures, coma, and even death.

A couple of important caveats:

- Make sure you have ruled out *pseudohyponatremia*, a false decrease in the serum sodium that is just a laboratory artifact. *It is most often caused by an excess of lipids in the blood.* In this case, the actual sodium concentration in the fluid component of the blood sample is normal, but because the lab measures the sodium in the *total* blood sample, fluid and lipid alike, the sodium may appear to be low when it is actually perfectly fine.

- You also need to consider the presence of other highly osmotic molecules that can dilute the serum sodium by pulling fluid out of the body's cells into the circulation; *the most common culprit is a high serum glucose.*

Once these possibilities are off the table—and except in situations of marked hyperlipidemia or hyperglycemia you rarely have to worry about them—you are ready to proceed.

A low sodium is best addressed by knowing your patient's volume status.

Hyponatremia with decreased extracellular volume ("hypovolemic hyponatremia"):
Patients with low extracellular volume will appear dehydrated. Clinically, the only clue may be a resting tachycardia and/or dry mucous membranes, but there may also be orthostatic hypotension or an absence of axillary sweat. These patients have lost both sodium and fluid, so you might reason that the sodium concentration should remain normal. However, with significant loss of fluid, the preservation of extracellular volume becomes more important than the preservation of the sodium concentration; osmolality and the sodium concentration are, of course, important, but volume loss can lead to hypotension, shock, and death far more quickly. Therefore, the body attempts to hold onto fluid by increasing the secretion of both aldosterone and ADH. As a result, water retention increases, resulting in dilution of the serum sodium, that is, hyponatremia.

Sodium loss can occur via the kidneys or, less often, via other routes.

- *Renal sodium loss* is usually due to the use of *diuretics* (eg, furosemide or hydrochloro-thiazide), but can also occur with *adrenal insufficiency, renal tubular acidosis,* and *certain salt-wasting nephropathies.*

- *Nonrenal sodium loss* can occur with *massive burns, excess perspiration* (eg, running a marathon on a hot day), or, more often, gastrointestinal (GI) fluid loss due to *diarrhea and/or vomiting, pancreatitis,* or *bowel obstruction.*

How can you tell if the sodium is being lost through the kidneys or by some other mechanism? The clinical picture may make the diagnosis obvious—for example, your patient is taking diuretics, or may have a severe gastroenteritis—but if it is not, check a *urine sodium concentration.*

- If the urine sodium is less than 25 mEq/L, then the kidneys are appropriately holding onto sodium. Therefore, nonrenal (eg, GI) sodium loss is likely the problem. Such patients often have a urine sodium that is undetectably low (ie, <10 mEq/L).

- If the urine sodium is more than 40 mEq/L, then the kidneys are inappropriately excreting too much sodium into the urine, and renal loss is probably the problem.

- In our experience, a urine sodium greater than 25 but less than 40 mEq/L is usually due to renal sodium loss (but this is not always the case).

Hyponatremia with increased extracellular volume ("hypervolemic hyponatremia"): These patients are fluid overloaded. They are hyponatremic because the excess fluid is diluting out the serum sodium. There are three major causes: *congestive heart failure, cirrhosis,* and *renal failure.* Edema is often present, a key tip-off that your patient is fluid overloaded. The clinical picture usually allows you to distinguish among these causes, but, as in the case of hypovolemic hyponatremia, a urine sodium may be helpful (see Figure 5.4).

Hyponatremia with normal extracellular volume ("euvolemic hyponatremia"): This is the most common type of hyponatremia. As many as 30% of hospitalized patients develop hyponatremia, and most have a normal extracellular fluid volume. Almost all of these patients have some form of what is called the *syndrome of inappropriate antidiuretic hormone* (SIADH for short). ADH, as we mentioned earlier, increases water retention, thereby concentrating the urine and diluting the serum. You should consider SIADH when your patient with hyponatremia is neither obviously hypovolemic nor obviously hypervolemic.

There are many reasons why ADH secretion may be inappropriately elevated. Among the more common causes are:

- Malignancies, most notoriously small cell carcinoma of the lung

- Central nervous system disorders (eg, meningitis)

- Pulmonary infections (eg, pneumonia)

- Drugs: chlorpropamide, nonsteroidal anti-inflammatory agents (NSAIDs), the selective serotonin reuptake inhibitors (SSRIs) used to treat depression and anxiety, multiple chemotherapeutic agents, and more can all increase the secretion of ADH.

The key to establishing the diagnosis of SIADH in a patient with euvolemic hyponatremia is to check the urine sodium and osmolality. In any patient with hyponatremia, the kidneys should be trying to put out a dilute urine (lower urine osmolality) in order to concentrate the serum. But in SIADH the urine osmolality is high (usually >300 mOsm/kg).

Why not just measure the serum ADH? The test is expensive and its accuracy is at best problematic. It is generally only used in research protocols.

Other endocrinopathies that can cause euvolemic hyponatremia—less commonly than SIADH—include adrenal insufficiency and hypothyroidism. Urine studies typically look similar to those in SIADH. It is often prudent to check a thyroid-stimulating hormone (TSH) and morning cortisol level in patients with euvolemic hyponatremia, especially if they have other signs or symptoms of adrenal insufficiency (eg, hypotension, hypoglycemia) or hypothyroidism (eg, constipation, weight gain). The workups for these conditions are discussed further in Chapters 19 and 7, respectively.

Drinking Your Way to Hyponatremia

Can you drink yourself into a state of hyponatremia? Yes, but it's not easy[a]; your kidneys, assuming they are healthy, do a pretty good job of getting rid of excess fluid. However, patients with *psychogenic*, or *primary*, *polydipsia* can consume sufficient fluid to cause hyponatremia. There are also descriptions of marathon runners drinking way beyond their thirst requirements and causing clinically significant hyponatremia. Expect such a patient to have very dilute urine (Uosm <100 mOsm/kg).

[a]Unless you are an infant.

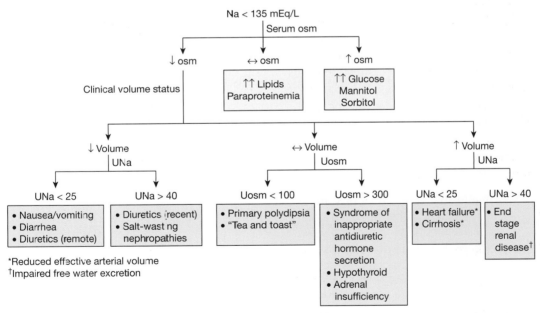

Figure 5.4 Flow chart for the laboratory workup of hyponatremia using clinical volume status, serum osmolality, urine osmolality, and urine sodium concentration. Remember that urine sodium tends to fall in response to high circulating levels of aldosterone (ie, states of intravascular volume depletion). Urine osmolality rises in response to high circulating levels of ADH. As always, the clinical picture is your most powerful diagnostic tool—the above cutoff values serve more as a rough guide than as a set of absolute rules. Importantly, hyponatremia can often be multifactorial; in these cases, the lab results may not perfectly fit any one of the above diagnoses. ADH, antidiuretic hormone.

Hypernatremia: As with hyponatremia, mild hypernatremia—especially if chronic or gradually progressive—typically does not cause symptoms. Significant symptoms of hypernatremia are often seen when the sodium reaches the high 150s (a number frequently cited is 158 mEq/L). The faster the hypernatremia develops, the more likely the patient is to be symptomatic.

An increased sodium concentration can occur when:

- *The patient is unable to consume adequate fluids.* Patients who are obtunded or comatose or who for whatever reason do not have access to water (eg, someone stranded on a desert island) can become hypernatremic.

- *Significant water loss exceeds sodium loss.* This can occur with severe diarrhea, excessive perspiration or fluid loss from extensive burns on the skin.

- *The kidneys cannot adequately conserve sodium.* This is usually due to inadequate secretion of ADH (the opposite of SIADH) or the failure of the kidneys to respond to ADH. The former is termed *central diabetes insipidus (DI),* the latter *nephrogenic DI.* Central DI can be caused by any process that interrupts the hypothalamic-pituitary axis, such as infiltrative diseases (eg, sarcoidosis), tumors, and strokes. Nephrogenic DI can result from numerous renal disorders, but can also be caused by medications, notably lithium (commonly used for bipolar disorder).

Diagnosing Diabetes Insipidus: Urine Osmolality and the Water Restriction Test

Polyuria is the most common presenting symptom in patients with DI. Whereas hypernatremia may be seen, it is not universally present. How, then, can you tell if your patient with polyuria has DI and not some other cause of increased urine output?

In the *water restriction test,* the patient is asked to refrain from drinking fluids for several hours (usually overnight), long enough to drive up the serum osmolality to more than 295 mOsm/kg and the serum sodium to more than 145 mEq/L. Hypertonic saline can be added if the desired thresholds are not achieved. In patients who do not have DI, ADH levels spike in response to the high serum osmolality, resulting in a corresponding spike in urine osmolality, usually to at least 500 mOsm/kg. In a patient with DI, the water restriction fails to produce a significant increase in urine osmolality.

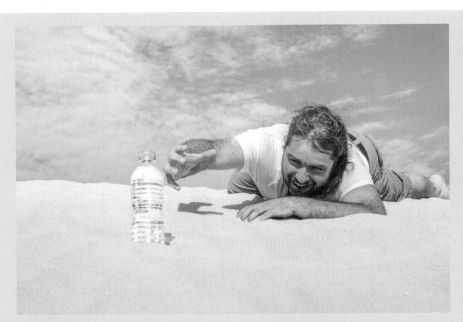

Figure 5.5 Do not torture your patients—a water restriction test can be quite unpleasant and isn't always necessary to make a diagnosis of diabetes insipidus (DI) or primary polydipsia. Many experts vastly shorten the time of fluid restriction or even avoid the test altogether in any patient with a baseline urine osmolality <100 mOsm/kg; in these patients, severe DI is likely and prolonged water deprivation can result in profound hypovolemia and hypernatremia. (Courtesy of tilialucida/ Shutterstock.)

In patients with a water restriction test suggestive of DI, central DI can be distinguished from nephrogenic DI by administering desmopressin (exogenous ADH). Expect urine osmolality to at least double in a patient with central DI because the kidneys are able to respond to the hormone. Urine osmolality should remain largely unchanged (usually <15% increase, and almost always <300 mOsm/kg) in a patient with nephrogenic DI.

Potassium: The serum potassium is maintained within a very narrow range. Normal values lie between 3.5 and 5.0 mEq/L. Although subtle deviations from normal usually cause no problems—many patients live with potassium levels that are chronically slightly low or high—sudden or significant changes can have profound effects, none of them good. A *low potassium* can cause severe weakness, ileus (functional—as opposed to mechanical—obstruction of the bowel), and cardiac arrhythmias. A *high potassium* can also cause significant cardiac arrhythmias and conduction blocks (hyperkalemia can do almost anything to the electrocardiogram [ECG]).

How the serum potassium can go awry: The bottom line when thinking about abnormal levels of potassium is to consider three potential sources of the imbalance:

- the kidneys,

- the GI tract, and

- the movement of potassium into and out of cells across their cellular membranes.

Excessive or impaired renal secretion as well as the loss of potassium via the GI tract are intuitively easy to understand. The third item on our list, transmembrane shifts, requires just a bit of thought. Unlike sodium, potassium is largely an *intracellular* cation. To keep sodium outside the cell and potassium inside, a transmembrane pump requires energy to exchange one ion for the other. Anything that affects this pump—eg, adrenergic stimulation—will affect how much potassium is in the bloodstream (and therefore measurable) versus inside the cells.

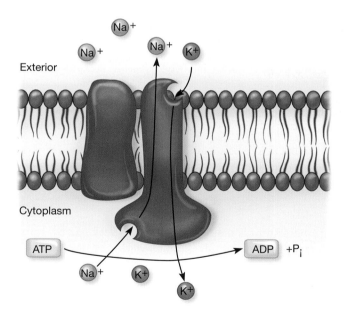

Figure 5.6 The sodium-potassium pump. (From Craven RF, Hirnle CJ, Henshaw CM. *Fundamentals of Nursing: Human Health and Function.* 8th ed. Wolters Kluwer; 2017.)

Our cells also contain transmembrane pumps that exchange potassium (K^+) for hydrogen ions (H^+). These pumps are critical in maintaining the acid-base balance in the bloodstream. For example, with metabolic acidosis (more on this in Chapter 9), excess hydrogen ions (H^+) enter the cells and—in order to maintain electrical neutrality—potassium ions depart (if one positive ion goes in, one must go out). The result is that more potassium ions enter the circulation, resulting in hyperkalemia. With metabolic alkalosis, the opposite happens. H^+ leaves the cells, forcing potassium to move intracellularly. The result is hypokalemia.

Important factors that can move potassium into or out of cells are shown in Table 5.1.

Table 5.1 Things That Move K^+ Into and Out of Cells

Factors That Move K^+ Out of Cells and Can Cause Hyperkalemia	Factors That Move K^+ Into Cells and Can Cause Hypokalemia
β_2-adrenergic antagonists	β_2-adrenergic agonists
α-adrenergic agonists	α-adrenergic antagonists
Acidosis	Alkalosis
Hyperosmolality*	Insulin
Cell lysis	
Intense or prolonged exercise	

* This is most often relevant in patients with diabetes who develop hyperglycemia and associated hyperosmolality. Potassium is dragged out of their cells along with water. These patients either don't secrete or don't respond to insulin, which would normally move the potassium back into the cells.

Hypokalemia: The leading causes of *hypokalemia*, the ones you should think of first, are:

- *Diuretics* (thiazides, such as hydrochlorothiazide or chlorthalidone; and loop diuretics, such as furosemide)

- *GI disorders* (especially diarrhea)

- *Hyperaldosteronism* (aldosterone enhances sodium reabsorption and potassium excretion by the kidneys; see Chapter 19)

- *Hyperglycemia* when it is associated with an osmotic diuresis

Hyperkalemia: The leading causes of *hyperkalemia* are:

- *Renal failure* (acute or chronic; the kidneys just can't excrete potassium appropriately)

- *Hypoaldosteronism* (sodium is excreted by the kidneys and potassium is reabsorbed)

- *Type IV renal tubular acidosis* (this is actually just a form of hypoaldosteronism)

- *Drugs that reduce K+ secretion*

  - "K+-sparing" diuretics such as spironolactone, eplerenone, and triamterene

  - NSAIDs

  - Angiotensin-converting enzyme (ACE) inhibitors and angiotensin receptor blockers (ARBs): angiotensin stimulates the synthesis of aldosterone, so anything that blocks the activity of angiotensin will decrease aldosterone levels

- *Massive cell death,* leading to the release of large quantities of intracellular K+ into the circulation

  - Tumor lysis syndrome is the classic example (see Chapter 20)

- What about *excess K+ intake?* In the absence of underlying kidney disease, it is extremely difficult to consume your way to hyperkalemia.

Pseudohyperkalemia

This may actually be the most common cause of hyperkalemia. When a blood sample is allowed to sit untended for too long, the cells in the sample can lyse, releasing their intracellular contents of potassium into the serum, causing a falsely high reading. Cell lysis causing a falsely high serum potassium can also occur with a traumatic blood draw or when the tourniquet is tied too tightly around the arm. When you see an elevated potassium in a healthy patient with no obvious cause, repeat the test before embarking on an extensive evaluation.

How to Evaluate Potassium Disorders: The clinical picture will almost always suggest the reason for a patient's altered potassium level. For example, you will generally know if your patient is suffering from diarrhea or is on a diuretic. But sometimes a more thorough investigation is needed.

Checking the *urine potassium*—which sounds like a reasonable way to distinguish altered renal excretion from other causes of a potassium disorder—can sometimes be helpful. If, in a

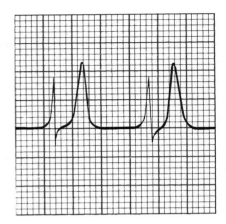

Figure 5.7 Potassium imbalances, particularly hyperkalemia, can do almost anything to the electrocardiogram. Here are the classic peaked T waves that can be an early indicator of significant hyperkalemia (and the more electrically erudite among you may have also noticed the absence of detectable P waves).

patient with hypokalemia, the potassium-creatinine ratio in a spot urine sample is less than 13 mEq/g, then you can be reasonably confident that the kidneys are not the cause of potassium loss; in other words, the kidneys are doing their best to hold onto whatever potassium comes their way. But this test isn't always as reliable as one might think, primarily because the kidneys are constantly adjusting to maintain the existing balance between potassium intake and excretion. A 24-hour urine collection for potassium may be more accurate.

Depending on the clinical scenario, you may want to order additional lab chemistries to rule out diabetes (a fasting glucose or hemoglobin A1c), renal failure (creatinine and BUN), and metabolic acidosis or metabolic alkalosis (a blood gas). An evaluation for hypo- or hyperaldosteronism is indicated in some patients (see Chapter 19), particularly in those with hypokalemia and hypertension, in whom hyperaldosteronism may be the culprit.

One final note: an ECG is actually the best indicator of the clinical severity of hypokalemia or hyperkalemia, more accurate than the actual serum potassium level itself.

Chloride: What can we say about chloride? It is truly the forgotten electrolyte. Looked at simply as a number in isolation, it tells you practically nothing. Its major diagnostic role is in helping sort out the potential causes of acid-base disturbances. For now we are going to leave it at that. Oh yes—normal serum values are 98 to 106 mEq/L.

CO_2: We think of CO_2 as a gas that we exhale as a by-product of our body's metabolism. So why do we classify it with the electrolytes? CO_2, as reported on the CMP, actually represents carbon dioxide *in all its forms* (technically, "total CO_2" or "TCO_2"). The vast majority of carbon dioxide in the blood exists in the form of HCO_3^- (bicarbonate). Only a very small percentage is free CO_2 gas dissolved in the serum (carbamate, the form of CO_2 carried by hemoglobin, also makes up a small percentage). When you see "CO_2" on a CMP or BMP, simply substitute "HCO_3^-" (bicarbonate) in your head. Bicarbonate is the key agent that buffers H^+ in the blood and therefore plays a critical role in maintaining acid-base balance.

The equilibrium equation you want to keep in mind is this:

$$CO_2 + H_2O \leftrightharpoons H_2CO_3 \leftrightharpoons HCO_3^- + H^+$$

And, to take this one step further, the pH of the blood is proportional to the ratio of the HCO_3^- to the Pco_2 (the partial pressure of CO_2 in the blood):

$$pH \propto HCO_3^-/Pco_2$$

Why are we telling you all this? Because you can't accurately interpret the bicarbonate (ie, the CO_2 on the CMP) without also knowing the pH and Pco_2. We are therefore going to ask that you be a little patient while we postpone our discussion of CO_2 until our chapter on blood gases chapter on blood gases (Chapter 9). Normal values range from 23 to 28 mEq/L (there is some variation by laboratory).

The Anion Gap

When you sum up the concentrations in the blood of the positive electrolytes (Na^+ and K^+) and compare it to the sum of the negative electrolytes (Cl^- and HCO_3^-), you will notice something strange. They don't match. The amount of positively charged electrolytes is greater than that of the negatively charged ions. This difference is called the anion gap. The formula for calculating it is simple:

$$\text{Anion gap} = (Na^+ + K^+) - (Cl^- + HCO_3^-)$$

The normal anion gap is between 8 and 16 mEq/L throughout most of the world, and between 4 and 12 mEq/L in the United States where, for reasons we don't understand, the K^+ is left out of the equation.

Since we know that positive and negative charges must be equivalent so they balance each other out, some other negatively charged molecules must fill that gap. These normally include proteins (primarily albumin) and various organic acids, such as phosphates and sulfates.

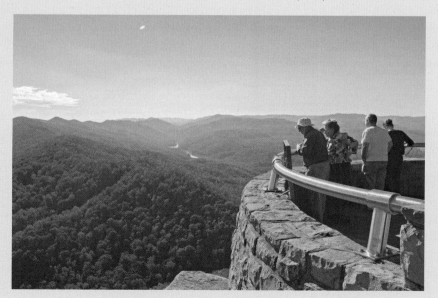

Figure 5.8 A picture of the famous Cumberland Gap in Kentucky. Compared to the anion gap, the view is better. (Courtesy of Kentucky Tourism.)

Assessing the anion gap is most useful in the setting of *metabolic acidosis*, a common circumstance in which the acid-base balance of the body is thrown off because the body is producing too much acid (by acid, we mean positively charged hydrogen ions, H+). We will discuss this situation more in Chapter 9. For now—especially for those of you who like adding things up and might be wondering why there appear to be more positive ions than negative ones—we just wanted you to know that an anion gap exists, is easily calculated, what it consists of, and that it is one of the many useful things the CMP brings to the table.

Measures of Kidney Function: The Creatinine, Blood Urea Nitrogen, and Glomerular Filtration Rate

The kidneys do a lot of things: remove metabolic waste from the body, regulate fluid balance, and maintain electrolyte and acid-base equilibria. They are also involved in vitamin D metabolism, regulation of blood pressure, and the release of hormones that regulate red blood cell production.

Among all the things the kidneys do, the CMP focuses its attention on just a single aspect of renal function: the ability of the kidneys to remove waste and excess fluid. And it does so, with reasonable although less-than-perfect accuracy, by reporting the *glomerular filtration rate (GFR)*. The GFR is the amount of blood that is filtered through the kidneys (the renal glomeruli) each minute.

Determining the GFR is a laudable goal—of all the things the kidneys do, this is the one with the most dire consequences should it go awry. When patients end up on dialysis or become candidates for renal transplantation, it is the GFR that has declined to the point where dangerous metabolic products can build up in the blood, fluid overload can develop, and electrolyte and acid-base disturbances can become dangerously severe.

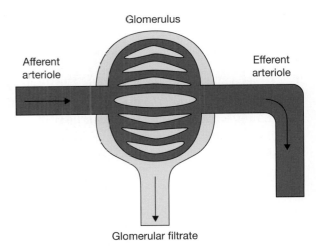

Figure 5.9 Glomerular filtration in a nutshell (or more precisely in a glomerulus). Blood enters each glomerulus (there are about one million in each kidney) via afferent arterioles, is filtered, and exits via efferent arterioles. As the filtrate passes through the renal tubules, various substances are secreted and reabsorbed. Measurements of the glomerular filtration rate, however, are concerned only with the first step. (From Christensen CR, Lewis PA. *Core Curriculum for Vascular Nursing.* 2nd ed. Wolters Kluwer; 2014.)

Creatinine: Measuring the GFR is not easy. You need a marker, ideally a substance that is passively filtered by the kidneys, one that is not actively secreted or reabsorbed. It should also be easy and inexpensive to measure. And, finally, it should be produced by the body at a steady rate and largely independent of body composition.

The serum *creatinine*, a metabolite of the amino acid creatine, which is found in most skeletal muscle, hits some of these markers, although it delivers only a glancing blow to others. Although the serum creatinine does vary with body composition and is, to a small extent, actively secreted, it still serves as a reasonably reliable measure of the GFR. Normal values of creatinine are 0.7 to 1.3 mg/dL. In individuals with little muscle mass, especially in someone with malnutrition or muscle wasting—such as can be associated with aging—the serum creatinine will usually overestimate the GFR. In addition, several medications, most commonly cimetidine and trimethoprim, can reduce creatinine secretion and thereby increase the serum creatinine in the absence of any actual reduction in GFR. In general, though, an elevated serum creatinine can be considered a reasonably reliable marker of renal dysfunction.

Blood Urea Nitrogen: Suppose you find that your patient has a newly elevated creatinine consistent with renal dysfunction. What is the cause? The BUN (normal values 8-20 mg/dL) may help you begin to answer this question.

Unlike creatinine, urea can be reabsorbed by the kidneys. Volume contraction leads to increased renal reabsorption of solutes as the kidneys attempt to retain more fluid. Urea is one of these solutes. So, with volume contraction, because urea is reabsorbed and creatinine is not, the BUN will increase more than the creatinine. Although the creatinine will increase somewhat as well, a ratio of BUN/creatinine more than 20 suggests that the cause of a diminished GFR *may* be (please note the emphasis on *may*) a result of volume contraction rather than an intrinsic renal disorder. This situation is referred to as *prerenal azotemia*.*

An increased BUN/creatinine ratio can also be caused by an increase in the blood urea concentration independent of any renal disease. Urea is produced from ammonia (NH_3), so anything that increases nitrogenous waste in the blood will preferentially increase the BUN. A high BUN can therefore occur with a high-protein diet, a large GI bleed, and massive cellular breakdown (as can be seen, for example, in patients with sepsis). It is also worth noting that a low-protein diet, malnutrition, and liver disease can cause a low BUN.

The Glomerular Filtration Rate: The CMP will always report the GFR. In general, a value of at least 90 mL/min/1.73 m²** is considered normal, but any value that is greater than 60 mL/min/1.73 m² is rarely cause for immediate concern.

It is important to know that the GFR is a *calculated* number, and an imperfect one. Most equations used to compute the GFR—and there are many—use the serum creatinine in their

---

*There is also a common entity called *postrenal azotemia*, which causes an elevated creatinine and BUN as a result of obstruction to urine flow *below* (distal to) the kidneys. Common causes include a blockage of the ureters due to prostatic hypertrophy or a pelvic malignancy. This diagnosis is typically made with imaging, usually a renal ultrasound showing swelling of the kidneys—*hydronephrosis*—from urine backup. The BUN/creatinine ratio tends not to help you rule this in or out.
**The GFR is adjusted for surface area, hence the meter-squared (m²) in the number.

calculations. The one that is most often recommended today is the CKD-EPI Creatinine Equation, which incorporates age, sex, and the serum creatinine. It also used to include the patient's race, but as we discussed earlier (see page 18), race has now been removed from the equation. Of all the readily available calculators, the CKD-EPI Creatinine Equation appears to be the most accurate for patients whose GFR is more than 60 mL/min/1.73 m². More recent equations have also incorporated cystatin C (see the box below) into the calculation, allowing for even greater accuracy.

Here is a version of the equation that does not include the cystatin C. Don't let the math scare you—you will not have to do the calculation yourself (we can only speak for ourselves, but our ability to calculate something raised to an exponent of -1.200 does not come naturally). Either the lab will do it or you can plug the relevant numbers into any of a number of calculators you can find online.

$$eGFRcr = 142 \times min(Scr/\kappa, 1)^\alpha \times max(Scr/\kappa, 1)^{-1.200} \times 0.9938\ Age \times 1.012\ [if\ female]$$

where

Scr = standardized serum creatinine in mg/dL

κ = 0.7 (female) or 0.9 (male)

α = -0.241 (female) or -0.302 (male)

$min(Scr/\kappa, 1)$ is the minimum of Scr/κ or 1.0

$max(Scr/\kappa, 1)$ is the maximum of Scr/κ or 1.0

Age (years)

Cystatin C

Cystatin C is not part of the CMP, but it is worth mentioning here because, when combined with a serum creatinine, it may provide the best overall measure of the GFR.

Cystatin C is a low-molecular-weight protein produced by all cells that contain nuclei. Its normal value is 0.51 to 0.98 mg/L. Like creatinine, it is freely filtered by the kidneys, but is less impacted by age, sex, and muscle mass, although it can be elevated by inflammation, malignancy, and infection with HIV. Most of the time your clinical decision-making will not require the precision that is obtainable by adding cystatin C to your calculation, but you should know that there is a *CKD-EPI Creatinine-Cystatin C Equation* that nephrologists sometimes rely upon to help guide their management.

The serum creatinine and BUN can be your first indications of underlying renal dysfunction and may provide clues to the potential causes of acute kidney injury. But to really nail down the cause of the problem you will usually need further testing. We will look at some of the next diagnostic steps in patients with acute kidney injury in Chapter 18.

Liver Function Tests

The term "liver function tests" is a misnomer. These blood tests are actually a measure of liver injury, not function. Normal levels = normal liver (most but not all of the time); elevated levels = injured liver (most but not all of the time).

The liver is the hub of metabolism and catabolism, so you can imagine, correctly, that there are a lot of things you can measure to assess the health of someone's liver. You will meet many of these tests later in this book. For now, let's just focus on the tests that the CMP offers you. And the information the CMP provides is remarkably helpful, sufficient to divide the potential causes of liver injury into two major categories that can guide your further evaluation:

- *Hepatocellular disease:* intrahepatic disease processes that affect the liver parenchyma directly, and

- *Biliary disease:* cholestatic extrahepatic disease processes of the biliary tree that affect the liver indirectly.

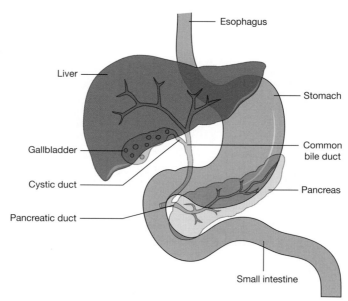

Figure 5.10 The liver and biliary system. Just a reminder.

The Transaminases (Alanine Aminotransferase and Aspartate Aminotransferase)

AST and ALT are enzymes that can be found throughout the body, but are most abundant in the liver. Elevation of the ALT is more specific for liver disease than elevation of the AST, but increased levels of either or both of these serum markers usually signify hepatocellular injury.

Normal values for both the ALT and AST range from 0 to 35 U/L. The most common causes of a significant *transaminitis* (a term often used as a shorthand when the AST and ALT are elevated) are *nonalcoholic fatty liver disease** (NAFLD, the most common liver disease in the developed world) and *alcoholic liver disease*. The relative and absolute values of the ALT and AST can help point you toward the likely diagnosis:

- With alcoholic liver disease, the AST is rarely more than 8 times normal, the ALT rarely more than 5 times normal. *The AST/ALT ratio is usually 2 or more* (see the box "The Alanine Aminotransferase and Aspartate Aminotransferase Ratio").

- With NAFLD, usually neither transaminase will exceed 4 times normal. *The AST/ALT ratio is usually 1 or less.*

- Values of both the ALT and AST can skyrocket to more than 25 times normal (think ALT and AST levels in the thousands) with acute *viral hepatitis, drug/toxin-induced liver damage,* and *ischemic hepatitis.*

Mild transaminase elevations (<5 times normal) are very common in the general, asymptomatic population, affecting somewhere in the neighborhood of 10% of people in the United States. Although persistently elevated transaminases mandate further evaluation, be aware that, with mild elevations, often either no cause will be identified or you will ultimately make a diagnosis of NAFLD.

Important Causes of Mild Transaminase Elevations

- No cause can be identified (still #1)
- NAFLD (#2, but closing fast)
- Alcoholic liver disease (acute or chronic alcoholic hepatitis)
- Hereditary hemochromatosis
- Drug-induced liver damage
- α_1-antitrypsin deficiency
- Autoimmune hepatitis
- Wilson disease
- Extrahepatic causes—eg, celiac disease, thyroid disorders, and rhabdomyolysis

*The term *nonalcoholic fatty liver disease* has recently been superceded by the less stigmatizing *metabolic dysfunction-associated steatotic liver disease (MASLD)*. Because most clinicians still use the older term, we will too for now just to keep things simple.

The Alanine Aminotransferase and Aspartate Aminotransferase Ratio

With most causes of hepatocellular injury, the ALT is elevated more than the AST. However, as mentioned earlier, in patients with alcoholic hepatitis, the reverse is usually true. In patients with an AST/ALT more than 2, alcoholic liver disease is the most likely diagnosis (specificity ~90%). If the ratio is more than 3, the specificity approaches 96%. If you prefer likelihood ratios (see page 15), an AST/ALT ratio more than 2 has an impressive likelihood ratio of 17 for alcoholic liver disease.

The AST may also sometimes—unusually—be higher than the ALT in some patients with NAFLD and in those with hepatic cirrhosis (eg, with hepatitis C and Wilson disease), but in these settings rarely is it more than twice the value of the ALT.

These simple guidelines are not hard and fast, and you will need to temper your rush to diagnosis by considering the clinical context.

Alkaline Phosphatase

Normal values of ALP range from 36 to 92 U/L. An elevation in the ALP disproportionate to a rise in either or both of the transaminases is a clue that biliary disease may be present.

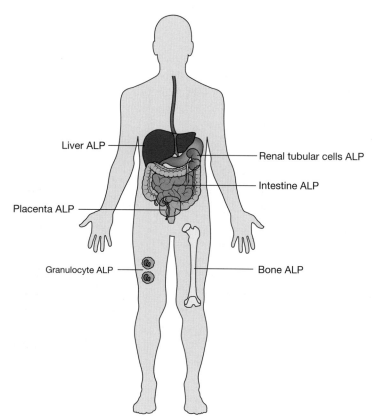

Figure 5.11 Sources of ALP in the body. The major ones are the liver, bone, and placenta. ALP, alkaline phosphatase.

ALP is actually a family of enzymes that can be found in many tissues, most notably the liver, bone, intestines, and placenta. In the liver, ALP resides in the sinusoidal and biliary surfaces of the liver cells, hence its utility as an indicator of biliary disease.

When we say that the ALP is disproportionately higher than the ALT and AST, what exactly do we mean? We can put numbers to this concept and use something called the *R index*, or *R factor*, to help estimate the likelihood of biliary versus hepatocellular disease:

R factor = ratio of (ALT/upper limit of normal of ALT)/(ALP/upper limit of normal of ALP)

If the ratio is more than 5, then hepatocellular disease is likely.

If the ratio is less than 2, then biliary disease is likely.

If the ratio is between 2 and 5, then the picture is mixed and you have more work to do.

Thus, for example, a patient with an ALT of 70 (upper limit of normal is 35) and an ALP of 368 (upper limit of normal is 92)—and yes, we know we've picked numbers that divide nicely—will have an R factor of 2/4 or 0.5; biliary disease is likely.

An Isolated Increased Alkaline Phosphatase

It is not uncommon to encounter a patient with an isolated increase in the ALP. Does this indicate biliary disease, or is the ALP coming from the bone or—in a pregnant patient—the placenta? You can order a *γ-glutamyl transpeptidase* (GGT, normal values 0-30 U/L) to help sort this out. GGT is an enzyme that is more specific than the ALP for liver disease, and if it is also elevated you are likely dealing with a biliary disorder. However, the GGT is not perfect either. Like the ALP, it too resides in small quantities elsewhere in the body, so if you want to get really specific, consider obtaining a *5'-nucleotidase* (normal values 2-17 U/L), an enzyme that is found only in the liver.

In asymptomatic patients (those without symptoms of liver disease, such as itching and jaundice) who have mild elevations in their ALP that is less than 2 times normal, you do not have to immediately and aggressively pursue a diagnosis; it is generally okay to follow these patients serially with ALP measurements and see whether the ALP is increasing or if there is any change in the patients' clinical condition that points you toward a diagnosis. What is going on with these patients?

An elevated ALP can sometimes be found in patients with type O or B blood types after they consume a fatty meal (the contribution here is from intestinal ALP; the ALP elevation typically lasts several hours), and older patients tend to have slightly elevated ALP levels. In neither of these situations is the increased ALP clinically important; that's why we follow them and pursue a workup only if the ALP levels continue to climb or if there are other clues pointing to an underlying disease (liver or otherwise).

Table 5.2 Some Important Causes of an Elevated Alkaline Phosphatase

Liver	Bone
Biliary obstruction: choledocholithiasis, malignancy (of the pancreas, gallbladder, or bile duct), infections (notably *Ascaris lumbricoides* and liver flukes)	Hyperthyroidism
Intrahepatic cholestasis: primary biliary cholangitis, primary sclerosing cholangitis, infiltrative diseases (such as sarcoidosis, lymphoma, and amyloidosis), intrahepatic cholestasis of pregnancy	Paget disease of bone
Can also be elevated with any type of liver parenchymal disease, so check the R factor	Hyperparathyroidism
	Healing fractures
	Osteomalacia
	Malignancy

Bilirubin

The bilirubin can increase with either hepatocellular or cholestatic disorders. It is a metabolic product of hemoglobin that has been released by dying red blood cells into the circulation where, in its *unconjugated* (aka indirect) form, it is bound to circulating albumin. It quickly reaches the liver where it is *conjugated* (aka direct bilirubin) to glucuronic acid and then secreted into the urine and the bile.

The vast majority of total measured bilirubin (normal 0.3-1.2 mg/dL) in a healthy adult is unconjugated; the normal value for the conjugated bilirubin is only 0 to 0.3 mg/dL. Bilirubin is responsible for the yellow discoloration of jaundice, which as a rule (one that is frequently violated) is only apparent when the bilirubin exceeds twice its normal value. Both conjugated and unconjugated bilirubin are elevated in most hepatocellular and biliary diseases in conjunction with an elevation in several or all of the other liver tests.

Unconjugated/Indirect and Conjugated/Direct Bilirubin

The terms *unconjugated/indirect* and *conjugated/direct* bilirubin are used interchangeably. The term "direct" stems from the ability of conjugated bilirubin to react directly with the testing reagent; "indirect" or unconjugated bilirubin must first be solubilized before it reacts. You should know, however, that these terms—conjugated and direct, and unconjugated and indirect—aren't exactly the same thing; it depends on the lab and the technique used to fractionate the bilirubin. However, for clinical purposes, you can use the terms interchangeably and no one will argue with you. So maybe you didn't need to know this after all.

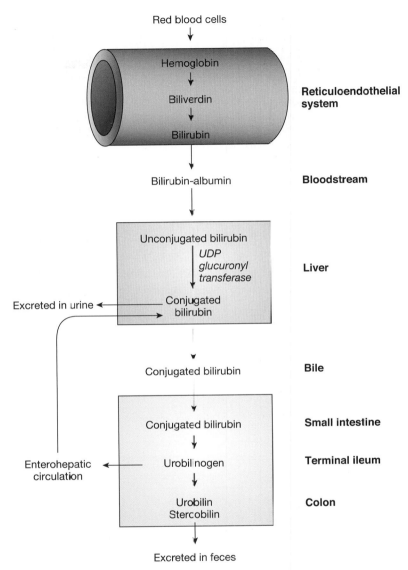

Figure 5.12 The pathway of bilirubin metabolism starting with hemoglobin, the source, and progressing to the end products, which include conjugated and unconjugated bilirubin. (From Costanzo LS. *Board Review Series: Physiology.* 7th ed. Wolters Kluwer; 2019.)

When the bilirubin is elevated in isolation, it can be helpful to fractionate it into its conjugated and unconjugated components (this typically requires ordering a separate liver function panel; see the box "The Liver Function Panel: Alone and Unafraid"):

- *Unconjugated or indirect hyperbilirubinemia* usually indicates either hemolysis or—in adults—Gilbert syndrome (see the box "Gilbert Syndrome"). You will learn how to evaluate suspected hemolysis on page 366.

- If more than 20% to 40% of the bilirubin is conjugated (remember that the conjugated bilirubin is normally present only in very small amounts), the patient should be considered to have *conjugated* or *direct hyperbilirubinemia*, which indicates either hepatocellular or biliary disease. When the percentage of conjugated bilirubin is particularly high, exceeding 50%, the cause most likely lies in the biliary tract. Look at the transaminases and ALP to guide your next steps in evaluating the patient.

The Liver Function Panel: Alone and Unafraid

Sometimes all you want to know is the state of your patient's liver without all the other stuff that comes with a full CMP. Perhaps, for example, you want to assess the progression of known liver disease, or you are monitoring the success of your treatment of hepatitis C. For these situations, you can order a liver function panel.

YourLab

Specimen Number 193–996–9516–0		Patient ID		Control Number	Account Number 90000999	Account Phone Number 336–436–8645	Route 00
SAMPLE REPORT	Patient Last Name						
Patient First Name 322755		Patient Last Name					
Patient SS#	Patient Phone		Total Volume				
Age (Y/M/D) 26 / 05 / 18	Date of Birth 01 / 24 / 97	Sex M	Fasting				
Patient Address				ABNORMAL REPORT	Additional Information		
Date and time Collected 07/11/23 00:00	Date Entered 07/12/23	Date and Time Reported		Physician Name	NPI	Physician ID	
Hepatic Function Panel (7)				Test Ordered			

TESTS	RESULT	FLAG	UNITS	REFERENCE INTERVAL	LAB
Hepatic Function Panel (7)					
Protein, Total, Serum	**5.4**	**Low**	g/dL	6.0 – 8.5	01
Albumin, Serum	4.3		g/dL	3.5 – 5.5	01
Bilirubin, Total	1.0		mg/dL	0.0 – 1.2	01
Bilirubin, Direct	0.32		mg/dL	0.00 – 0.40	01
Alkaline Phosphatase, S	**123**	**High**	IU/L	39 – 117	01
AST (SGOT)	32		IU/L	0 – 40	01
ALT (SGPT)	23		IU/L	0 – 44	01

Figure 5.13 A sample liver function test (LFT) report.

As you can see from the illustration shown, this panel typically consists of several tests available on the CMP: the AST, ALT, ALP, bilirubin, total protein, and albumin (and sometimes—but not on the example just mentioned—the protein/albumin ratio). The liver function panel has the added advantage that it reports the direct bilirubin, whereas the CMP typically gives only the total bilirubin. Different labs may offer variations on this basic theme. Some may include, for example, a GGT or a prothrombin time (this makes sense because the liver manufactures factors that affect blood coagulation as measured by the prothrombin time international normalized ratio [INR; see Chapter 20]).

Gilbert Syndrome

Gilbert syndrome is a common, benign condition caused by impaired glucuronidation of bilirubin. The result is an unconjugated hyperbilirubinemia. It can be inherited or appear sporadically. The bilirubin rarely rises above 4 mg/dL, although fasting, fever, impaired sleep, and other stressors can increase it further. Patients are almost always asymptomatic, although jaundice can develop if the bilirubin rises sufficiently high. Gilbert syndrome is usually detected incidentally on bloodwork done for some other reason. The CBC, liver transaminases, and ALP are all normal. No further evaluation or treatment is needed.

Jaundice in the Newborn

Mild unconjugated hyperbilirubinemia—although often high enough to cause jaundice—is common in newborns. The causes appear to be multifactorial: (1) the short half-life of fetal red blood cells, (2) a low level of circulating albumin to bind circulating bilirubin, (3) the decreased ability of the neonatal liver to conjugate bilirubin, and (4) increased enterohepatic circulation (see Figure 5.12) due to fewer intestinal bacteria available to convert bilirubin to urobilinogen.

ABO or Rh blood type incompatibility between the mother and baby can lead to hemolysis and extremely high levels of bilirubin; at these levels bilirubin is a dangerous neurotoxin and urgent treatment is needed.

Elevated bilirubin and mild jaundice can also occur in completely healthy infants who are breastfed (with adequate intake of breast milk). The mechanisms here are varied and complex and beyond the scope of this book. Suffice to say that "breast milk jaundice" is considered benign and self-limited, although it can persist for weeks. This is in contrast to the hyperbilirubinemia and jaundice seen with "breastfeeding failure jaundice," thought to be the result of reduced biliary elimination in the stool of breastfed infants who are not getting sufficient nutrition; treatment here *is* required and, as you might expect, entails increased nutritional support (eg, increased frequency/duration of breastfeeds or supplementation with formula).

 Total Protein, Albumin, and Globulins

Total Protein

The total protein lives up to its billing: it is a measure of all the proteins circulating in the blood. The total protein normally lies between 6.0 and 7.8 g/dL. The two major types of protein are the *albumin* (normally ~60% of the total) and a large assemblage of proteins referred to collectively as *globulins* (the other 40%).

- An elevated total protein is almost always due to an elevation in the globulin fraction. A high albumin is usually only seen with markedly decreased intravascular volume from severe dehydration.

- A low total protein can be caused by nutritional deficiencies, severe liver disease, and protein loss via the GI tract (protein-losing enteropathies such as Crohn disease and celiac disease) or via the kidneys (nephrotic syndrome).

The ratio of *albumin/globulin* is also reported on the CMP and can give you a quick assessment as to which of these components, if any, is preferentially increased or decreased. The normal ratio, obviously, is slightly greater than 1.

Albumin

The normal level of albumin is 3.5 to 5.5 g/dL. It is made in the liver and has two major functions:

- It helps to maintain oncotic pressure within the circulation, effectively pulling blood into the vessels and keeping it from leaking out.
- It transports many enzymes and hormones through the circulation (as well as many drugs and medications the patient might be taking).

Low levels of albumin can be seen in any of the conditions that can produce a low total serum protein. It also occurs normally during pregnancy. Although many patients with malnutrition may have low albumin, a low albumin in and of itself does not necessarily indicate poor nutritional status. As we discuss in Chapter 22, albumin is a *negative acute phase reactant*, meaning that levels *decrease* in states of inflammation and/or acute illness (eg, infection, cancer).

The Globulins

The sum total of the globulins normally ranges from 2.5 to 3.5 g/dL. They can be divided into several categories based on how they move during *serum protein electrophoresis* (SPEP; more on this test in Chapter 20; for now, see Figure 5.14), which separates out the circulating proteins by differences in their electrical charge. There are four major categories of globulin:

- Alpha 1 (α1)
- Alpha 2 (α2)
- Beta (β)
- Gamma (γ)

The α1-, α2-, and β-globulins include a huge variety of proteins, many of which can be increased during various inflammatory processes. However, it is the fourth category, the *γ-globulins*, that is usually most useful to look at. It consists of the immunoglobulins (antibodies) that are an essential part of the immune system.

The γ-globulins can be increased in two basic ways: diffusely as a *broad band* or narrowly as a single, *monoclonal spike*.

- A broad, polyclonal γ-band (see Figure 5.14C) is what you often see with an infection or inflammatory reaction. It represents a large population of many different antibodies that move slightly differently during electrophoresis. Hence the band is broad.
- A single, narrow spike signifies a monoclonal immunoglobulin. This is most often due to multiple myeloma, Waldenström macroglobulinemia, or monoclonal gammopathy of undetermined significance (MGUS). The type of monoclonal immunoglobulin that is present can be determined by a second test called *immunofixation*, in which labeled antibodies that bind to specific antibodies in the blood sample are allowed to interact with the electrophoretic gel (we discuss immunofixation further in Chapter 20).

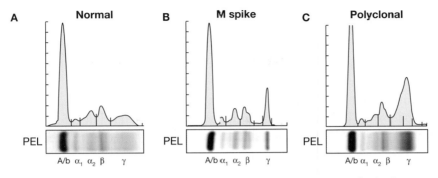

Figure 5.14 A. A normal serum protein electrophoresis. B. An M spike in the γ-globulins as one might see in multiple myeloma. C. A broad increase in the γ-globulins, as could be seen with a systemic inflammatory reaction.

Monoclonal Gammopathies

A diagnosis of *multiple myeloma* requires the presence of a monoclonal γ-globulin spike more than 3 g/dL (referred to as an M protein). The M protein may consist of IgG (most commonly), IgA, IgE, or just pieces of an intact immunoglobulin, the κ- or λ-immunoglobulin light chains. The abnormal protein is produced by a clone of plasma cells in the bone marrow; these clonal plasma cells must make up at least 10% of the cells in the marrow in order for multiple myeloma to be diagnosed (alternatively, the finding of a mass-like peripheral collection of clonal plasma cells called a *plasmacytoma* may also be used to support the diagnosis).

Other laboratory abnormalities you will often see in multiple myeloma include an elevated white blood cell count, which may include an abnormal number of plasma cells; an elevated creatinine; a normocytic anemia; and hypercalcemia that is primarily the result of calcium released into the circulation by lytic bone lesions.

Waldenström macroglobulinemia is diagnosed when the immunoglobulin spike consists of a monoclonal IgM protein.

MGUS is diagnosed when the M protein spike is less than 3 g/dL and there are fewer than 10% plasma cells in the marrow as well as an absence of other clinical features of multiple myeloma. MGUS carries a small risk of progressing to either of the above plasma cell dyscrasias; which one depends on the class of the immunoglobulin spike. We will talk more about MGUS in Chapter 20.

Other causes of a monoclonal spike in the gamma region include primary amyloidosis, light chain deposition disease, and POEMS syndrome (*polyneuropathy, organomegaly, endocrinopathy, monoclonal protein, and skin changes*).

Calcium

We have arrived at the last of the tests included in the CMP. Hopefully you now have a good sense of the remarkably broad reach of this panel.

Calcium is critical for muscle activity, blood clotting, bone health, and many enzymatic reactions. Approximately 99% of the calcium in the body is contained in the bones. Normal serum calcium values are 9.0 to 10.5 mg/dL.

The serum calcium (Ca++) is regulated primarily by parathyroid hormone (PTH, produced by the parathyroid glands) and vitamin D. These two hormones (yes, vitamin D is considered a hormone) act on:

1. the bones (the body's major reservoir of calcium)

2. the kidneys

3. the GI tract

PTH and vitamin D increase the serum calcium (see the following figure), thereby maintaining normal serum calcium levels in the face of renal and GI calcium excretion and calcium deposition in the bone. A third hormone, *calcitonin*, blocks bone resorption and thereby decreases the serum calcium.

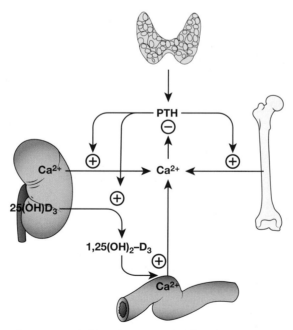

Figure 5.15 Calcium homeostasis is largely maintained by the actions of parathyroid hormone (PTH) and vitamin D on the kidneys, bones, and intestines.

Fortunately, the differential diagnosis of both hypercalcemia and hypocalcemia is relatively straightforward. As with the other tests on the CMP, the calcium is just the beginning of your evaluation. Other tests are needed to determine the cause of any abnormalities in the serum calcium level.

Total Calcium and Ionized Calcium

Before digging into the causes of what appears to be an abnormal calcium in a patient, you want to make sure that what looks like an abnormal calcium really is an abnormal calcium. To do this, you must take into account the impact of the serum albumin on the measured serum calcium.

The serum calcium consists largely of two components:

1. the *ionized form*, which is the active form of calcium that is actually regulated by PTH and vitamin D. Under normal circumstances, this makes up 40% to 45% of circulating calcium.

2. the *bound fraction*, most of which consists of calcium bound to albumin. This form of calcium is not biologically active.

The calcium that the CMP reports is the total calcium, not the active, ionized portion. Normally, the total calcium is an adequate surrogate for the ionized calcium—after all, we know how much of the total calcium is typically made up of ionized calcium. But what happens when the balance of bound and ionized calcium is thrown off?

Any change in the albumin changes the relative amounts of bound calcium and ionized calcium. Take a look at this picture:

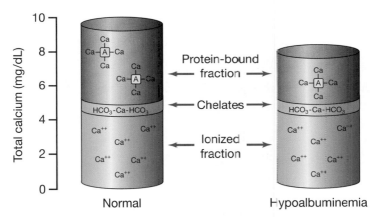

Figure 5.16 All you need to remember is that lowering albumin lowers the total calcium *but not the ionized calcium*. Put another way: the lower the albumin, the higher the ratio of ionized calcium to protein-bound calcium. Thus, in patients with a low serum albumin and low total calcium, the ionized calcium—what we actually care about—may actually be normal. Similarly, those with high albumin and high calcium may also have a normal ionized calcium (From Marino PL. *Marino's The ICU Book.* 4th ed. Wolters Kluwer Health; 2014.)

Our normal range for total calcium should really shift based on a patient's albumin—for example, the normal range should be lower for a patient with a low albumin. But instead of shifting the normal range, we can simply "correct" a patient's total calcium for their albumin to determine if the calcium is clinically abnormal (ie, reflects an abnormal ionized calcium). Here is the formula:

$$\text{Corrected calcium} = \text{measured calcium} + (0.8 \times [4.0 - \text{serum albumin}])$$

Thus, if the measured calcium is 8.0 mg/dL (normal 9-10.5 mg/dL) and the serum albumin is 2.5 g/dL (normal 3.5-5.5 g/dL), then the corrected calcium is 9.6 mg/dL—normal. Although this equation is helpful in giving an estimate of the calcium, it is not always very accurate (especially among patients with chronic kidney disease), and today many clinicians faced with a low total measured calcium order an *ionized calcium level* (bonus: no math necessary). This is a separate test that you will have to order in addition to the CMP.

Hypercalcemia

Mild hypercalcemia is usually asymptomatic and detected on a routine CMP obtained for some other reason. When severe, however, hypercalcemia can lead to renal, musculoskeletal, GI, neuropsychiatric, and cardiac symptoms. (The classic mnemonic is "[kidney] *stones, bones* [musculoskeletal pain], *groans* [constipation/GI distress], psychiatric *overtones*." Catchy, but not an exhaustive list.)

- The most common cause of hypercalcemia in the *outpatient* setting is *hyperparathyroidism*.

- In the *inpatient* setting, the most common cause is *malignancy*. Malignancies can elevate the calcium by any of several mechanisms (see the box "PTHrP and Hypercalcemia of Malignancy"), including the release of PTH-related peptide (PTHrP).

- Other causes include:
  - *granulomatous diseases*, such as sarcoidosis, which increase the serum calcium via the production of 1,25 $(OH)_2$-vitamin D by macrophages within the granulomas
  - *prolonged immobilization*, due to bone resorption
  - *Paget disease of the bone*, due to increased bone turnover
  - *hyperthyroidism*
  - *adrenal insufficiency*
  - consumption of large amounts of calcium—for example, calcium-containing antacids; this is referred to as *milk-alkali syndrome* (discussed further in Chapter 9)
  - *various medications*, notably the thiazide diuretics and lithium

As you can tell from this short list, once you have confirmed the presence of actual hypercalcemia, the next test you will want to order is a PTH (normal values 10-65 pg/mL). If this is normal, then you will want to check vitamin D levels and a PTHrP.

A Few Words About Hyperparathyroidism

When, in your evaluation of hypercalcemia, you find an elevated PTH, you are usually dealing with *primary hyperparathyroidism,* a disorder of the parathyroid glands themselves. However, in patients with chronic renal failure, the kidneys and not the parathyroid glands may be responsible for an elevation in the PTH. This is called *secondary hyperparathyroidism* and occurs for two main reasons:

1. Impaired renal excretion of phosphate. Phosphate builds up in the circulation, where it binds ionized calcium. The parathyroid glands respond to the lowered concentration of ionized calcium by increasing their activity in order to maintain normal serum levels of ionized calcium.

2. Impaired activation of vitamin D, a process that normally occurs in the kidneys (not so much when they aren't working). The low levels of activated vitamin D lead to low calcium, stimulating PTH release.

In time, the continuous hyperactivity of the parathyroid glands in patients with renal disease may cause them to become autonomous and refractory to the usual feedback inhibition. This state of affairs is called *tertiary hyperparathyroidism.*

Hypocalcemia

The evaluation of hypocalcemia is equally straightforward. Mild hypocalcemia is usually asymptomatic and is often discovered incidentally on a CMP. Muscle cramps and perioral tingling are common initial symptoms. When hypocalcemia is severe, tetany, seizures, serious cardiac arrhythmias, and laryngospasm can develop.

In some patients, hypocalcemia may first be suspected when an ECG is obtained; hypocalcemia is the most common cause of a prolonged QT interval, a fertile ground for life-threatening polymorphic ventricular tachycardia.

In many cases, the cause will be obvious clinically. Among the more common are:

- *Low PTH*: the most common cause of a low PTH is irradiation or surgery to the neck damaging the parathyroid glands.

- *Low vitamin D* (or resistance to vitamin D): this is most common in persons with low ultraviolet (UV) light exposure and limited vitamin D in their diet.

- *Hypomagnesemia* (see the box "And Let's Not Forget Magnesium"): this deficiency can cause hypocalcemia via its impact on end-organ responsiveness to PTH or via decreased PTH secretion.

- Other less frequent causes:

  - *Parathyroidectomy:* shortly after surgery, patients can develop severe hypocalcemia (hungry bone syndrome).

  - *Severe, acute pancreatitis*: hypocalcemia in this setting may predict a poor prognosis from their inflammatory disorder.

- *Rhabdomyolysis*

- *Diffuse osteoblastic metastases* of the bones

- *Medications*: for example, bisphosphonates, which are used to treat osteoporosis

- *GI malabsorption*: for example, celiac disease

As with hypercalcemia, you can see from the causes that the next steps in your evaluation will include obtaining a serum PTH and vitamin D, plus a serum magnesium.

Vitamin D Metabolism and Measurement

We have two sources of vitamin D: (1) our diet and (2) the UV light of the sun,[a] which manufactures vitamin D by its actions on a substrate (7-dehydrocholesterol) present in the skin. These inactive precursors are hydroxylated in the liver to 25-hydroxy vitamin D, which is still inactive until it is hydroxylated one more time in the kidneys to create 1,25-dihydroxy vitamin D. This last step is promoted by PTH and inhibited by high serum concentrations of serum calcium.

When you want to know the body's vitamin D status, the test you want is the *25-hydroxy vitamin D* (normal values are often given as 30 to 80 ng/mL, but no one really knows for sure what a normal vitamin D level should be); this is the main circulating reservoir of the hormone and best reflects the body's total vitamin D stores. The active hormone, 1,25-dihydroxyvitamin D, which can be measured, circulates in low concentrations and only reflects vitamin D activity rather than what you generally want to know, which is how much vitamin D the body contains.

[a]Sunscreen with a sun protection factor (SPF) of 15 or greater reduces the vitamin D created by this pathway by almost 100%.

Where's the Phosphate?

Good question. Phosphate is not part of the CMP, although it probably should be since its hormonal regulation is so closely wedded to that of calcium. Phosphate is also controlled by PTH and vitamin D, the one significant difference being that PTH *decreases* phosphate reabsorption in the kidneys, in contrast to its effect on calcium.

Phosphate likes to live inside cells. It is critical for the body's energy (the P in ATP stands for phosphate) and the activity of many enzymes. Normal values are 3.0 to 4.5 mg/dL.

- *Hypophosphatemia* can cause weakness and ultimately neurologic symptoms and respiratory failure. It is most often caused by the movement of phosphate into cells (eg, with alkalosis or insulin therapy) or by medications that bind phosphate in the gut (such as calcium or antacids).

- *Hyperphosphatemia* is most often the result of a shift of phosphate* out of cells (eg, with acidosis or cellular lysis) or less commonly is caused by hypoparathyroidism, vitamin D toxicity, or impaired renal excretion due to advanced chronic kidney disease. It is usually asymptomatic unless there is concomitant hypocalcemia.

And Let's Not Forget Magnesium

After potassium, magnesium is the second most abundant cation inside cells. It, too, is not included in the CMP, but you will find yourself checking it often as part of your evaluation of hypocalcemia.

Normal values of magnesium are 1.5 to 2.4 mg/dL.

- *Hypomagnesemia* is quite common in the general population, but is usually asymptomatic until severe. Initial symptoms may include nausea, vomiting, muscle cramps, and weakness. Medications—proton pump inhibitors and diuretics—are among the most common causes of a low magnesium. It can also result from poor dietary intake or diarrhea.

- *Hypermagnesemia* rarely causes any problems unless there is underlying kidney disease. Overuse of magnesium-containing antacids can sometimes lead to hypermagnesemia.

Parathyroid Hormone–Related Peptide and Hypercalcemia of Malignancy

PTHrP is secreted by some tumors and is responsible for the majority of cases of hypercalcemia caused by malignancy. PTHrP bears some structural similarity to PTH (it is larger than PTH) and, just like PTH, it increases the release of calcium from bone and increases renal and GI reabsorption of calcium. PTHrP should be undetectable in healthy individuals.

The underlying culprits are usually advanced solid tumors (classically squamous cell lung cancer) and non-Hodgkin lymphoma. If you have a patient with cancer, hypercalcemia, and a normal or low PTH, you will want to order a PTHrP.

Less common causes of hypercalcemia of malignancy include osteoclastic metastases and tumor production of 1,25-dihydroxyvitamin D; rarely, tumors may produce PTH itself.

---

*In medicine, the terms *phosphorus* and *phosphate* are generally used interchangeably. Some labs call it one thing, some another. Most clinicians will refer to phosphate when they are discussing this subject, and we will too.

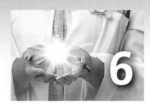

6 The Lipid Panel

A typical lipid panel is shown in Figure 6.1. It includes measurements of the total cholesterol (TC), high-density lipoprotein (HDL), low-density lipoprotein (LDL), triglycerides (TG), and—sometimes—very-low-density lipoprotein (VLDL) and non-HDL cholesterol. This panel is drawn in a serum separator tube; a single tube provides sufficient blood to measure both a comprehensive metabolic panel (CMP) and lipid panel.

The goal of the lipid panel is to determine the concentration of circulating lipids primarily to assess their contribution to a patient's overall cardiovascular risk. These are actionable numbers: they help to determine who might benefit from therapy (eg, a cholesterol-lowering agent such as a statin) as well as providing a measure of the efficacy of ongoing treatment (which could include lifestyle modification and/or medication).

Before we proceed any further, we need to stress that lipid levels are only one piece in the management of atherosclerotic cardiovascular disease. Any assessment of cardiovascular risk must take into account all contributors to cardiovascular disease, including lifestyle, hypertension, diabetes, family history, smoking history, and more. There are many calculators available that do just that, and you should make sure that you have one of them (eg, the one offered by the American Heart Association/American College of Cardiology) on your desktop or phone for quick access.

Patient Report   **YourLab**

Specimen ID: **244-988-9010-0**   Acct #: **90000999**   Phone: Rte: **00**

SAMPLE REPORT, 303756

Patient Details   **Specimen Details**   **Physician Details**
DOB: **02/14/1987**   Date collected: **08/31/2023 0000 Local**
Age(y/m/d): **036/06/17**   Date received: **08/31/2023**
Gender: **F**   Date entered: **08/31/2023**
Patient ID: Date reported: **08/31/2023 0000 ET**

Clinical Info: ABNORMAL

Lipid Panel

Lipid Panel

Cholesterol, Total	**201**	**High**	mg/dL	100-199	01
Triglycerides	**154**	**High**	mg/dL	0-149	01
HDL Cholesterol	**32**	**Low**	mg/dL	>39	01
VLDL Cholesterol Cal	28		mg/dL	5-40	
LDL Chol Calc (NIH)	**141**	**High**	mg/dL	0-99	

Figure 6.1 A typical lipid panel report.

Lipid metabolism is complicated, and even today there is much we still do not know. The traditional lipid panel shown earlier has been around for some time now. Although it offers an incomplete assessment of a patient's lipid levels—there are subtleties upon subtleties—it nevertheless provides information that has been proven to be clinically useful.

 ## Total Cholesterol, Triglycerides, and the Lipoproteins

Cholesterol and TGs are independent risk factors for cardiovascular disease. They are carried in the circulation by lipoproteins, which in turn are classified according to their density. The lipoproteins you need to know are LDL, VLDL, and HDL.

- *LDL ("Bad")* carries cholesterol and is the major atherogenic lipoprotein. It has long been the key therapeutic target in the management of patients with hyperlipidemia.

- *VLDL ("Bad")* primarily carries TGs and is also atherogenic, but less so than LDL. Both LDL and VLDL deposit cholesterol in the walls of blood vessels.

- *HDL ("Good")* removes cholesterol from the vasculature and is therefore protective against cardiovascular disease. Although a high HDL is considered protective, there is no firm evidence that a low HDL is harmful.

- *TGs ("Sort of Bad")* are fats. Their levels can fluctuate throughout the day, so a slightly high level is not concerning. Levels can be elevated after a fatty meal, alcohol consumption the night before, or in the setting of uncontrolled diabetes. Persistently elevated fasting TGs more than 500 mg/dL typically warrant pharmacologic treatment because of the

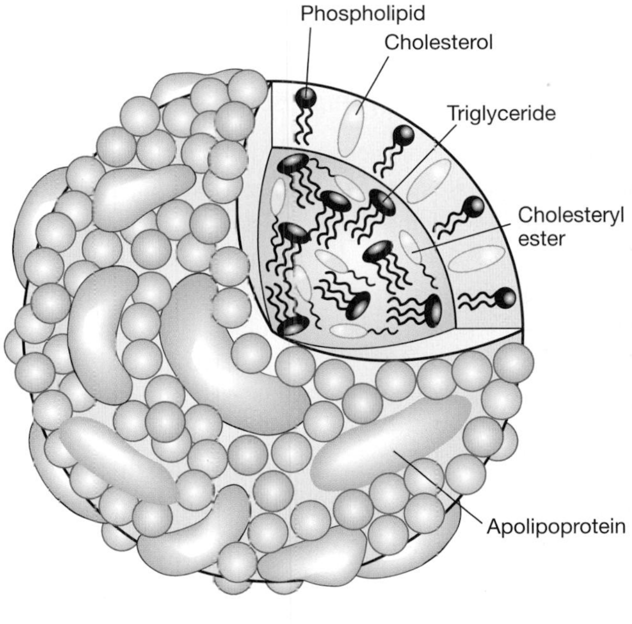

Figure 6.2 The structure of a typical lipoprotein. The "density" of lipoproteins refers to the ratio of proteins to lipids: the higher the relative protein content of the lipoprotein, the higher the density. (From Bishop ML, Fody EP, Schoeff LE. *Clinical Chemistry: Principles, Techniques, and Correlations*. 8th ed. Wolters Kluwer; 2018.)

Phospholipid
Cholesterol
Triglyceride
Cholesteryl ester
Apolipoprotein

associated risk of cardiovascular disease. Levels over 1,000 mg/dL are associated with high risk of pancreatitis.

- *TC ("It Depends")* is made up of a combination of LDL, HDL, and TGs. A high TC is not necessarily a bad thing, depending on whether it reflects a high HDL (a good thing) or a high LDL or TGs (bad things).

The LDL reported on the lipid panel is not measured directly, but rather is calculated using the following formula:

$$LDL = TC - (HDL + [TG/5])$$

The calculated LDL can be an inaccurate gauge of the true LDL when there are high levels of TGs, so a more direct measure is often preferable. A *direct LDL* can be ordered separately if therapeutic decisions are hanging on a precise measure of the LDL.

The *non-HDL cholesterol*, which is often included in the lipid profile, is also a calculated number. It is just what it sounds like: the TC minus the HDL. It therefore includes the LDL and VLDL as well as other cholesterol carriers such as intermediate-density lipoprotein (IDL) and lipoprotein(a). Whereas LDL has traditionally been the number that triggers therapeutic decisions, the non-HDL cholesterol may actually provide a more accurate measure of risk than the LDL alone.

What to Do With These Numbers

We don't strictly define normals for these lipid tests, but take the view that basically the lower the better (for all but HDL, where we aim high). There are numerous guidelines to help us determine when to be concerned, when to consider treatment, and so on. These guidelines keep evolving as we learn more and more.

Calculators and Guidelines

As of this writing, most experts would agree that an LDL cholesterol greater than 190 mg/dL mandates an evaluation for familial hypercholesterolemia and—in almost all cases—initiation of cholesterol-lowering therapy. Below that level, clinicians rely on calculators for guidance.

These calculators incorporate much more than just the LDL; they factor in the HDL cholesterol (remember: the higher the better with HDL), blood pressure, sex, age, smoking history, and coexisting diabetes mellitus, and then present you with the patient's risk, reported as a percentage chance of having a cardiovascular event over the next 10 years.* Once you have this number, there are then recommendations, issued by many different organizations, as to what to do with that number. Whatever the result, it should be incorporated into shared decision-making with your patient as to what is the next best course of action—for example, lifestyle interventions, medications, or further testing such as coronary artery calcium scoring to better define the patient's risk.

---

*Why 10 years? Because that's what we have the most data for. We'd really like to know lifetime risk, particularly for our younger patients, but we just don't know enough to accurately calculate risk over such a long (hopefully very long) period of time.

Apolipoprotein B

Apolipoprotein B (ApoB) is the major protein component of the VLDL and LDL lipoproteins. It is essential for the initiation and evolution of atherosclerotic plaques. There is one ApoB molecule per particle. Thus, measuring the ApoB tells you the *total number of particles* carrying cholesterol, a value that may be more closely associated with atherogenic risk than LDL. Some clinicians are starting to incorporate ApoB measurements into their cardiovascular assessments, and it may someday be included in the standard lipid panel (some experts believe it may replace the other tests entirely!).

Fasting Versus Non-fasting?

Does your patient need to fast before getting a lipid panel? In most cases, the answer is no. Non-fasting LDL levels are only 5 to 10 mg/dL higher than fasting LDL levels. The TGs are more sensitive, but even they are only approximately 25 mg/dL higher in the non-fasting state. In neither of these instances is the difference likely to affect management (but if it will, have your patient fast). Fasting can be helpful in patients who are at risk of having a high TG level—for example, those with diabetes or other components of metabolic syndrome. The typical "fast" means no food after midnight and an early morning blood draw.

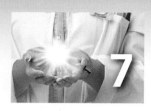

Thyroid Function Tests

7

Clinicians can hardly resist blaming everything that goes wrong on the thyroid gland (patients often do too). It is nearly impossible to count the number of cellular processes that are affected by the thyroid hormones. To name just a couple: stimulating messenger RNA synthesis and protein synthesis. So, yes, these hormones are pretty fundamental. Thyroid hormones are the energizers of the body—too little and everything slows down or even grinds to a halt, too much and everything speeds up and goes haywire. If a patient is tired or depressed, it could be the thyroid. If a patient is hyperactive or manic, that too could be the fault of the thyroid.

Of course, most of the time it *isn't* the thyroid, but because it almost always *could be*, the thyroid profile is one of the most commonly ordered laboratory tests. But much of the time (and we've seen estimates as high as *99% of the time*), if you are evaluating the possibility of thyroid dysfunction, you do not need to order the full set of thyroid function tests. You only need to order one test: the thyroid-stimulating hormone (TSH).

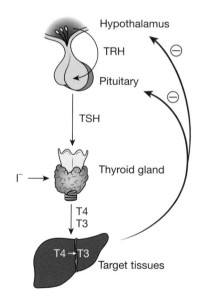

Figure 7.1 The pathway of thyroid hormone regulation. TRH is produced by the hypothalamus in the brain when levels of circulating thyroid hormone are low. TRH stimulates the pituitary gland to release TSH, which in turn stimulates the thyroid gland to synthesize and release the two thyroid hormones: a lot of T4 and a little bit of T3. The thyroid hormones exert negative feedback on the pituitary and hypothalamus. The numbers after each T represent the number of iodine moieties in each molecule (the synthesis of thyroid hormone is the only process in the body that requires iodine). T3 is the more potent of the two thyroid hormones and is primarily synthesized peripherally by conversion from T4. Most tissues in the body can convert T4 to T3, but the liver and kidneys handle the bulk of the work. T3, triiodothyronine; T4, thyroxine; TRH, thyrotropin-releasing hormone; TSH, thyroid-stimulating hormone; I-, iodide.

Thyroid-Stimulating Hormone

As you can see from Figure 7.1, the production and release of the thyroid hormones, thyroxine (T4) and triiodothyronine (T3), can be compromised by dysfunction at any of several levels: the hypothalamus, pituitary gland, thyroid gland, or even some process in the periphery that conveys resistance to thyroid stimulation or that blocks conversion of T4 to the more highly active T3. *However, the vast majority of the time, the source of thyroid dysfunction is the thyroid gland itself.*

You can screen for both hypothyroidism and hyperthyroidism by ordering a TSH. A normal TSH (in nonpregnant adults) is 0.5 to 5.0 µU/mL.

The TSH will be high if the thyroid gland is underperforming (hypothyroidism), because decreased negative feedback on the pituitary gland and hypothalamus will stimulate the production of more TSH to drive the thyroid gland to produce more thyroid hormone. Conversely, the TSH will be low in hyperthyroidism due to enhanced feedback suppression from the elevated levels of thyroid hormone. The system is finely tuned, and the body adjusts to even subtle fluctuations in thyroid hormone levels. So, for example, for patients who are on thyroid hormone replacement therapy, the TSH is typically the only test you need in order to monitor the adequacy (too much, too little, just right) of your treatment.

Why not measure the T4 and T3 instead of the TSH? The TSH is actually a more sensitive indicator of thyroid dysfunction, particularly when the gland is starting to fail. The thyroid gland may be able to generate normal or near-normal levels of hormone even as its function is declining, but in this setting it takes extra TSH to drive the gland. Thus, the TSH may rise even as the actual thyroid hormones themselves cling precariously to normal.

Most commercial labs appreciate the value of the TSH and offer what is termed a *thyroid cascade*. If you order this test—and you should—the lab will run just the TSH, and only if it is abnormal will it run additional tests. These can include a free T4, total T3, and—depending on the clinical circumstances—thyroid peroxidase (TPO) antibodies.

 ## Thyroxine (T4) and Triiodothyronine (T3)

Although the thyroid hormones in the circulation are largely bound to proteins—primarily *thyroid-binding globulin* but also *albumin* and others—it is the little bit of free hormone that is physiologically active. Ideally, when we do need to measure the thyroid hormones themselves, we would like to know the values of their active—free, unbound—concentrations. However, you will find that most of the time we actually order a "*free*" T4 and "*total*" T3. Why? Measuring free T4 is easy and accurate, but the test for free T3 is not nearly as reliable, so we opt for measuring the total T3.

Normal values for free T4 are 0.9 to 2.4 ng/dL, and for total T3 are 70 to 195 ng/dL.

Why should you care what the free T4 and total T3 are if you have already measured the TSH? Most of the time you don't. However, there are some circumstances where knowing one or both of these values can be helpful:

- A free T4 can be useful in determining the degree of hypothyroidism. Some patients have what is termed *subclinical hypothyroidism* in which the TSH is elevated (usually mildly so) but the free T4 is normal; evidence suggests that many of these patients do not require treatment. But if the free T4 is low, then treatment is almost always appropriate.

- If you have a patient in whom you strongly suspect hypothyroidism but their TSH is normal, you should check the free T4. A normal TSH in the setting of a low free T4 is considered "inappropriately normal"—after all, the TSH should be high if the pituitary and hypothalamus are working properly to compensate for an underactive thyroid. Therefore, the combination of a normal (or low) TSH and low free T4 indicates hypothyroidism caused by a problem with either the pituitary or hypothalamus (referred to as secondary and tertiary hypothyroidism, respectively; both are far less common than primary hypothyroidism, ie, thyroid gland dysfunction).

- The TSH rises modestly with age. This is normal and not pathologic. If you have an elderly patient with a slightly elevated TSH (around 5-8 μU/mL), this likely does not indicate actual hypothyroidism. Checking the free T4 can confirm that this is the case.

Why measure both the free T4 and total T3? Isn't it sufficient to check just the free T4 since it comprises the bulk of circulating thyroid hormone? The answer is yes. Most of the time you do not need to check the total T3. However, some patients—not many—with severe hyperthyroidism (thyrotoxicosis) actually have isolated T3 thyrotoxicosis, and you will need the total T3 to make that diagnosis. In cases of hypothyroidism, you almost never need to check the total T3.

Thyroid Peroxidase Antibodies and Subclinical Hypothyroidism

TPO is an enzyme involved in the iodination of tyrosine, a key step in the synthesis of thyroid hormone. *Anti-TPO antibodies* are responsible for the autoimmune destruction that accompanies almost all cases of *Hashimoto disease*. In patients with subclinical hypothyroidism (see earlier), you may want to consider ordering TPO antibodies. If they are elevated, it indicates an increased risk of progressing to frank hypothyroidism. You may then choose to monitor the TSH at regular intervals so you can intervene should symptomatic hypothyroidism develop.

 ## The Differential Diagnoses of Hypothyroidism and Hyperthyroidism

Hypothyroidism

By far and away the major cause of hypothyroidism in the United States is Hashimoto thyroiditis, also known as chronic autoimmune thyroiditis.* An elevated TSH pretty much

---

*Worldwide, iodine deficiency may be even more common.

gives the game away and is all you need in most patients to make the diagnosis. There are, of course, other causes, such as various medications (lithium and amiodarone are two common culprits), but a careful medication history will reveal these possibilities.

Hyperthyroidism

Hyperthyroidism presents a more complex set of potential diagnoses. Most patients with hyperthyroidism will prove to have *Graves' disease*, but other causes include *toxic adenoma(s)* and the *early stages of destructive thyroiditis*. In the latter, the inflammatory process causes the thyroid gland to release its store of preformed hormones, producing hyperthyroidism; after a short time the patient develops hypothyroidism. Graves' disease is caused by autoantibodies directed against the thyrotropin (TSH) receptor, appropriately called *thyroid receptor antibodies (TRAb)*. These antibodies stimulate the TSH receptor and increase the synthesis of thyroid hormones. If you are unsure of the cause of your patient's hyperthyroidism, ordering TRAb should be part of the evaluation.

> **Thyroid Tests and Biotin**
>
> Biotin is a common supplement used to prevent hair loss. It can interfere with the assays used to measure thyroid function, causing a falsely low TSH or falsely high free T4 and total T3. Patients should discontinue their biotin at least 2 days before having any of these tests.

> **Thyroid Tests in Critically Ill Individuals**
>
> It is difficult to assess thyroid function in very sick patients, particularly those in the hospital. Often the T4 and T3 are low. The TSH may also be low (an abnormally high TSH, or "rebound elevation," may be seen during recovery from severe illness). This condition used to be called "sick euthyroid syndrome," because it was believed that these patients actually had normal thyroid function. More recently, it has been determined that they may have temporary hypothalamic or pituitary dysfunction causing these abnormalities. Why would our bodies do this? It's unclear, but it is theorized that lowering thyroid activity protects an ailing body from excessive catabolism. Thyroid hormone replacement is not recommended. The best management is treatment of the underlying condition (ie, whatever caused the critical illness in the first place), after which thyroid tests should begin to normalize.

There are other thyroid tests that can help determine the precise cause of thyroid dysfunction, and we'll get to the most important of these in Chapter 19. For now, the important thing to remember is that the TSH is your best screening tool for most things thyroid, and ordering a thyroid cascade is usually the best way of starting your evaluation of a patient with suspected hypo- or hyperthyroidism.

Table 7.1 Thyroid Tests at a Glance

Disease State	TSH	Free T4	Total T3[a]
Primary hypothyroidism	High	Low	Low or normal
Secondary or tertiary hypothyroidism	Low or normal	Low	Low or normal
Subclinical hypothyroidism	High	Normal	Normal
Hyperthyroidism	Low (usually)[b]	High	High
Critical illness	Low (usually)	Low	Low

T3, triiodothyronine; T4, thyroxine; TSH, thyroid-stimulating hormone.
[a]Remember that, in most cases, the TSH and free T4 are all you need to check.
[b]Rare TSH-secreting pituitary tumors cause hyperthyroidism with high TSH and high free T4.

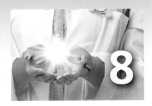 # 8 The Urinalysis

It is time we leave the blood and explore some of the body's other fluids that are routinely analyzed. In this section we are going to tackle the urinalysis, which typically consists of a *urine dipstick* and, sometimes, *urine microscopy*. The dipstick offers a quick, easily performed assessment of several important characteristics of the urine, and often it is all you need to make a diagnosis. Microscopy is more time consuming but allows for direct visualization of elements such as cells, casts, bacteria, and crystals—these results may help confirm or refute findings on the dipstick.

Let's march down the urine dipstick test by test. We will discuss relevant aspects of urine microscopy as they come up.

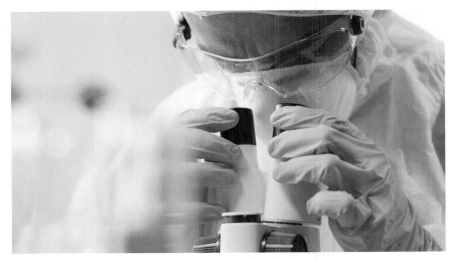

Figure 8.1 Urine microscopy is a bit of a lost art among clinicians, but thankfully the lab continues to pick up our slack. (Courtesy of DC Studio/Shutterstock.)

The Urine Dipstick

The urine dipstick can screen for and help diagnose disorders anywhere in the urinary tract (from the kidneys, down through the ureters, past the prostate [in men], and into the bladder and urethra) as well as screen for several metabolic disorders (eg, diabetes).

YourLab

Specimen Number 238–988–9004–0		Patient ID		Control Number	Account Number 90000999
SAMPLE REPORT	Patient Last Name				
Patient First Name 003772		Patient Last Name			
Patient SS#	Patient Phone		Total Volume		
Age (Y/M/D) 24 / 06 / 13	Date of Birth 02 / 12 / 99	Sex F	Fasting		
Patient Address				ABNORMAL REPORT	Additional
Date and time Collected 08/25/16 00:00	Date Entered 08/25/23	Date and Time Reported		Physician Name	NPI

Test Ordered

Urinalysis, Complete

TESTS	RESULT	FLAG	UNITS
Urinalysis, Complete			
Urinalysis, Gross Exam			
Specific Gravity	1.016		
pH	6.5		
Urine-Color	Yellow		
Appearance	**Cloudy**	**Abnormal**	
WBC Esterase	**2+**	**Abnormal**	
Protein	Negative		
Glucose	Negative		
Ketones	Negative		
Occult Blood	Negative		
Bilirubin	Negative		
Urobilinogen, Semi-Qn	1.0		mg/dL
Nitrite, Urine	Negative		
Microscopic Examination	See below:		
Microscopic was indicated and was performed.			
WBC	**6-10**	**Abnormal**	/hpf
RBC	0-2		/hpf
Epithelial Cells (non-renal)	0-10		/hpf
Casts	None seen		/1pt
Mucus Threads	Present		
Bacteria	Fow		

Figure 8.2 A typical urinalysis report. Note the highlighted abnormal results. hpf, high power field.

What Is Normal? What Is Abnormal?

If you look at the picture of a typical urine dipstick (see Figure 8.3), you will see that each test is marked off by a series of boxes with evolving colors. The left column shows what a negative test should look like, and the farther to the right you go the colors tend to deepen as the degree of deviation from normal becomes greater and greater. These colorimetric reactions correlate reasonably but imperfectly with the results of more sophisticated quantitative methods of testing.

For most of the tests on the dipstick, a negative reading is considered normal. However, the pH and specific gravity do not have clearly defined normal and abnormal levels. These tests can be normal throughout their range or can indicate a specific problem within the appropriate context. For example, a particular pH might be perfectly normal in a healthy patient, but might suggest a predisposition to certain types of kidney stones in a patient with recurrent flank pain. A low specific gravity might reflect that the kidneys are properly removing excess fluid from the body, or instead that they are unable to concentrate the urine in a patient with renal disease. It's all in the context.

How to Obtain a Urine Specimen

How should a urine sample be obtained? Unlike the blood tests we have discussed so far, a urinalysis provides more than just a snapshot in time. What you see in a urine sample is everything from the previous void up to the time you obtain your sample, that is, the contents of the bladder. It is therefore a summation of data accumulated over hours. The longer the time from the previous void, the greater the sensitivity. Thus, a first morning sample will typically give the highest diagnostic yield. Obtaining a fresh morning specimen is not always necessary or practical, but is always worth considering. In addition, when you suspect infection, you want to obtain a *clean-catch* urine specimen. This is done by gently sterilizing the urethral orifice with a towelette before the patient voids. Next, have the patient void just a bit and discard these initial milliliters of urine. Now have your patient continue voiding and collect the actual sample you are going to test. This technique is referred to as a midstream catch.

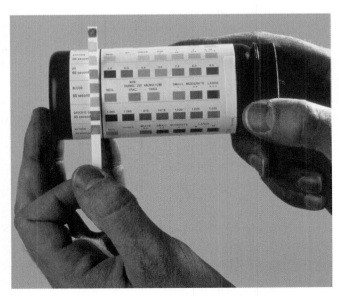

Figure 8.3 A urine dipstick. You can only use each dipstick once. Pay attention to the expiration date! (From Saturn Stills/ Science Source.)

There are many different dipsticks with a varying number of tests. The following are usually included in the results:

Leukocyte esterase (normal: negative)

Nitrites (normal: negative)

Urobilinogen (normal: 0.2-1)

Protein (normal: negative or trace)

pH ("normal" depends on clinical context; range 5.0-8.5)

Blood (normal: negative)

Specific gravity ("normal" depends on clinical context; range 1.000-1.030)

Ketones (normal: negative)

Bilirubin (normal: negative)

Glucose (normal: negative)

The most common reason to use a urine dipstick is to check for a possible urinary tract infection (UTI). The first two tests, leukocyte esterase and nitrites, do just that. Remember that most of the time you will recognize a UTI clinically (dysuria, urinary urgency, and/or urinary frequency with uncomplicated cystitis; fever and flank pain with pyelonephritis), and the urine dipstick then primarily serves to confirm—or sometimes challenge—your suspicions.

Leukocyte Esterase

The urine dipstick measures the enzyme *leukocyte esterase*, which is present in white blood cells. The urine should normally contain virtually no cellular elements at all. We say *virtually* because it is not unusual for the occasional white blood cell (or red blood cell for that matter) to somehow find its way into the urine. Under the microscope, normal is defined as 0 to 2 white cells per high-power field. The presence of white blood cells in the urine is referred to as *pyuria*. More than a couple of white blood cells in the urine is abnormal, and the more the white blood cells, the greater the likelihood that your patient may have an infection or inflammation somewhere in the urinary tract. The intensity of the color change on the urine dipstick correlates with the number of white blood cells in the urine.

Some antibiotics, including nitrofurantoin and tetracycline, can interfere with the leukocyte esterase test and cause a false-negative result. Urine microscopy is helpful in these situations.

The Limits of Pyuria

Pyuria does not point unequivocally to infection. A positive leukocyte esterase on the dipstick (as well as white blood cells on microscopy) may be seen, for example, in patients with renal stones, genitourinary malignancies, or chronic painful bladder syndrome (formerly known as chronic interstitial cystitis).

Pyuria is especially common in hospitalized patients in whom it is not a reliable marker of infection. Using a relatively high cutoff of 25 white blood cells per high-power field, only about 50% of these patients will prove to have a positive culture or any other identifiable pathologic process. Most of these patients are asymptomatic, affirming the general recommendation not to perform a urinalysis unless there are symptoms of a UTI.

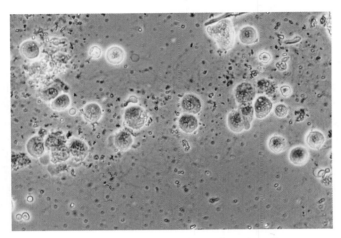

Figure 8.4 A whole lot of leukocytes in the urine. (From McClatchey KD. *Clinical Laboratory Medicine*. 2nd ed. Lippincott Williams & Wilkins; 2002.)

Nitrites

Many gram-negative urinary pathogens, including the most common urinary pathogen, *Escherichia coli*, produce an enzyme that reduces urinary nitrates to nitrites. These can be detected on the urine dipstick. This is one test where the intensity of the color does *not* correlate with what is being tested, in this case the number of bacteria in the urine.

False negatives can be caused by the presence of ascorbic acid (vitamin C) in the urine. Also, if the urine has not been retained in the bladder for at least several hours (four is the number usually cited)—in other words, if there has been insufficient time to allow any bacteria to convert nitrates to nitrites—the test may fail to pick up an infection. Infection may also be missed if the urine specimen is very dilute. Finally, and most importantly, several urinary pathogens do not convert nitrates to nitrites and will go undetected by this test; examples include *Candida* species, streptococcal species, enterococci, and *Haemophilus* species. In these instances, you may be saved by the urinary leukocyte esterase, which may light up on the dipstick. And, of course, any bacteria may be visualized on urine microscopy or identified on urine culture.

When both the urinary leukocyte esterase and nitrites are positive, the likelihood of infection is extremely high; when both are negative, the chance of infection is vanishingly small.

> ### Screening for Asymptomatic Urinary Tract Infections
>
> With few exceptions, screening asymptomatic patients for a urinary infection is not recommended. Treatment of most patients with laboratory evidence of a UTI but without symptoms (also called "asymptomatic bacteriuria") has not been shown to improve outcomes and exposes patients needlessly to antibiotic therapy. The major exceptions include pregnancy, patients scheduled for a urologic procedure, and recent recipients of renal transplants.

Urobilinogen and Bilirubin

We've already met *bilirubin*, a metabolic product of hemoglobin, in our discussion of the comprehensive metabolic panel (see Figure 5.12 if you want to review bilirubin metabolism). Bilirubin is normally excreted into the bile and then into the gastrointestinal (GI) tract. Biliary obstruction—for example, in patients with choledocholithiasis—can cause conjugated (direct) bilirubin to back up into the circulation. Because it is soluble, it will be filtered by the kidneys and pass into the urine. Any bilirubin in the urine should be considered abnormal.

Bacteria in the GI tract convert bilirubin into *urobilinogen*, some of which is reabsorbed by the GI tract. Urobilinogen eventually is either metabolized by the liver or excreted in the urine. Some urinary urobilinogen is normal—you will notice that the lowest reading on the urine dipstick is not zero.* High levels can be seen with elevated concentrations of circulating bilirubin, which can occur with hemolysis, bacterial overgrowth in the GI tract, and severe liver disease.

Protein

A normal urine specimen should contain very little protein. However, when the renal glomeruli are damaged, protein can begin to leak into the urine. Albumin and other small-molecular-weight proteins are typically the first to appear. The presence of albuminuria is a hallmark of early renal disease and is an important part of the evaluation of patients with diabetes mellitus and hypertension.

It is common to use the terms *albuminuria* and *proteinuria* interchangeably. Much of the time this is fine, because the bulk of the protein will be albumin, but not all of the time.

The urine dipstick is very good at detecting albumin, but not so good at detecting globulins and other non-albumin proteins. For example, secretion of immunoglobulins or their light chains in patients with multiple myeloma may be missed by a urine dipstick.

The urine dipstick test for protein tends to miss very low levels of proteinuria (<10-20 mg/dL). False positives can occur if there is radiocontrast material in the urine, significant hematuria, or a urinary pH >8. The degree of color change on the dipstick, while

---

*If bilirubin excretion into the GI tract is completely blocked—for example, by a large pancreatic malignancy—then urobilinogen cannot be produced and the urobilinogen level in the urine will, in fact, be zero. The urine dipstick, however, does not distinguish between no urobilinogen and the usual low amounts normally present.

somewhat indicative of the amount of albumin in the urine, cannot be relied on for perfect accuracy.

Any urine protein value on the dipstick above "trace" should generally be quantitated; the gold standard test is a *24-hour urine collection* (see the box below).

How to Do a 24-Hour Urine Collection

A 24-hour urine collection, while a logistic nuisance to your patient, can be a powerful tool in quantifying the amount of any given substance excreted in the urine. Quantification of proteinuria is probably the most common use of the 24-hour urine collection, but many other substances can be measured, such as hormones (eg, cortisol in suspected adrenal insufficiency or, conversely, Cushing syndrome) and minerals (eg, copper in suspected Wilson disease).

An incomplete collection can make interpretation problematic at best. Here is how it should be done:

The patient is given a several liter plastic jug to take home. Standard practice is to collect and discard the first void of the day after the patient awakens. All subsequent urine specimens are collected and stored until the same time the next morning. The first void of that next morning is then collected and the container is sealed, labeled, and delivered to the lab. It is useful to order a 24-hour urinary creatinine excretion along with whatever substance you are testing for in order to confirm that the sample represents a true 24-hour urine specimen. A 24-hour urinary creatinine excretion between 15 and 20 mg/kg (using the patient's actual body weight) confirms an adequate sample, with lower or higher numbers indicating under- or over-collection, respectively.

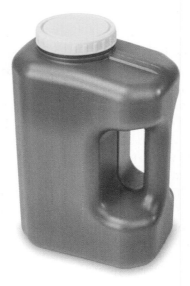

Figure 8.5 A typical 24-hour urine collector.

With all due respect to the 24-hour urine collection, it is now more common to order a *spot urine protein/creatinine ratio* on a random urine specimen to quantify proteinuria. Because the body's excretion of creatinine is fairly consistent, this test does not require a 24-hour collection. Just divide the protein in the sample (measured in mg/dL) by the creatinine in the sample (in g/dL) to get the ratio expressed as mg/g. And here's the really good news—the lab will often do this calculation for you! This test is much easier for the patient (truly, no one enjoys collecting and storing a day's worth of urine) and most of the time correlates well with the results of a 24-hour collection*:

- Very small amounts of protein (<30 mg/d on a 24-hour collection or <30 mg/g of creatinine on a spot urine) are considered normal.

- Values of 30 to 300 mg/d or 30 to 300 mg/g are referred to as *moderately increased proteinuria* (previously called microalbuminuria).

- Values above 300 mg/d or >300 mg/g of creatinine are referred to as *severely increased proteinuria* (previously called macroalbuminuria).

These categories are important and help determine everything from future screening intervals to pharmacologic intervention (eg, starting an angiotensin-converting enzyme inhibitor or angiotensin receptor blocker to slow the progression of renal dysfunction).

Benign Causes of Proteinuria

Transient proteinuria is a common finding, especially in younger patients, usually a result of exercise or fever. Repeat testing will identify this issue. *Orthostatic proteinuria*—increased excretion of protein in the upright position—is also common, and can be ruled out by comparing a sample checked when the patient has been upright for several hours (high protein) to a sample checked when the patient has been recumbent for several hours (low or undetectable protein).

---

*There are exceptions. On average, people excrete 1 to 2 g of creatinine in their urine daily. For those who excrete <1 g—this is often seen in young adults—the protein/creatinine ratio may overestimate the degree of proteinuria. Conversely, in patients with high muscle mass who produce a lot of creatinine, the protein/creatinine ratio may underestimate the degree of proteinuria. Because the correlation between the spot urine and the 24-hour urine collection is not perfect, it is often prudent to also obtain a 24-hour urine collection as part of the evaluation of patients with proteinuria, especially if the results of the spot protein/creatinine ratio do not seem to fit with the clinical context.

Nephrotic Syndrome

Proteinuria >3.5 g/24 hr is the defining feature of nephrotic syndrome and, as such, is often referred to as "nephrotic range proteinuria." Other findings of nephrotic syndrome include a low serum albumin (often <3.0 g/dL) and peripheral edema. Renal failure may be present. Hyperlipidemia (see Chapter 6) and lipiduria are common, and patients also have a greatly increased risk of thromboembolic disease (thought to be related, at least in part, to the loss of antithrombin III in the urine). Cells and casts in the urine are few in number. The cause is always a disease of the glomeruli; examples include advanced diabetic kidney disease and lupus nephritis. Minimal change disease, a so-called "primary" nephrotic syndrome, is a common culprit in children.

pH

The urine pH can range from approximately 4.5 to 8; the dipstick starts at 5 and stops at 8, a reasonably comprehensive range.

The pH will vary depending upon how much of an acid load the body needs to dispose of, so any value can be perfectly normal. Our daily metabolism always produces some acid that needs to be unloaded, so it is not surprising that the average pH is acidic, around 6. The pH tends to be on the lower end (more acidic) in patients who eat a high-protein diet, and higher (more basic) in vegetarians.

Where the urine pH comes in most handy is in diagnosing the cause of a metabolic acidosis. As we will discuss in Chapter 9, a metabolic acidosis can be caused by increased acid generation (eg, diabetic ketoacidosis), loss of bicarbonate (eg, severe diarrhea), or diminished renal excretion of acid (eg, renal failure, renal tubular acidosis). In the nonrenal causes, the urine pH will be low as the kidneys try to reestablish a healthy acid-base balance by excreting the excess acid. When the kidneys are the cause of the problem, however, the urine pH will usually be inappropriately high.

In patients with kidney stones, the urine pH can also be important to know, as different types of stones form preferentially in either acidic or basic environments (see Chapter 18).

Blood

Normal urine does not contain red blood cells.

If you look carefully at Figure 8.6, you will notice that the second and third boxes on the dipstick report non-hemolyzed trace amounts of hemoglobin creating a mottled pattern, typically green on a yellow background. These indicate the presence of intact red blood cells in the urine. The next test, moving rightward on the dipstick, is hemolyzed trace; here the

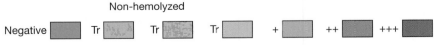

Figure 8.6 Close-up view of the dipstick test for blood on a urine dipstick.

mild yellow-green coloration is uniform and can be due to hemolyzed or intact red blood cells. And from there the progression goes from small (+) to moderate (++) to large (+++). Does it matter if the result indicates hemolyzed or intact red blood cells? Not really—any positive result requires your attention.

Urine microscopy is particularly valuable—and complements the dipstick well—in patients with hematuria.

- The urine dipstick test for blood will detect intact hemoglobin whether it resides inside red blood cells or is freely circulating (eg, released by hemolyzed red blood cells). The dipstick will also react with myoglobin, which is released from damaged muscle cells such as in rhabdomyolysis. So how can you tell hemoglobin from myoglobin in patients who have a positive dipstick? The easiest way is to look under the microscope; red blood cells will be seen in patients with actual hematuria but not in those with myoglobinuria.

- When hematuria is present on dipstick, the finding of *dysmorphic red blood cells* on urine microscopy suggests glomerular disease. The irregular shape of the red blood cells is thought to result from their being squeezed through a damaged glomerulus. Distinguishing glomerular from non-glomerular (eg, bleeding from the bladder or urethra) hematuria is key in determining the direction and extent of the rest of your diagnostic workup.

We should add that hematuria is a common finding in patients who are menstruating. If this is a possibility, do not forget to ask.

Specific Gravity

This test is a measurement of the density of the urine compared to water. It correlates roughly with *urine osmolality*, largely a function of how much sodium, potassium, and urea is in the urine.

Urine specific gravity, like urine osmolality, will vary from moment to moment depending on the body's fluid and electrolyte status, and can be perfectly normal wherever the result lands. The specific gravity varies not just with the number of particles in the urine, but with their size as well. Thus, the presence of radiocontrast media or glucose in the urine will elevate the specific gravity. Low specific gravity indicates dilute urine; whether or not that dilute urine is physiologically appropriate depends on the clinical context.

Ketones

If you have ever fasted for 24 hours and then tested your urine with a dipstick, you have probably seen the ketones light up in one of the boxes marked "large." This test has really nothing to do with assessing renal function, but rather with assessing the body's overall metabolic state. It's on the urine dipstick because, well, it can be!

Ketones are derived from the breakdown of fat and are used for fuel when adequate glucose is not available. Thus, individuals eating a ketogenic diet (ie, avoiding dietary carbohydrates) will have ketones in their urine. Any disease that can cause ketones to build up in the serum—for example, diabetic or alcoholic ketoacidosis—can cause ketones to appear in the urine.

The three major ketones that the body excretes are *acetone*, *acetoacetate*, and *β-hydroxybutyrate*. β-Hydroxybutyrate is usually the ketone that is present in the highest concentration, especially in patients with alcoholic or diabetic ketoacidosis. However, the urine dipstick only detects acetoacetate (and acetone, but to a far lesser extent). Therefore, it is unwise to rely on a urine dipstick to rule out diabetic or alcoholic ketoacidosis. If either is suspected, direct measurement of β-hydroxybutyrate in the serum should be performed.

Glucose

Normal urine should contain no (or very little) glucose. Very small amounts may be present in some healthy patients who happen to have a lower threshold for excreting glucose in their urine.

In general, the dipstick will not register positive for glucose until the plasma glucose exceeds 180 mg/dL.* The detection of urinary glucose ("glucosuria") used to be the way clinicians diagnosed diabetes mellitus (or—and this is not an urban legend—by tasting the urine for sweetness), and even today the dipstick may unexpectedly uncover diabetes in a patient whose urine is being tested for some other reason. But our blood tests are far superior for diagnosing and monitoring diabetes and have largely replaced the urine dipstick for these purposes.

 # Urine Microscopy: More to See

Urine microscopy provides a description of anything that can be visualized in the urine under the microscope, not just cells or organisms. Findings may include crystals, casts, squamous epithelial cells, or mucus.

Crystals

Crystals come in many shapes and sizes depending on their chemical composition. In patients with kidney stones they may allow you to identify the exact nature of the stone. Occasionally, scattered crystals may be present in the absence of underlying disease and may reflect a predilection to the formation of certain types of stones. We'll discuss the role of the laboratory in diagnosing kidney stones (nephrolithiasis) and evaluating their cause in Chapter 18.

---

*One important exception: patients with diabetes and/or heart failure taking sodium-glucose cotransporter-2 (SGLT-2) inhibitors (eg, empagliflozin), which work by blocking the renal reabsorption of glucose, are expected to have significant glucosuria regardless of their serum glucose.

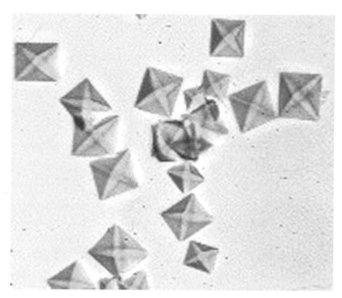

Figure 8.7 Calcium oxalate crystals in the urine of a patient with nephrolithiasis. (From Bergin J. *Medicine Recall*. Wolters Kluwer Health; 2007.)

Casts

Casts are clusters of urinary particles (eg, cells, fat, or even microorganisms) embedded in a protein matrix.* They look like rectangular tubes because they are formed in the renal tubules. There are several types of casts that are important to know about:

- *Hyaline casts*—These casts are translucent and typically do not indicate any serious underlying pathology. They can be found in perfectly healthy individuals, particularly after exercise.

- *Granular casts*—Containing degenerated renal tubular cells, these casts are indicative of renal tubular injury. They can be pigmented in patients with rhabdomyolysis.

- *Red blood cell casts*—These can be seen along with dysmorphic red blood cells (see page 100) when there is acute glomerular injury.

- *White blood cell casts*—Most often associated with pyelonephritis, these casts can also be seen with acute interstitial nephritis, granulomatous diseases such as sarcoidosis, and athero-embolic disease.

---

*The major protein in casts is called the Tamm-Horsfall protein; it is made by renal tubular cells and plays a role in combating UTIs.

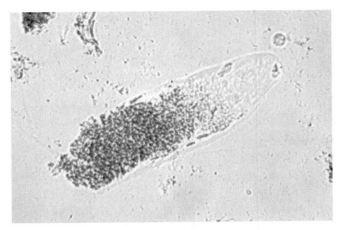

Figure 8.8 A half-granular, half-hyaline cast. (From Mundt LA, Shanahan K. *Graff's Textbook of Urinalysis and Body Fluids.* 2nd ed. Wolters Kluwer/Lippincott Williams & Wilkins; 2011.)

Squamous Epithelial Cells

Squamous epithelial cells line the distal urethra and, of course, the surrounding skin. They are a common finding on urinalysis and generally do not indicate any underlying pathology. The finding of many squamous epithelial cells in the urine (no exact cutoff) may be indicative of sample contamination (ie, improper specimen collection). Depending on the clinical scenario, you may want to repeat a urinalysis with a clean-catch specimen—you may find, for example, that the bacteria seen on the first specimen disappear along with the squamous cells.

Mucus

The lab report will often indicate the presence of "mucus strands" or "mucus threads" on the urinalysis. A little mucus is a common finding in the urine. A lot can indicate an infection (but is still nonspecific). In either case, we can't recall an instance when this finding was helpful in either diagnosis or management.

9 Blood Gases

A blood gas measures, as you might guess, the most important gases in the bloodstream: *carbon dioxide* (CO_2) and *oxygen* (O_2). It also tells us the *pH of the blood* (how acidic or basic the blood is), the *hemoglobin oxygen saturation* (also called the oxyhemoglobin saturation), the *bicarbonate concentration* (HCO_3^-), and the *lactate concentration*. We'll go over how these values can give us an accurate snapshot of a patient's oxygenation, ventilation (the process by which the lungs and atmosphere exchange air), and acid-base status. Because a blood gas can be drawn and analyzed within minutes, it is an especially powerful tool.

A complete blood gas assessment is rarely if ever performed in the outpatient setting. As we will discuss later, there is a simple and inexpensive tool for measuring oxygenation outside the hospital, the pulse oximeter,* but whereas this gives you only a single reading—the oxygen saturation—a complete blood gas determination provides a wealth of data that can be essential to successfully managing ill patients, especially those in an intensive care setting.

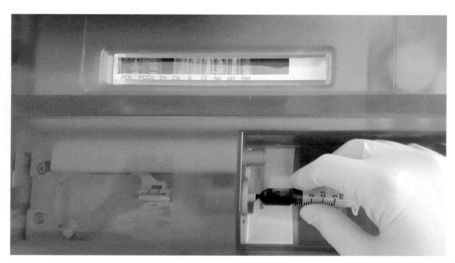

Figure 9.1 Various versions of this machine can be found in hospitals throughout the world. It can spit out results of an arterial blood gas in seconds. (Courtesy Chamaiporn Naprom/Shutterstock.)

One quick warning—we are going to be getting pretty deep into the weeds in this section. But this information is important to understand because it is particularly applicable to those patients who are the most ill. We've done our best to make everything as clear and simple as we can. If we can understand it, we are pretty certain you can, too.

---

*It is used in the hospital, too.

Arterial Versus Venous Blood Gases

A blood gas can be drawn from an artery (ABG) or a vein (VBG).

ABG and VBG measure the same substances, but the normal ranges are not the same. The difference is *where* in the body they are being measured: an artery, where the oxygen content is high, or a vein, where the oxygen content is low.

- ABG: An ABG is typically drawn from either a radial or femoral artery (other possible sites include the brachial, axillary, or dorsalis pedis arteries). The radial artery is the most common site.

- VBG: A VBG may be drawn from a:

  1. peripheral vein (the most common site; our discussion will focus mainly on the peripheral VBG),

  2. central vein (usually the superior vena cava, from a central line), or

  3. pulmonary artery (from a Swan-Ganz/pulmonary artery catheter).

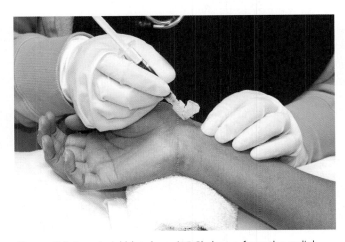

Figure 9.2 An arterial blood gas (ABG) drawn from the radial artery. Use a regular syringe and needle. Feel for the pulse and go in at an angle between 30° and 45° in line with the artery, aiming proximally. The artery is not deep; it is easy to go right through the artery so advance the needle slowly. A flash of blood in the syringe will indicate success. Once the syringe is filled, put the sample immediately on ice* (unless you are certain the analysis can be run in fewer than 20 minutes) and get it to the lab as quickly as you can. The ABG should be run within a few minutes of the blood draw. Make sure to apply pressure to the puncture site for several minutes. (Courtesy Kim M Smith/Shutterstock.)

---

*Why ice? Because, unless the sample is chilled, within ~20 minutes you will see a decrease in the partial pressure of oxygen (Po_2) and an increase in the partial pressure of carbon dioxide (Pco_2) due to metabolism by cells within the sample. Cooling the sample slows this process down.

The big difference between an ABG (taken from oxygen-rich blood) and VBG (taken from oxygen-depleted blood) is that the ABG is a reliable measure of tissue oxygenation, whereas the VBG is not. What about all the other values on the report? For these, the results of a VBG better correlate with those of an ABG:

Partial pressure of CO_2 (Pco_2): Peripheral venous Pco_2 ($Pvco_2$) is approximately 3 to 8 mm Hg higher than arterial Pco_2 ($Paco_2$).

pH: Peripheral venous pH is approximately 0.02 to 0.04 pH units lower (more acidic) than arterial pH.

Bicarbonate (HCO_3^-): Peripheral venous HCO_3^- concentration is approximately 2 to 3 mEq/L higher than arterial HCO_3^-.

Aside from the oxygen level, then, the differences between an ABG and VBG are small and relatively consistent. Thus, a peripheral VBG can give us a reliable measurement of Pco_2, pH, and HCO_3^- and reasonably reflect a patient's acid-base status (more on this to come).

When Do You Order an ABG Versus a VBG?

Order a VBG when you want to assess the Pco_2 and/or pH but aren't concerned about oxygenation (or if you already have all the information you need about oxygenation). A VBG is usually far easier and less painful to obtain than an ABG—think of the difference between a superficial pin prick and a deep piercing stab—with less risk of bleeding or hematoma.

Order an ABG when you want to assess oxygenation in addition to the Pco_2 and/or pH. An ABG is the test of choice in shock or critical illness.

For the remainder of this section we will be focusing on the ABG, but remember that our discussion of everything that follows—with the key exception of oxygenation—applies both to ABG and VBG.

 # Oxygenation

Although our bodies can fuel themselves for short periods of time in the absence of oxygen via anaerobic metabolism, it is an inefficient and unsustainable process that also produces harmful by-products such as lactic acid. For most patients who comfortably walk into our office or are even just sitting comfortably without evidence of respiratory distress, we can assume their oxygenation is adequate. But for critically ill patients, especially if they are in respiratory distress, we need to know the oxygen level in their blood.

Oxygen within the circulation exists in two forms, both of which are measured directly on the ABG:

1. *Oxygen bound to hemoglobin.* We measure this as the percent of hemoglobin that is saturated by oxygen, or *oxyhemoglobin saturation.* The shorthand is So_2, or Sao_2 when we are talking about arterial blood specifically.

2. *Free oxygen dissolved in the plasma.* We measure this as the partial pressure of oxygen. The shorthand is Po_2, or Pao_2 when we are talking about arterial blood specifically.

Normal ranges for Pao_2 and Sao_2 on the ABG vary widely depending on the patient and situation, at least in part because tissue hypoxia may occur at different levels of Pao_2 and Sao_2 in different clinical scenarios. That said, in a healthy patient at rest, it's reasonable to consider a Pao_2 more than 80 mm Hg and an Sao_2 more than 95% as normal. Although there is no definitive line at which supplemental oxygen is needed, a Pao_2 less than 55 mm Hg or an Sao2 less than 85% is almost always concerning.

Levels of free oxygen and oxyhemoglobin tend to rise and fall together—that is, if one goes up so does the other. At any given time, exactly how much of the oxygen in the blood is bound to hemoglobin versus how much is dissolved in the plasma depends on factors such as pH, temperature, and CO_2 level.

Temperature Corrected Blood Gas Values

An ABG report will typically list measured values and "temperature corrected" values. What does "temperature corrected" mean? Oxygen and carbon dioxide both bind hemoglobin with less affinity at higher temperatures. As a result, as body temperature increases, levels of free oxygen and carbon dioxide (Pao_2 and $Paco_2$, respectively) increase, and the pH decreases (we will go over why later in this chapter). The blood gas machine automatically adjusts for this by providing a "temperature corrected" pH, Pao_2, and $Paco_2$.

This can be confusing: the machine measures the ABG with the sample at 37 °C, regardless of the patient's temperature. The person running the test enters the patient's actual temperature into the machine, then the machine calculates what the pH, Pao_2, and $Paco_2$ would be at the patient's body temperature—these are the "temperature corrected values." Usually the difference between the measured and temperature corrected values is minimal. In a patient with a temperature less than 36 °C or more than 38 °C, we recommend using the temperature corrected values as they are likely more accurate.

Causes of a falsely low Sao_2 or Pao_2 on an ABG:

- Leaving the sample out for too long at room temperature
- Mislabeling a VBG as an ABG

Causes of a falsely high Sao_2 or Pao_2 on an ABG:

- Too many air bubbles in the sample (these should be grossly visible)

Regardless of the exact balance between free oxygen and oxyhemoglobin, *oxyhemoglobin always makes up the vast majority of the oxygen content of the blood*. So why not just forget about Pao_2 and only measure Sao_2? In fact, we often do just that, particularly if all we are interested in is oxygenation and do not need all the other tests that come with a complete ABG. We can do this with a pulse oximeter.

The Pulse Oximeter

A *pulse oximeter* is an inexpensive, noninvasive device that can be clipped onto a finger (less commonly a toe or an ear) that provides a continuous reading of a patient's Sao_2.

Unlike the complete ABG, pulse oximeter is available for easy outpatient use. It gained widespread public attention during the COVID-19 pandemic through its use at home to allow infected patients to keep an eye on their respiratory status.

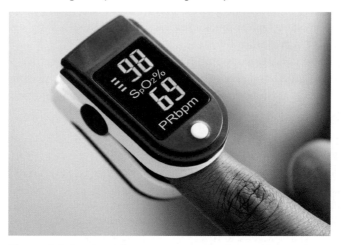

Figure 9.3 A pulse oximeter worn on the finger. (Courtesy Andrey_Popov/Shutterstock.)

The pulse oximeter uses light emitted at two different wavelengths to measure the proportion of red blood cells whose hemoglobin is bound to oxygen, that is, the oxyhemoglobin saturation. A properly functioning pulse oximeter has a characteristic accompanying waveform (see Figure 9.4). A flat or irregular waveform may indicate improper device positioning (try a different finger), motion artifact (ask your patient to stop moving), or malfunction of the device (replace the pulse oximeter or cord).

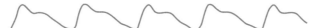

Figure 9.4 The normal waveform of a pulse oximeter.

So how does the pulse oximeter stack up against the ABG?

Table 9.1 Pulse Oximetry Versus ABG

Advantages vs ABG	Disadvantages vs ABG
Noninvasive	Cannot measure Pa_{O_2}
Continuous monitoring	Cannot measure Pa_{CO_2}
Immediate results	Less accurate at low Sa_{O_2} (<~90%)
Inexpensive	Cannot detect hyperoxemia[a]
	Cannot detect abnormal hemoglobins[b]

ABG, arterial blood gas.
[a]Too much oxygen in the blood.
[b]Methemoglobin, carboxyhemoglobin, sickle hemoglobin, sulfhemoglobin.

Pulse oximetry is so common, useful, and easy to perform that an Sao_2 by pulse oximeter is increasingly considered a fifth vital sign (measured along with blood pressure, temperature, heart rate, and respiratory rate). *Continuous* pulse oximetry is also commonly used; patients likely to benefit from continuous pulse oximetry include those hospitalized for respiratory or cardiac illness (especially if they are hypoxemic on admission)—in other words, anyone whose oxygenation you need to keep a close eye on in case of any sudden changes. An example would be an older, otherwise healthy patient who is hospitalized for pneumonia with mild hypoxemia and is requiring a small amount of supplemental oxygen.

When Pulse Oximetry Betrays Us: Abnormal Hemoglobins (Dyshemoglobins)

In carbon monoxide poisoning, carbon monoxide binds hemoglobin with more affinity than oxygen, displacing the oxygen in the process. This can lead to a rapid, life-threatening decline in Sao_2. Unfortunately, a typical pulse oximeter cannot tell the difference between carboxy-hemoglobin (hemoglobin bound to carbon monoxide) and regular oxyhemoglobin[a]—so a patient with 60% oxyhemoglobin and 40% carboxyhemoglobin would have an Sao_2 reading on pulse oximetry of 100%. Therefore, you need to consider the possibility of carbon monoxide poisoning in a cyanotic, obtunded patient who presents with a normal pulse oximeter reading. If there is any concern at all for carbon monoxide poisoning, order an ABG, which can detect and differentiate between carboxyhemoglobin and oxyhemoglobin.

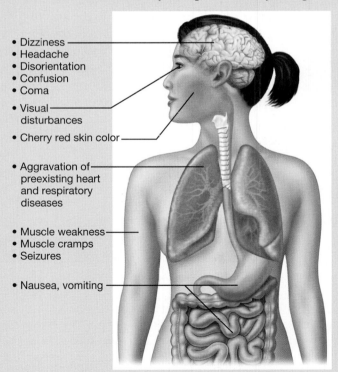

• Dizziness
• Headache
• Disorientation
• Confusion
• Coma

• Visual disturbances

• Cherry red skin color

• Aggravation of preexisting heart and respiratory diseases

• Muscle weakness
• Muscle cramps
• Seizures

• Nausea, vomiting

Figure 9.5 The signs and symptoms of carbon monoxide poisoning. (From Donnelly-Moreno LA. *Timby's Fundamental Nursing Skills and Concepts.* 12th ed. Wolters Kluwer; 2021.)

The pulse oximeter runs into similar problems with other abnormal hemoglobins (dyshemoglobins), including methemoglobin (oxidized hemoglobin; a rare side effect of topical anesthetics, some antimalarial medications, and various toxic chemicals and dyes) and sulfhemoglobin (caused by some medications, including dapsone and metoclopramide). Rarely, even sickle hemoglobin—which carries oxygen normally but can get stuck in the vasculature, leading to vaso-occlusive crises in patients with sickle cell disease—may cause spuriously high or low pulse oximeter readings. Bottom line: if you think a patient may have hypoxemia in the setting of a dyshemoglobinemia, check an Sao_2 on an ABG.

[a]There are some special pulse oximeters that can estimate levels of carboxyhemoglobin and other dyshemoglobins such as methemoglobin. They can be useful as an initial screening tool but aren't nearly as accurate as an ABG.

When Pulse Oximetry Doesn't Quite "Nail" the Sao_2

Nail polish can cause falsely low pulse oximeter readings by up to 3% or 4%. This is presumably due to absorption of light at specific frequencies by some colors of nail polish, particularly blue, black, and brown. Red nail polish seems to be safe. Clipping the pulse oximeter onto the sides of the finger (instead of over the nail) or to another site fixes the issue, as does removing the nail polish.

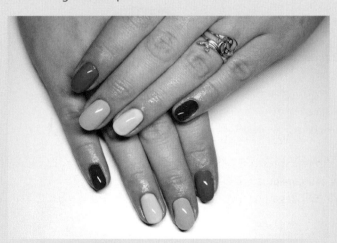

Figure 9.6 Be careful which finger you choose here for your pulse oximeter. (Courtesy MikhailPopov/Shutterstock.)

More importantly, pulse oximetry may record higher readings in patients with dark skin, potentially missing severe or even life-threatening hypoxemia. This is disturbingly common: as many as one in every nine Black patients with hypoxemia can be misdiagnosed by pulse oximetry. Presumably the increased pigment in the skin affects the strength and accuracy of the signal picked up by the oximeter. If you have reason to suspect hypoxemia in a patient with darkly pigmented skin and the pulse oximeter reading is normal, consider getting an ABG for an accurate reading.

When is pulse oximetry not sufficient? An ABG is usually necessary in cases of:

- severe hypoxemia (ie, an Sao_2 significantly less than 90%, where pulse oximetry is less accurate),

- concomitant ventilation (CO_2) problems,

- suspected presence of abnormal forms of hemoglobin (eg, carbon monoxide poisoning or methemoglobinemia; see the box "When Pulse Oximetry Betrays Us: Abnormal Hemoglobins (Dyshemoglobins)"), or

- critical illness; intubated patients in particular often require ABGs every few hours in order to adjust ventilator settings to maintain normal oxygen and carbon dioxide levels.

The Alveolar-Arterial (A-a) Gradient

The A-a gradient is useful for differentiating among the different causes of hypoxemia. It is defined as the difference between the amount of oxygen in the alveoli and the amount dissolved in the arterial blood. Here's the formula:

$$\text{A-a} = PAo_2 - Pao_2$$

A capital "A" is used to denote an alveolar reading and a small "a" the arterial reading.

The Pao_2 is of course reported on the ABG. But how do you know what the partial pressure of oxygen is in the alveoli? If you think it must reflect the partial pressure of oxygen in the atmosphere, you are correct, but you need to do a little bit of calculating to arrive at precisely the right number. Here is the equation you need, but don't panic—although this may seem like a lot of work, you can do this in seconds on the calculator on your cell phone, and the information is well worth the small investment in time.

$$PAo_2 = Fio_2 (P_{atm} - P_{H_2O}) - (Paco_2/R)$$

where P_{atm} is the atmospheric pressure (760 mm Hg at sea level), P_{H_2O} is the partial pressure of water (45 mm Hg), R is a constant called the respiratory quotient (you can generally use 0.8), and Fio_2 is the fraction of oxygen in the inspired air (21%, or 0.21, with the patient on room air). A commonly cited normal value for the PAo_2 at sea level on room air is 104 mm Hg.

A normal A-a gradient is 5 to 10 mm Hg for a young healthy patient breathing room air; the normal range increases significantly with age and for patients receiving supplemental oxygen. We can account for age by approximating a normal A-a gradient as $2.5 + 0.21 \times$ age in years.

When you are evaluating a patient with hypoxemia and you aren't sure of the cause, it can be helpful to distinguish those causes that are associated with a normal versus increased A-a gradient:

- The only causes of hypoxemia producing a *normal* A-a gradient are those where not enough oxygen is getting to the alveoli in the first place—either a problem with the air we are breathing in (eg, at high altitudes where there is a low pressure of inspired oxygen) or a problem with the actual amount of air we are breathing (not breathing fast or deeply enough, ie, hypoventilation).

- Problems with the lung parenchyma (eg, emphysema, pneumonia, fibrosis) or cardiopulmonary circulation (eg, intracardiac or intrapulmonary shunt) produce an abnormally elevated A-a gradient.

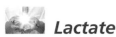 Lactate

Lactate is the conjugate base of—and thus a surrogate measurement for—lactic acid. The normal range is 0.5 to 1.6 mEq/L. Take the lower limit with a large grain of salt, because only an abnormally elevated lactate is clinically significant. Measurements on the ABG, VBG, and standalone serum tests all correlate very closely (the venous lactate is on average only about 0.3 mEq/L higher than the arterial lactate), so you can use any of these tests to check the lactate.

Why Do We Care About Lactic Acid, and Why Is It on the Blood Gas Report?

Lactic acid is a product of anaerobic metabolism, the pathway by which tissues that are not getting enough oxygen can still generate energy. Lactate therefore pairs well with measures of oxygenation; both tell us something important about the oxygen supply to the tissues. *Clinically, we use lactate as a marker of tissue hypoxia, which occurs in disease states such as hypovolemia, heart failure, sepsis, or any type of shock.*

Consider checking a lactate when you are concerned about an acute clinical change such as a sudden drop in blood pressure or acutely altered mental status, especially in a patient who is already severely or critically ill. It's a way of asking, *Is my patient getting worse or even developing shock?* However, obtaining a lactate is not the end of the story; you will generally *not* be able to establish any one specific diagnosis with a lactate alone, but will next need to look for the underlying cause of the patient's decompensation.

Is an Elevated Lactate Always Worrisome?

Lactic acidosis that is caused by systemic hypoxia and/or hypoperfusion is called *type A lactic acidosis*, which is the scary type and is always cause for concern. Lactic acidosis caused by anything else is called *type B lactic acidosis*, which is (usually) less scary. The lactate elevation in type B lactic acidosis is typically mild to moderate (rarely >6 mEq/L). The mechanisms underlying type B lactic acidosis are heterogeneous and may involve poor lactate clearance, impairment of cellular metabolism caused by various toxins (including mitochondrial dysfunction), or localized (rather than systemic) ischemia.

Here are some of the most common causes of type B lactic acidosis:

- Liver disease (especially with progression to cirrhosis)

- Diabetes (lactic acidosis is usually mild in the absence of ketoacidosis)

- Chronic alcoholism

- Malignancy

- HIV infection

- Thiamine deficiency

- Medications: β-agonists (injection of intravenous [IV] epinephrine, high-dose inhaled albuterol), metformin, salicylates (aspirin), acetaminophen (Tylenol), antiretroviral therapy (ART), propofol, linezolid

Patients with type B lactic acidosis may have elevated lactate levels in the absence of systemic hypoxia or hypoperfusion. However, it still may be helpful to trend their lactate over time; the trend is often more important than any one isolated value. For example, a patient with hepatic encephalopathy caused by cirrhosis whose lactate jumps from 3.8 mEq/L (that patient's "baseline lactate") to 6.5 mEq/L may have developed shock. Also note that, while not necessarily indicative of sepsis or shock, a new type B lactic acidosis (such as can be caused by metformin, a very common drug used in the treatment of type 2 diabetes mellitus) may warrant a change in management, because accumulation of lactic acid in and of itself can be harmful.

ʟ-Lactate and ᴅ-Lactate

Lactate exists in two structurally related forms ("isoforms"): ʟ-lactate and ᴅ-lactate. The vast majority of lactate found in humans is ʟ-lactate, which is the only form detected on the blood gas (or when we order a stand-alone serum lactate). Excessive ʟ-lactate is responsible for all of the forms of lactic acidosis discussed earlier. Rarely, ᴅ-lactate can accumulate, causing a **ᴅ-lactic acidosis**. This is most often seen in patients whose small intestines have been resected and have so-called **short bowel syndrome**.

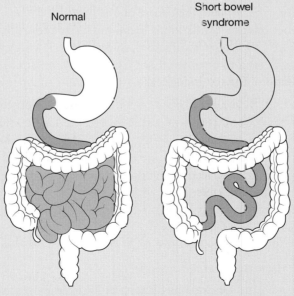

Figure 9.7 Patients with short bowel syndrome are at risk of developing ᴅ-lactic acidosis.

In these patients, carbohydrates normally absorbed by the small intestines make it all the way to the colon, where they are converted by bacteria to both L-lactate and D-lactate. The body can readily metabolize the L-lactate (we have enzymes for this) but not the D-lactate, so D-lactate accumulates. Signs of D-lactic acidosis are relatively nonspecific and include drowsiness, slurred speech, and headache. If you are concerned for possible D-lactic acidosis—perhaps in a patient with a history of small bowel resection with unexplained metabolic acidosis—you'll need to order a separate test for D-lactate.

 ## CO_2 and Ventilation

The blood gas directly measures the amount of CO_2 dissolved in the plasma. This is called the partial pressure of CO_2, or P_{CO_2}. The VBG measures P_{CO_2} in venous blood (P_{VCO_2}) before it has traveled through the right side of the heart to the lungs, where we dump CO_2 and pick up O_2. The ABG, on the other hand, measures CO_2 levels after this exchange (P_{aCO_2}). Hence CO_2 levels are slightly higher (3-8 mm Hg) on the VBG than on the ABG.

CO_2 is a by-product of normal metabolism. It would quickly build up to dangerous levels if we did not blow some of it off in the breath. The amount of CO_2 we breathe off is directly related to our *minute ventilation*, defined as the total volume of air we breathe in or out (the number is the same either way) over the course of 1 minute:

$$\text{Minute ventilation} = \text{RR} \times V_T$$

where RR is the respiratory rate (breaths/minute) and V_T is the tidal volume, a term for the volume of air inhaled (or exhaled) over the course of one breath.

A patient with a higher minute ventilation is breathing faster and/or more deeply and will therefore breathe off more CO_2 (hyperventilation), lowering the P_{CO_2}. A patient taking slow and/or shallow breaths will tend to breathe off less CO_2 (hypoventilation), raising the P_{CO_2}.

Unless minute ventilation changes dramatically—for example, if a person goes from breathing 20 times per minute to 4 times per minute—the effects on oxygenation are small compared to those on the P_{CO_2}.

Hypercapnia

Abnormally high P_{CO_2} is called *hypercapnia* (P_{aCO_2} >45 mm Hg or P_{VCO_2} >~50 mm Hg). There are a few key causes to remember:

- Hypoventilation

  Breathing may be too slow, too shallow, or both. Why would this happen?

  1. **Won't breathe**: decreased respiratory drive

     – Some common causes include medication or illicit drug overdose (eg, opioids, barbiturates), primary central nervous system disease (encephalitis, stroke, central sleep apnea), and metabolic alkalosis (discussed later).

2. **Can't breathe**: neuromuscular weakness
   – Causes include diaphragmatic paralysis from cervical spinal cord or phrenic nerve injury, amyotrophic lateral sclerosis, Guillain-Barré syndrome, myasthenia gravis, myopathy or myositis from any cause.

• Dead Space

This is just what it sounds like. Ventilation is normal—enough air gets to and from the lungs—but some alveoli are not being properly perfused with blood, so the air in those alveoli just sits there without gas exchange occurring. Those spaces are useless ("dead") and cannot contribute to removing CO$_2$ from the body. Another term for this phenomenon is "ventilation without perfusion." Anything that disrupts the normal architecture of the lungs (and therefore the capillaries that perfuse the alveoli and facilitate gas exchange) can cause pathologic dead space and hypercapnia.
   – Common causes include chronic obstructive pulmonary disease (COPD), pneumonia, pulmonary fibrosis, pulmonary embolism, and pulmonary hypertension.

Hypocapnia

Abnormally low Pco$_2$ is called *hypocapnia* (Paco$_2$ <35 mm Hg or Pvco$_2$ <~40 mm Hg). The main cause of hypocapnia is *hyper*ventilation. Common drivers of hyperventilation include anxiety, pain, intense exercise, anemia, and pregnancy (hypocapnia is typically mild in the last case).

Hyperventilation with resultant hypocapnia can also occur as a compensatory mechanism, either in response to metabolic acidosis (see page 118) or to hypoxemia. In the latter case, the so-called "hypoxic respiratory drive" increases minute ventilation in an attempt to improve oxygenation. But, as we stated earlier, minute ventilation tends to drive CO$_2$ levels more than O$_2$ levels, so although hyperventilation may improve oxygenation a bit, it does so at the cost of a significant drop in Pco$_2$.

Hyperventilation During an Acute Asthma Attack

Hyperventilation due to hypoxemia is common in an acute asthma exacerbation, in which case hypocapnia should actually be taken as a reassuring sign that the patient's hypoxic respiratory drive and respiratory muscle strength are intact. A hypoxemic patient with asthma who stops hyperventilating—that is, whose Pco$_2$ returns to normal—should prompt immediate concern for impending respiratory failure.

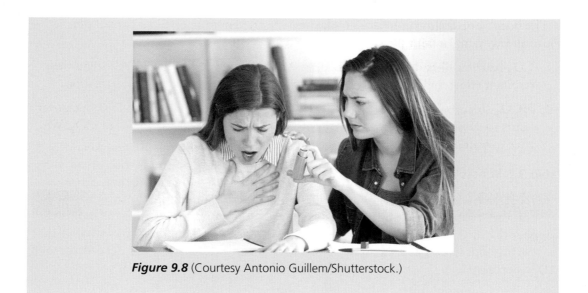

Figure 9.8 (Courtesy Antonio Guillem/Shutterstock.)

Our bodies are exquisitely sensitive to changes in P_{CO_2}. For example, if you've ever found yourself hyperventilating, you may recall feeling dizziness, numbness, or tingling after only seconds of hypocapnia. Hypercapnia can be even worse, leading to fatigue, confusion, and eventually death. Receptors throughout the body (including those in the lungs, peripheral circulation, and central nervous system) are constantly sensing CO_2 levels and sending signals to adjust respiratory drive to maintain a normal CO_2. Why is this tight regulation of CO_2 so important? It turns out that CO_2 plays a key role in our body's delicate system of acid-base balance, our next topic.

 ## Acid-Base Balance

It is now time to discuss how you can use the pH, P_{CO_2}, and HCO_3^- on your blood gas to determine a patient's acid-base status, which can in turn clue you in to the presence or absence of specific respiratory and metabolic problems. This makes the blood gas an extremely powerful diagnostic tool.

Why is acid-base balance so important? The body is only really happy when the extracellular arterial pH is at or very close to 7.4. Throw the pH out of balance in either direction and the body begins to malfunction (predictably, the further the pH from 7.4, the worse the consequences): enzymes cease to do their jobs, nerves start to misfire, muscles (including cardiac myocytes) can't contract properly, and the mitochondria can't generate appropriate amounts of adenosine triphosphate (ATP) for energy. Understanding acid-base disorders is essential for understanding and managing critically ill patients.

Even small deviations from the normal pH can be hazardous. *Acidemia is defined as an arterial pH less than 7.35; alkalemia is defined as an arterial pH more than 7.45.*

The body has a built-in mechanism called a buffer system to maintain a normal pH. You're already familiar with the key components:

1. **CO_2 (carbon dioxide)** acts as an acid, *decreasing* the pH. Changes in CO_2—and the resultant effects on pH—happen over minutes as we adjust our minute ventilation.

2. **HCO_3^- (bicarbonate)** acts as a base, *increasing* the pH. Changes in HCO_3^- happen over hours to days, since we can't simply breathe bicarbonate off like we can with CO_2. We have to wait for our kidneys to do their work.

Table 9.2 Buffers and pH

Buffer Component	Effect on pH	Regulating Organ	Effect Timeframe
HCO_3^-	↑	Kidneys	Hours to days
CO_2	↓	Lungs	Minutes

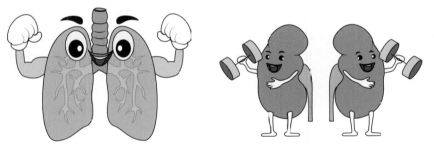

Figure 9.9 Our lungs (CO_2) and kidneys (HCO_3^-) are constantly working to maintain a normal blood pH.

CO_2 and HCO_3^- exist in an equilibrium that ultimately determines the blood pH.

$$CO_2 + H_2O \leftrightharpoons H_2CO_3 \leftrightharpoons HCO_3^- + H^+$$

You can see, even if just intuitively, how increasing the CO_2 concentration drives the equation to the right and generates more H^+ ions, whereas increasing the HCO_3^- drives the equation to the left, consuming more H^+ ions.

The pH can be calculated using the Henderson-Hasselbalch formula*:

$$pH = 6.1 - \log_{10} \left(\frac{[HCO_3^-]}{0.03 \times pCO_2} \right)$$

---

*Note: you will not have to do this calculation. The lab will do this for you (whew!). We include this here as an aid to understanding only.

> **Calculated Versus Measured Bicarbonate**
>
> Neither the VBG nor ABG directly measures the bicarbonate. Instead, they measure the pH and the P_{CO_2}, then calculate the bicarbonate using the Henderson-Hasselbalch formula. This is the bicarbonate you see on the ABG and VBG reports. On the other hand, the basic metabolic panel (BMP) more or less *directly measures* the bicarbonate concentration (see Chapter 5).
>
> So which should we rely on—the measured (BMP) or calculated (ABG/VBG) bicarbonate? The good news is that we rarely have to choose, because measured and calculated values tend to agree fairly closely the vast majority of the time. In cases where there is a significant difference (say, greater than 3 mEq/L), it may be due to poor sample handling or delayed time to analysis. Some discordance can also be seen in critical illness. The convention in this case is generally to use the measured bicarbonate on the BMP. You might also consider re-drawing either the blood gas or the BMP if there are concerns about sample handling.

Acid-Base Disorders

We call any process affecting the CO_2 a *respiratory process*.
Any process affecting the HCO_3^- is called a *metabolic process*.
Any process increasing the pH (via either CO_2 or HCO_3^-) is called an *alkalosis*.
Any process decreasing the pH is called an *acidosis*.

So it makes sense that there are four possible acid-base disorders:

1. Respiratory alkalosis

2. Respiratory acidosis

3. Metabolic alkalosis

4. Metabolic acidosis

More than one of these processes can be going on simultaneously in the same patient (we'll go over this in detail later). Whatever acid-base processes are happening, the net result is the pH you see on your blood gas: acidemia, alkalemia, or a normal pH.

Compensation: Increase or decrease the CO_2, and the kidneys can compensate by adjusting the HCO_3^-. Increase or decrease the HCO_3^-, and the lungs can compensate by adjusting the CO_2. Because CO_2 and HCO_3^- have opposite effects on pH, an increase in one will lead to a compensatory increase in the other. A decrease in one will lead to a compensatory decrease in the other. In other words, CO_2 and HCO_3^- tend to rise and fall together.

Since both the CO_2 and the HCO_3^- will change with any acid-base disorder—one as the primary disorder, the other as compensation in an effort to restore the normal pH—how do we know which is the primary problem and which is the body's attempt to compensate? There are just *two steps you need to know to determine the primary acid-base disorder from a blood gas:*

1. **Look at the pH** (remember that normal is 7.40 on an ABG or 7.36 on a VBG). If it is high, the primary process is an alkalosis. If it is low, the primary process is an acidosis.

2. **Look at either the HCO_3^- or the CO_2** (it shouldn't matter which, since the vast majority of the time both are high or both are low).

a. If HCO_3^- and CO_2 are abnormal *in the same direction* as the pH, the primary process is metabolic. Thus, for example, the HCO_3^- is low with a metabolic acidosis (low pH), and the CO_2 decreases to compensate. Similarly, the HCO_3^- is high with a metabolic alkalosis (high pH), and the CO_2 increases to compensate.

b. If HCO_3^- and CO_2 are abnormal *in the opposite direction* as the pH, the primary process is respiratory. Thus, the CO_2 is high with a respiratory acidosis (low pH), and the HCO_3^- increases to compensate. Similarly the CO_2 is low with a respiratory alkalosis (high pH), and the HCO_3^- decreases to compensate.

What if HCO_3^- and CO_2 are abnormal in opposite directions from one another (ie, CO_2 is high and HCO_3^- is low, or vice versa)? There must be two processes going on, both driving the pH in the same direction. You will rarely see this pattern, but if you do, know that you cannot tell which process (respiratory or metabolic) is the primary problem based on numbers alone.

Table 9.3 If you can reason your way through each value on this table then you understand all the fundamental acid-base concepts you will need moving forward

Acid-Base Disorders			
Disorder	pH	HCO_3^-	Pa_{CO_2}
Normal	7.40	24	40
Metabolic acidosis	↓	↓	↓
Metabolic alkalosis	↑	↑	↑
Respiratory acidosis	↓	↑	↑
Respiratory alkalosis	↑	↓	↓

Why does it matter which type of acid-base disorder a patient may have? The simple reason is that it helps us identify the source of the problem and guides our choice of therapy. Let's make all this a lot more concrete by following along one patient's odyssey in order to master each type of acid-base disorder.

Akio's Story: A Primer on Acid-Base Disorders

Respiratory Alkalosis: Akio is a 62-year-old male with a history of heart failure who is brought into the emergency room with a broken right leg following an automobile accident.

He is conscious and appears to be breathing rapidly. An ABG is checked in the emergency room:

pH 7.49

HCO_3^- 22 mEq/L

$Paco_2$ 29 mm Hg

The pH is high, indicating that the primary acid-base disorder is an alkalosis. Because both his HCO_3^- and CO_2 are low—abnormal in the *opposite* direction as the pH—the primary process is respiratory. He has a *respiratory alkalosis*, the result of a decreased CO_2 (hypocapnia), which raises the pH.

You already know the main cause of hypocapnia: hyperventilation. In Akio's case, the hyperventilation is very likely due to pain and anxiety. But why is his HCO_3^- slightly low?

In respiratory alkalosis, the kidneys compensate by excreting HCO_3^- over several hours to days. This process of "unloading" base returns the pH toward normal (but not all the way). This means that a patient with a *chronic respiratory alkalosis*—one going on for at least several days—will tend to have lower pH (closer to normal) and a lower HCO_3^- than someone with an *acute respiratory alkalosis* whose kidneys have not had time to get rid of as much HCO_3^-. Online calculators are available to help you determine whether a respiratory alkalosis is acute or chronic.

Respiratory Acidosis: Akio receives pain medication and calms down. Soon after, he is taken to the operating room for repair of a displaced right femoral fracture, which goes well. After waking up from the surgery, he endorses ongoing pain and gets a hefty dose of morphine. An hour later, his nurse notices that he appears somnolent and seems to be breathing slowly. His pulse oximeter reading has gradually been ticking down: 90% → 88% → 85% ....

Here's his latest ABG:

pH 7.26

HCO_3^- 26 mEq/L

$Paco_2$ 59 mm Hg

The low pH tells us we are dealing with an acidosis. The high CO_2 and HCO_3^-—abnormal in the *opposite* direction as the pH—tell us that the cause must be respiratory. Akio now has a *respiratory acidosis*, a result of the increased $Paco_2$ (hypercapnia) that lowers the pH.

We already know what causes hypercapnia: hypoventilation (central nervous system pathology, neuromuscular weakness) and dead space (COPD, pneumonia, pulmonary fibrosis, pulmonary embolism, pulmonary hypertension). Akio is very likely experiencing decreased respiratory drive ("won't breathe") from an opioid overdose.

In respiratory acidosis, the kidneys compensate by—you guessed it—retaining HCO_3^- over several hours to days. A patient with a *chronic respiratory acidosis* will tend to have a higher pH (closer to normal) and a higher HCO_3^- than someone with an *acute respiratory acidosis* whose kidneys have not had time to retain more HCO_3^-.

Don't Be Fooled by Chronic Respiratory Acidosis!

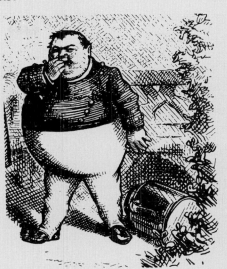

Figure 9.10 Rendering of Dickens' character Mr Pickwick, after whom "Pickwickian syndrome," now known as obesity hypoventilation syndrome, was named. Patients with chronic obstructive pulmonary disease and obesity hypoventilation syndrome may chronically retain CO_2 with resulting compensatory retention of HCO_3^-. (Thomas Nast's drawing of the fat boy in "The Pickwick Papers" from an American edition of the Posthumous Papers of the Pickwick Club, London, 1837; New York, 1873.)

Chronic respiratory acidosis is very common, especially in hospitalized patients. COPD and obesity hypoventilation syndrome (OHS), for example, cause chronic CO_2 retention. This can result in chronically elevated CO_2 levels as high as 60 or even 70 mm Hg. The normal compensatory response is retention of HCO_3^- by the kidneys. As a result, it isn't uncommon to see a HCO_3^- of 40 mEq/L or even higher in such patients. Do not fall into the trap of interpreting either the HCO_3^- or the $Paco_2$ in isolation. If you are worried that your patient has a new or acute acid-base derangement, it is imperative you do two things:

1. Check a blood gas, ideally an ABG for the most direct and accurate measurement of arterial pH and $Paco_2$. If an ABG is not feasible to obtain, a VBG is fine (but remember to convert your numbers to arterial values if you do this). If there is a primary respiratory acidosis, determine if it is acute or chronic as earlier.

2. Compare the new blood gas to those from prior encounters/hospitalizations to get an idea of how close the patient is to their recent baseline. If the pH is lower than before, the patient may have either chronic progression/worsening of disease or a new superimposed process (eg, COPD exacerbation, pneumonia, sedative overdose).

Metabolic Alkalosis: Akio receives naloxone for his opioid overdose and his respiratory status and alertness quickly improve. He does well overnight, but the next morning complains that he had some difficulty sleeping because he became short of breath while lying flat (orthopnea). His legs appear mildly edematous and a chest x-ray is consistent with pulmonary edema.

The team is concerned for a heart failure exacerbation, so they begin aggressive diuresis with IV furosemide. His orthopnea and edema gradually improve. Here's a follow-up ABG after 2 days of diuresis:

pH 7.48

HCO_3^- 33 mEq/L

$Paco_2$ 44 mm Hg

The pH is high—he has an alkalosis—with a high HCO_3^- and a high CO_2 (both abnormal in the *same* direction as the pH). Akio now has a *metabolic alkalosis*, a result of increased HCO_3^-, which raises the pH. The primary problem here is not with the respiratory system.

When you're trying to remember the causes of metabolic alkalosis, think of two organ systems—gastrointestinal (GI) and renal—then consider what would lead to the loss of acid (H^+) or the retention of base (HCO_3^-). Finally, consider whether an abnormal potassium may be playing a role.

1. GI Causes of Metabolic Alkalosis

    We can lose acid through *vomiting* (a loss of gastric acid). On the other hand, we can retain too much base by *ingesting large amounts of antacids or other basic substances.* The latter cause is uncommon; a patient is more likely to develop a metabolic alkalosis in this way if the basic substance is combined with calcium, leading to the so-called *milk-alkali syndrome* (*MAS*; see the box on page 123).

2. Renal Causes of Metabolic Alkalosis

    When the kidneys are responsible, a loss of acid is the primary mechanism of metabolic alkalosis. *Excess aldosterone (as in primary hyperaldosteronism), loop diuretics, and thiazide diuretics* all cause the secretion of both H^+ and K^+ into the urine. Diuretics may also induce hypovolemia, leading to so-called "contraction alkalosis" (see the box on page 123). Akio's metabolic alkalosis is most likely due to the acid- and volume-depleting effects of aggressive diuresis. Finally, there are genetic disorders that mimic thiazide and loop diuretics—*Gitelman and Bartter syndromes*, respectively—that have the same effects.

3. Hypokalemia as a Cause of Metabolic Alkalosis

    Our cells have pumps that can exchange K^+ and H^+. This is a handy tool for regulating plasma pH and potassium concentration while keeping the electrical charge of the cell the same. However, this coupling of K^+ and H^+ can cause problems. In *hypokalemia*, K^+ is pumped out of cells to nudge the plasma K^+ up to normal. In exchange, H^+ is pumped into the cells and out of the circulation with a resulting increase in the plasma pH. Note that, based on this mechanism, not only does hypokalemia cause alkalemia but alkalemia also causes hypokalemia.

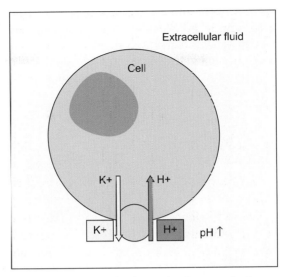

Figure 9.11 Hypokalemia can lead to metabolic alkalosis via H^+/K^+ exchange.

Contraction Alkalosis

You'll hear this term a lot on inpatient medical wards. The general idea is that anything that causes volume loss (or volume "contraction") without a proportional loss in HCO_3^- results in an increase in the plasma HCO_3^- concentration, that is, a metabolic alkalosis. Chloride losses also factor into the pathophysiology. Diuretic use (especially loop and thiazide diuretics) is the most common cause of contraction alkalosis.

In clinical practice, we can use contraction alkalosis to help guide diuretic therapy: a new metabolic alkalosis in a hospitalized patient who has been on diuretics (say, for a heart failure exacerbation) may be an indicator that the patient is sufficiently "dry." Other less common causes of contraction alkalosis include cystic fibrosis (loss of sweat that is high in Cl^- and low in HCO_3^-) and congenital chloride diarrhea.

Milk-Alkali Syndrome

MAS is caused by ingestion of large amounts of base ("absorbable alkali," eg, some antacids) taken in conjunction with calcium. The pathophysiology starts with hypercalcemia, which causes both renal vasoconstriction and salt wasting. Ultimately, the patient becomes hypovolemic with resulting contraction alkalosis, worsened by the ingested alkali. The classic presenting triad includes hypercalcemia, metabolic alkalosis, and acute kidney injury. Patients may be completely asymptomatic; any symptoms tend to be related to hypercalcemia (eg, vomiting, constipation, confusion, kidney stones) and can be acute, subacute, or chronic.

MAS was first recognized in the early to mid-20th century in patients prescribed antacids along with copious milk consumption to treat peptic ulcer disease. Although the incidence of MAS decreased as ulcer treatment evolved, the syndrome began to resurface again in the 1990s as more patients (particularly middle aged and older women) began taking high doses of calcium carbonate supplements for osteopenia or osteoporosis. Treatment consists of withdrawal of the offending agent and aggressive IV fluid administration.

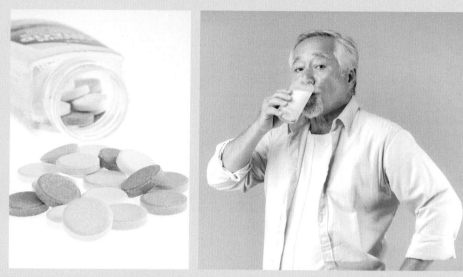

Figure 9.12 On the way to milk-alkali syndrome? (Courtesy Gerald Bernard/Shutterstock; HappyTime19/Shutterstock.)

The clinical history is often sufficient to tell us the cause of a metabolic alkalosis: has the patient been vomiting? Was a diuretic started or increased recently (as in Akio's case)? When the cause of a metabolic alkalosis is unclear, the next test to check is a urine electrolyte panel; specifically, we care about the *urine chloride*.

The body pulls in chloride (along with sodium and water) from the urine in states of hypovolemia. So we expect a low urine chloride (<20 mEq/L) when the patient is hypovolemic, such as can occur with vomiting or diuretic use (*in between* doses of diuretics, not while the diuretic is still acting on the kidneys). We would expect Akio's urine chloride, for example, to be low, provided it has been at least a few hours since the last dose of furosemide.

In contrast, a normal or high urine chloride (>20 mEq/L) is expected in hypervolemia or in cases where chloride is *currently* being pathologically dumped into the urine. We see high urine chloride in primary hyperaldosteronism and in Gitelman and Bartter syndromes (which act like continuous loop and thiazide diuretics, respectively).

Wide swings in a patient's urine chloride over hours to days may indicate surreptitious diuretic abuse, since urine chloride rises after diuretic administration then falls when the effect wears off.

We compensate for metabolic alkalosis by hypoventilating. The resulting CO_2 retention brings the pH down (closer to normal). We can adjust our minute ventilation very quickly, so compensation tends to occur over minutes. The lower the pH (closer to normal) and the higher the CO_2, the better the respiratory compensation.

Table 9.4 Causes of Metabolic Alkalosis

Etiology	Mechanism	Volume Status	Urine Cl^- (mEq/L)
Vomiting	GI H^+ losses	Low	<20
Loop/thiazide diuretics	Renal H^+ losses ±Hypovolemia	Low to normal	Recent use: <20 Remote use: >20
Bartter or Gitelman syndrome	Renal H^+ losses ±Hypovolemia	Low	>20
Contraction alkalosis • Excessive diuresis • Cystic fibrosis • Congenital chloride diarrhea	Loss of fluid with both • High Cl^- • Low HCO_3^-	Low	Usually <20
Mineralocorticoid excess • Primary hyperaldosteronism (Conn syndrome) • Renal artery stenosis • Cushing syndrome • SAME[a]	Renal H^+ losses	High	>20
Excessive HCO_3^- ingestion/ infusion	HCO_3^- excess • Risks: hyper-calcemia, renal insufficiency, hypovolemia	Variable	Variable
Milk-alkali syndrome	Hypercalcemia + HCO_3^- excess	Low	<20
Hypokalemia	Intracellular H^+ shift	Variable	>20
Post-hypercapnic alkalosis	Chronic renal HCO_3^- retention → rapid lowering of P_{CO_2}	Variable	Usually <20

GI, gastrointestinal; SAME, syndrome of apparent mineralocorticoid excess.
[a]Although SAME is most commonly a genetic disease, an acquired form can be seen with excess consumption of licorice.

Metabolic Acidosis: Akio's team backs off on his diuretic regimen and his metabolic alkalosis improves, but he isn't out of the woods yet. Over the next 2 days, he develops abdominal pain with worsening, profuse, watery diarrhea. His stool tests positive for *Clostridium difficile* (a common hospital-acquired infection; see Chapter 16). Despite initiation of appropriate antibiotic treatment, his blood pressure slowly begins to drop—he may be developing septic shock.

Here's what his ABG looks like now:

pH 7.33

HCO_3^- 14 mEq/L

$Paco_2$ 26 mm Hg

And here are his most recent electrolytes:

Na^+ 137

K^+ 4.0

Cl^- 104

Akio's pH is low—he has an acidosis. Because his HCO_3^- and CO_2 are also low, the cause must be metabolic. He has a *metabolic acidosis* due to decreased HCO_3^-, which lowers the pH. This can happen due to base loss, acid retention, or excess acid generation.

In practice, it is most helpful to divide metabolic acidosis into two categories: *normal anion gap* and *high anion gap* (this is why we also gave you Akio's electrolytes).

As a reminder from Chapter 5, the anion gap is the difference between the positive ions (cations) and negative ions (anions) measured on the BMP or comprehensive metabolic panel (CMP). In the United States, we typically don't include potassium in the calculation.

$$\text{Anion gap} = Na - (Cl + HCO_3^-)$$
$$\text{Akio's anion gap} = 137 - (104 + 14) = 19 \text{ mEq/L}$$

The normal range for the anion gap is 4 to 12 mEq/L. Hence Akio has a high anion gap. There must be some extra unmeasured anions floating around.

High anion gap metabolic acidosis (HAGMA): This disorder is caused by the accumulation of acids that break apart (dissociate) into H^+ ions and an unmeasured anion. Common causes of HAGMA can be summarized by the mnemonic *GOLDMARK*:

1. *G*lycols: ethylene glycol (antifreeze—don't consume it) and propylene glycol (a preservative in cosmetics and a solvent in many medications—safe in normal doses but dangerous in excess)

2. *O*xoproline: a toxic metabolite of acetaminophen that can build up in rare cases of acetaminophen toxicity which are distinct from the usual picture of acetaminophen overdose (which more commonly causes liver failure and lactic acidosis)

3. *L*-lactate: this is what builds up in lactic acidosis, such as in sepsis or shock

4. *D*-lactate: a less common form of lactate that can accumulate in short bowel syndrome (see page 113)

5. *Methanol ingestion*: a toxic alcohol that can cause vision loss

6. *Aspirin* (acetylsalicylic acid, or ASA) overdose

7. *Renal failure*: either acute or chronic. Look for an elevated blood urea nitrogen (BUN) and creatinine on the BMP or CMP.

8. *Ketoacidosis*: ketone buildup leads to production of unmeasured anions. Types of ketoacidosis include diabetic ketoacidosis, alcoholic ketoacidosis, and starvation ketoacidosis.

Given Akio's infection and hypotension, his HAGMA is most likely due to lactic acidosis in the setting of worsening shock.

Fine-Tuning the Anion Gap

The negatively charged molecules (anions) that normally "fill" the anion gap (maintaining electrical neutrality of the blood) include albumin and, to a lesser extent, organic acids such as phosphates and sulfates. Since albumin makes up most of the normal anion gap, a patient with a low albumin will have a smaller anion gap. Although many hospitalized patients are hypoalbuminemic, most have an albumin close enough to normal not to decrease the anion gap significantly. But if you want to be precise, or in cases where a patient's albumin is less than~3.0 g/dL, you should correct the measured anion gap for albumin:

$$\text{Albumin-corrected anion gap} = \text{anion gap} + [2.5 \times (4 - \text{albumin})]$$

Osmolar Gap: Diagnosing Toxic Ingestions in High Anion Gap Metabolic Acidosis

Some of the toxins that can cause a HAGMA—such as methanol and ethylene glycol—are "osmotically active." This means that they cannot cross a semi-permeable membrane and, as a result, they "drag" water with them wherever they go. We can exploit the fact that they are osmotically active to track them down.

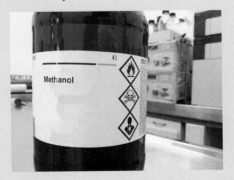 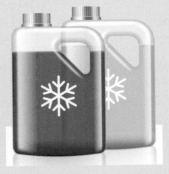

Figure 9.13 Two sources of a high anion gap metabolic acidosis with an elevated osmolar gap include methanol and antifreeze. (Courtesy DavidBautista/ Shutterstock; La Gorda/Shutterstock.)

The normal range of *serum osmolality* is 275 to 295 mOsm/kg H_2O. Normally, the main contributors to serum osmolality are sodium (Na^+), glucose, and BUN; ethanol (alcohol) also contributes to osmolality if it is present. We can calculate what the osmolality "should be" based on the known major contributors:

Calculated osmolality (mOsm/kg H_2O) = $2 \times Na^+$ + glucose/18 + BUN/2.8 + ethanol/3.7

If there aren't any rogue (unmeasured) osmotically active substances floating around, then the measured osmolality should be about the same as the calculated osmolality. Calculating the difference is straightforward:

Osmolar gap (mOsm/kg H_2O) = measured osmolality − calculated osmolality

If the measured osmolality is more than ~10 mOsm/kg H_2O higher than the calculated osmolality, we say that the patient has a high *osmolar gap*. In the right clinical context (say, a HAGMA in a patient who drank antifreeze), this is a sign of poisoning with an osmotically active toxin.

Normal anion gap metabolic acidosis (NAGMA): This disorder is caused by the loss of base or by the accumulation of acid that does *not* produce unmeasured anions. NAGMA tends to manifest with hyperchloremia, and therefore is sometimes referred to as *hyperchloremic metabolic acidosis.*

Use *HARDASS* (please, it's just a mnemonic) to remember common causes of a NAGMA:

1. *H*yperalimentation: also called total parenteral nutrition, or IV nutrition. Multiple components of the infused solution (including some amino acids) likely play a role in the pathophysiology of the acidosis.

2. *A*ddison disease (primary adrenal insufficiency): hypoaldosteronism reduces renal H^+ excretion.

3. *R*enal tubular acidosis (RTA): see the box "Renal Tubular Acidosis."

4. *D*iarrhea: this can lead to GI losses of HCO_3^- (as opposed to vomiting, which primarily causes acid loss). This is by far *the most common cause of NAGMA* (unfortunately, the constraints of the mnemonic consign it to fourth place in the listing).

5. *A*cetazolamide: a diuretic used most commonly as a glaucoma medication. The mechanism of acidosis is inhibition of the enzyme carbonic anhydrase, which decreases HCO_3^- reabsorption in the kidneys.

6. *S*pironolactone: inhibits aldosterone with a resulting reduction in renal H^+ excretion, just as occurs with regular hypoaldosteronism.

7. *S*aline: patients receiving large amounts of IV normal saline (0.9% NaCl) can develop a NAGMA. The pathophysiology is complex, but at least in part involves hyperchloremia (induced by the high concentration of chloride in the solution) leading to movement of HCO_3^- into cells.

Renal Tubular Acidosis

There are four RTAs, and they are all pretty common. RTA can be inherited but also can have multiple secondary causes. What they all have in common is that they cause a hyperchloremic, non–anion gap metabolic acidosis. The problem lies in the renal tubules; the glomerular filtration rate is normal or near-normal. Type 1, or distal RTA, results from a defect in H+ secretion by the distal tubule. Type 2, or proximal RTA, results from a defect in HCO_3^- reabsorption by the proximal tubule. Type 3 is a little bit of types 2 and 1 combined. Type 4, which is very common in patients with diabetes mellitus, is also called hyperkalemic RTA and is caused by a deficiency of or resistance to aldosterone. Like type 1 RTA, the problem is the result of impaired H+ secretion.

Figure 9.14 This short section deals with how to determine if a patient has more than one metabolic acid-base disorder (eg, both a high anion gap and normal anion gap metabolic acidosis). Consider it "advanced"—depending on your level of training and on your clinical role, you may want to skip this section for now and focus on the basics. (Courtesy GAS-photo/Shutterstock.)

At first glance it appears that Akio does not have a NAGMA. After all, his anion gap is high. But it turns out that it is possible to have both a HAGMA *and* a NAGMA at the same time (eg, from ketoacidosis and diarrhea). It's even possible to have a HAGMA and a metabolic alkalosis at the same time (eg, from lactic acidosis and vomiting). How could we tell in either case?

A bit of arithmetic—commonly called the *add-back method*—will give you the answer.

1. Calculate the anion gap. You know how to do this already.

2. Calculate how much higher the anion gap is than normal:

$$\text{Delta Gap} = \text{anion gap} - 12$$

3. Add that "Delta Gap" back to the patient's HCO_3^-. Imagine that you are giving back all of the HCO_3^- that was used up (buffering excess H+) during the process causing the

HAGMA. This will give you what the patient's HCO_3^- *would be* without the HAGMA process.

$$\text{``}HCO_3^- \text{ without HAGMA''} = \text{Delta Gap} + \text{measured } HCO_3^-$$

4. If the "HCO_3^- without HAGMA" is low (<22 mEq/L), the patient also has a normal anion gap metabolic acidosis (NAGMA). If it is high (>26 mEq/L), the patient also has a metabolic alkalosis. If it is normal (22-26 mEq/L), the patient has a pure HAGMA.

Let's practice with Akio:

1. Data we have from Akio's labs: Anion gap = 19 mEq/L, HCO_3^- = 14 mEq/L
2. Delta Gap = 19 − 12 = 7 mEq/L
3. HCO_3^- without HAGMA = 7 + 14 = 21 mEq/L

Because the HCO_3^- without the HAGMA is low (21 mEq/L) Akio must also have a NAGMA. We can determine the most likely cause clinically: his recent profuse diarrhea.

- -

We compensate for metabolic acidosis (regardless of anion gap) by hyperventilating. We get rid of acid by blowing off CO_2, bringing the pH up (closer to normal). As you already know, respiratory compensation happens very quickly. In the absence of a coexisting respiratory problem, we expect that in metabolic acidosis the Pco_2 will decrease by 1.2 mm Hg for every 1 mEq/L of HCO_3^- below normal. The shortcut formula for expected $Paco_2$ in a patient with metabolic acidosis is called *Winter formula*:

$$\text{Expected } Paco_2 = 1.5 \times HCO_3^- + 8 \ (\pm 2)$$

The "±2" indicates that a measured $Paco_2$ that is within 2 mm Hg of what you calculate (the "expected $Paco_2$") is normal, that is, indicative of appropriate respiratory compensation. A measured $Paco_2$ that is higher than expected means that the patient isn't blowing off enough CO_2 to appropriately compensate for the metabolic acidosis; in other words, there is also a respiratory acidosis. If the measured $Paco_2$ is lower than expected, the patient is blowing off too much CO_2 and the patient also has a respiratory alkalosis.

How is Akio doing with respiratory compensation?

$$\text{Expected } Paco_2 = 1.5 \times 14 + 8 = 29 \pm 2 \text{ mEq/L}$$

$$\text{Measured } Paco_2 = 26 \text{ mEq/L}$$

His measured $Paco_2$ is lower than his expected $Paco_2$ by 3 mEq/L. He is blowing off too much CO_2 and has a coexisting respiratory alkalosis! Perhaps poor Akio is in pain again, or he may be anxious about everything that has happened during his hospital stay.

Akio responds to fluids and treatment of his *C. difficile* infection. It's been a long and difficult journey, but he finally returns home where he makes a full recovery. Things certainly could have gone more smoothly, but your knowledge of blood gas and acid-base physiology saw him to a happy ending.

Here's a summary of the steps for analyzing any metabolic acidosis:

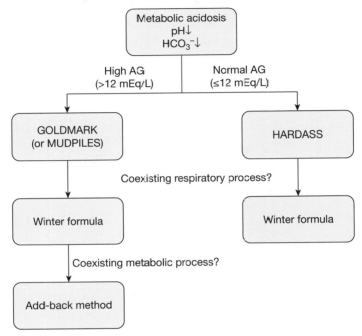

Figure 9.15 Following these few steps will allow you to diagnose any metabolic acidosis and determine if there are any coexisting respiratory or metabolic disorders. AG, anion gap.

Numbers on a Blood Gas You Can (and Should) Generally Ignore

1. Electrolytes: for the most part, we don't recommend using the electrolytes reported on a blood gas (Na^+, K^+, Cl^-, Ca^{2+}) to guide clinical management. Use the BMP or CMP instead, as these provide more accurate measurements that are less prone to error. However, if the situation is emergent and an ABG or VBG is all that is available, these numbers are better than nothing (eg, a patient with an arrhythmia and severe hyperkalemia on an ABG should get treated for presumptive hyperkalemia; do not wait for the BMP).

2. Pvo_2: the partial pressure of venous oxygen has no known clinical utility.

3. Hgb: hemoglobin is notoriously inaccurate on a blood gas. Use the hemoglobin on the complete blood count (CBC) instead.

4. Base excess: the blood gas analyzer uses pH and Pco_2 to calculate a theoretical amount of acid needed to bring 1 L of blood to a normal pH. The idea is presumably to give the clinician a quick idea of whether there is a metabolic derangement going on: metabolic alkalosis (positive base excess) or metabolic acidosis (negative base excess). The assumptions and calculations built into this result are more confusing than helpful. Ignore base excess. Instead, use the principles you've learned in this chapter to determine which acid-base derangements are present (if any).

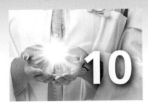

Cerebrospinal Fluid (CSF)

10

The cerebrospinal fluid (CSF) sits between the two inner layers of the meninges (the arachnoid and the pia) in the subarachnoid space, where it serves to cushion and nourish the central nervous system (CNS; the brain and spinal cord).

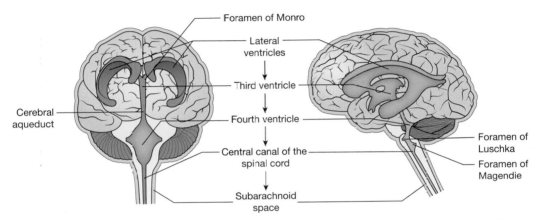

Figure 10.1 The CSF flows from the ventricular system into the central canal of the spinal cord and then into the subarachnoid space surrounding the cord and brain. CSF, cerebrospinal fluid.

The subarachnoid space is its own compartment in the body. It is separated from the blood by the aptly named blood-CSF* barrier, a term that has always seemed to us to carry an almost mythic significance, like the neutral zone in Star Trek. But really it just refers to the special properties of the vasculature of the CNS that allow it to regulate the movement of various substances between the CSF and the blood. Without the blood-CSF barrier, any infection or inflammatory response in the bloodstream could spill over into the CSF, wreaking havoc on the CNS.

But if the CNS is sequestered from the rest of the body—including the blood—how can we run any laboratory tests on it? What if we need to check for CNS disease, such as infection or malignancy? The answer, of course, is to sample the CSF directly.

---

*You will more often hear the term blood-brain barrier, but since the entire CNS is involved and not just the brain, the more accurate term is blood-CSF barrier.

Lumbar Puncture

We sample the CSF by doing a lumbar puncture (LP) and withdrawing a small amount of CSF.

What Are the Indications for Lumbar Puncture/Cerebrospinal Fluid Analysis?

An LP is appropriate when you are concerned about (or are uncertain about) underlying CNS disease, including:

- Infection (meningitis, encephalitis)—by far the most common reason for doing an LP
- Malignancy (cancer of the brain, meninges, or spinal cord)
- Autoimmune disease (eg, multiple sclerosis, neurosarcoidosis)
- Subarachnoid hemorrhage
- Idiopathic intracranial hypertension (pseudotumor cerebri)
- Normal pressure hydrocephalus (NPH)

Sometimes the diagnosis can be established without doing an LP. For example, a patient who arrives at the hospital with a sudden-onset, severe ("thunderclap") headache might get an emergency computed tomography (CT) of the head demonstrating a subarachnoid hemorrhage. That patient does not need an LP because the diagnosis has already been established.

The LP is an invasive test. It should only be performed if the results will change management.

How Is a Lumbar Puncture Done?

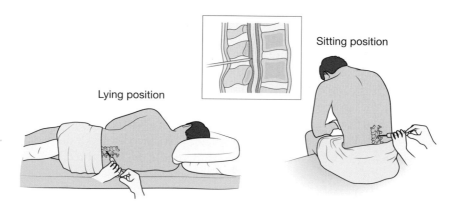

Sitting position

Lying position

Lumbar puncture

Figure 10.2 Here is where the needle goes when you do a lumbar puncture. Patients can be lying on their side or sitting up.

The goal is to sample the CSF while minimizing pain and other complications, such as post-LP headache, bleeding, or infection. It is imperative to avoid hitting the spinal cord with the needle. The cord extends down to vertebrae L1-L2 where it terminates in the conus medullaris. Therefore, a needle is inserted into the subarachnoid space at a spinal level *below* L1-L2, avoiding the cord, usually between either L3-L4 or L4-L5. Many clinicians use the highest point of the posterior iliac crest as a landmark to indicate the level of the L4 vertebra. In order to open up the space between the vertebral spinous processes, the patient is asked to flex the back and neck as shown in the picture. The procedure is done using sterile technique and can be completed in just a few minutes by an experienced clinician.

A typical CSF collection kit contains everything you need to obtain CSF under local anesthesia using sterile precautions. Several tubes are needed to run—potentially—a whole host of tests. You don't want to forget anything: this is not a test your patient will enjoy repeating just because you forgot to order something important.

When Is a Lumbar Puncture Contraindicated?

There are no "absolute contraindications," that is, conditions under which an LP can *never* be performed. This is because there are some circumstances under which an LP is emergent and potentially lifesaving (eg, suspected bacterial meningitis, which can be rapidly fatal if undiagnosed and untreated) regardless of the risk of complications. That said, it's generally wise to avoid an LP in the following scenarios:

1. *A space-occupying intracranial lesion*

   This is the most important contraindication to an LP; it is also the closest to an absolute contraindication. A patient with a brain tumor or abscess is at very high risk of brain herniation with an LP. The space-occupying lesion produces a very high intracranial pressure (ICP), which can literally push the brain downward if even a small amount of CSF is removed from the spinal canal below. Brain herniation is often fatal. The risk of herniation increases dramatically if a mass effect or midline shift of the brain is seen on a CT scan of the head. If you have even moderate suspicion that your patient has a space-occupying intracranial lesion (eg, based on symptoms such as new seizures or signs such as papilledema), check a CT or magnetic resonance imaging (MRI) of the brain before considering an LP. Significantly increased ICP may also be caused by obstructive hydrocephalus or cerebral edema, both of which are relative contraindications to LP.

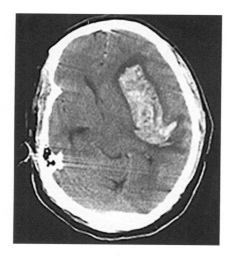

Figure 10.3 An MRI of the brain showing a large intracerebral bleed causing a mass effect that is disrupting the cerebral anatomy and practically effacing the ventricles. A lumbar puncture could lead to brain herniation in this patient. MRI, magnetic resonance imaging. (Reprinted with permission from Lois ED, Mayer SA, Boble JM. *Meritt's Neurology.* 14th ed. Wolters Kluwer; 2021.)

2. *Spinal epidural abscess (at or near the site of an LP)*

   Sticking a needle through a spinal epidural abscess runs the risk of spreading the infection into the subarachnoid space. It is also wise to avoid doing an LP at a site that appears superficially infected (eg, overlying cellulitis).

3. *Coagulopathy or anticoagulation*

   The risk of bleeding complications from an LP is low. However, if serious bleeding does occur, the spinal cord can be compromised and the clinical consequences dire. For these reasons, many clinicians avoid an LP in patients who are significantly thrombocytopenic (platelets <~50,000/μL) or have markedly abnormal coagulation studies (we go over these in Chapter 20). Guidelines and institution-specific policies vary, but certain antiplatelet agents (eg, clopidogrel) and anticoagulants need to be held for hours to days prior to performing the LP depending on the medication's pharmacokinetics. Aspirin is usually OK to continue through the procedure. If the LP is urgent or emergent and there's no time to hold the blood thinner(s), reversal agents (such as prothrombin complex concentrate for warfarin) can be used.

4. *Congenital abnormalities of the spine or brainstem*

   An LP is not feasible with certain abnormalities of the spine. In the case of a congenital Arnold-Chiari malformation, the cerebellum sits abnormally low, so an LP is usually avoided in order not to cause any further downward herniation. Common, acquired anatomic abnormalities such as lumbar spinal osteophytes (ie, due to osteoarthritis) may make an LP more challenging to perform but do not represent true contraindications; many such patients can undergo successful LP with the help of image guidance (eg, fluoroscopy).

Testing and Interpreting the Cerebrospinal Fluid

Now that you've obtained a sample of CSF, what do you do with it? There are many tests that you can and often will want to run in specific situations—for example, rapid antigen assays, polymerase chain reaction (PCR), antibody tests, VDRL (if you're concerned about neurosyphilis), and immunofixation—but we will reserve talking about these until later. For now, we are going to focus on the bread-and-butter CSF studies that will be run on almost all patients who require an LP:

- Appearance and opening pressure

- Cell count and differential

- Glucose, protein, and lactate

- Gram stain and bacterial cultures

- Cytology (not universally ordered, but important enough to include here)

Gross Appearance and Color

Even prior to running any tests, the gross appearance of the CSF can give you some helpful information. Normal CSF is clear and colorless. Many pathologic processes affecting the CSF—both infectious and noninfectious—can cause it to appear cloudy, thick, or opaque. A CSF that is anything but clear and colorless should prompt suspicion for underlying CNS pathology.

Xanthochromia refers to a yellowish appearance of the CSF and can be seen with an intracranial bleed, most notably a *subarachnoid hemorrhage*. The yellow tinge is the result of the breakdown of hemoglobin into bilirubin, which reliably occurs within 6 to 12 hours of the onset of bleeding and persists for weeks afterward. If it has been at least 12 hours since the onset of symptoms and you do *not* see xanthochromia in a patient's CSF (ie, the CSF is clear and colorless), you can be confident that the patient does not have a subarachnoid hemorrhage.

Xanthochromia is highly concerning for subarachnoid hemorrhage in the right clinical context (eg, in a patient with a sudden-onset, severe "thunderclap" headache). However, it can occasionally be seen in cases where the CSF protein is very high (see page 143) or in severe systemic hyperbilirubinemia (when the serum bilirubin is >~10 mg/dL). Sometimes, xanthochromia can be seen with a *traumatic tap* (when a capillary or venule is nicked during the LP—see the box "Differentiating Subarachnoid Hemorrhage from a Traumatic Tap").

Opening Pressure

Because the CSF flows within an enclosed space (the subarachnoid space), it exerts a pressure that we can measure by simply sticking a needle in that space. We call the measurement of the CSF pressure the "opening pressure." This will be the first actual measurement you will make on the CSF. The normal opening pressure is 70 to 200 mm H$_2$O.

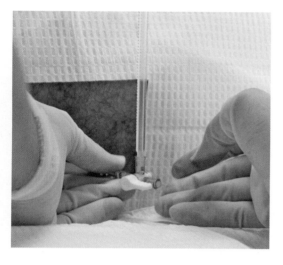

Figure 10.4 Measuring the opening pressure with a manometer during a lumbar puncture. It's important that the patient lies flat—changes in position may produce significant changes in opening pressure. Once the needle is secured in the subarachnoid space, attach a manometer to the stopcock and measure the height of the fluid column. This is your patient's opening pressure. (From Freer JM. *The Washington Manual of Bedside Procedures*. Wolters Kluwer; 2016.)

Intracranial Hypertension: We refer to *increased* opening pressure as *intracranial hypertension*. When severe, it can cause visual disturbances, severe headache, and tinnitus. However, these symptoms are not universally present, especially when the pressure elevation is mild.

Anything that increases CSF secretion, decreases reabsorption, or otherwise increases the volume of the contents of the subarachnoid space (eg, a mass, cerebral edema, or a severe inflammatory reaction) can cause intracranial hypertension. Once you understand this principle, it's easy to remember which disorders can lead to an increased opening pressure. Some of the most common and important disorders include:

1. *Most causes of hydrocephalus.* Exceptions include NPH (this one shouldn't be too hard to remember) and hydrocephalus ex vacuo (the appearance of hydrocephalus resulting from brain destruction or atrophy, usually seen in dementia or stroke).

2. *Idiopathic intracranial hypertension* (also called pseudotumor cerebri)

3. *An abscess or tumor of the brain or spinal cord* (including leptomeningeal metastasis)

4. *Cerebral edema*

5. *Bacterial, fungal, or tuberculous meningitis.* Intracranial hypertension is probably related to severe reactive inflammation. It is rare for a viral meningitis or encephalitis

to produce an elevated opening pressure; when this does occur, the elevation tends to be mild. Remembering that viruses are much smaller than bacteria and fungi can help remind you that viruses tend not to cause elevated opening pressure.

6. *Venous sinus thrombosis.* The mechanism here is blocked CSF outflow.

Intracranial Hypotension: The CSF pressure can also be *too low.* When it is below 4 mm Hg, we call it intracranial hypotension. It is an important cause of headaches that worsen when patients stand up and which resolve when they lie down. The most common cause is continued CSF leakage after an LP, but it can also occur from anything that damages the meninges, such as trauma (eg, a motor vehicle accident) or connective tissue disorders (eg, Ehlers-Danlos syndrome).

Cell Count and Differential

Think of this test as a complete blood count (CBC) that is run on the CSF. You'll notice many parallels between this section and our discussion of the CBC (see Chapter 4), which is no coincidence—the same principles apply. Like the CBC, the CSF cell count and differential measures red blood cells (RBCs) and white blood cells (WBCs).

Unlike the blood, normal CSF does not contain a significant number of RBCs or WBCs (it is "acellular"): more than 5 RBCs/µL or 5 WBCs/µL is considered abnormal. In young children and neonates, up to approximately 20 RBCs/µL or WBCs/µL may be normal. *The cell count and differential is simple, inexpensive, and often the CSF test with the highest diagnostic yield. It should almost always be sent after a diagnostic LP.*

Red Blood Cells: There are three main causes of elevated RBCs in the CSF:

1. *Traumatic tap.* In some patients, performing an LP can be difficult, and even with relatively straightforward ones it is easy to nick a small blood vessel on your approach to the CSF. The spectrum of bleeding from a traumatic tap is extremely wide, ranging from just a few RBCs to hundreds of thousands.

2. *Subarachnoid hemorrhage.* Remember to look for accompanying xanthochromia.

3. *Viral or necrotizing encephalitis,* especially herpes simplex virus-1 (HSV-1) encephalitis.

Differentiating Subarachnoid Hemorrhage From a Traumatic Tap

About 10% to 20% of all LPs are traumatic taps. How can you tell if xanthochromia is the result of a traumatic tap or a subarachnoid hemorrhage? Both a subarachnoid hemorrhage and a traumatic tap result in RBCs in the CSF. However, the RBCs typically do not begin to break down into hemoglobin (pink) and bilirubin (yellow) until they have been in the CSF for at least 2 hours. So, theoretically, a traumatic tap should produce bright or even dark red blood, whereas a subarachnoid hemorrhage that is at least 2 hours old should produce xanthochromia. Unfortunately, you'd be surprised how difficult it can be in practice to confidently distinguish various shades of muddy brown, yellow, pink, and pale red on visual inspection.

So how else can we differentiate a subarachnoid hemorrhage from a traumatic tap? One commonly employed method is checking for *blood clearing*. Typically, multiple tubes of CSF (usually four) are drawn during an LP. If the RBC count decreases by more than 65% from tube 1 to tube 4, a traumatic tap is much more likely than a subarachnoid hemorrhage.

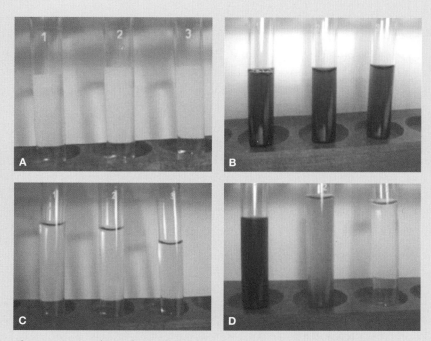

Figure 10.5 A. Three clear tubes drawn in a patient with normal CSF. B. Three bright red tubes in a patient with either a traumatic tap or SAH less than ~2 hours old. C. Three yellow tubes in a patient with SAH more than ~2 hours old. D. The CSF gradually becomes clearer following a traumatic tap. CSF, cerebrospinal fluid; SAH, subarachnoid hemorrhage. (From Mundt LA, Shanahan K. *Graff's Textbook of Urinalysis and Body Fluids*. 3rd ed. Wolters Kluwer; 2016.)

White Blood Cells: The finding of elevated WBCs in the CSF (>5 WBCs/μL) is called a *pleocytosis* and can be seen in both infectious and noninfectious processes affecting the CNS.

When the CSF WBC count is elevated, *how* elevated is the most important question:

- In *viral CNS infections* (meningitis or encephalitis), the CSF WBC count is usually elevated but less than 250 cells/μL.

- In *bacterial CNS infections*, the CSF WBC count is often more than 1,000 cells/μL.

- In *noninfectious CNS disease* such as thrombosis, bleeding (subarachnoid hemorrhage or traumatic tap), malignancy, or autoimmune disease, the CSF WBC count can be normal or only mildly elevated (usually <100 cells/μL).

- Although the mechanism is unclear, *infections outside the CNS* may occasionally cause a mildly elevated CSF WBC count, usually less than 100 cells/μL.

The higher the CSF WBC count above 100 cells/μL, the greater the likelihood that the patient has a CNS infection.

The normal CSF WBC differential is not well defined because the presence of a significant number of WBCs in and of itself is abnormal. In general, of the very few "normal" WBCs present in CSF, we expect most will be lymphocytes and monocytes. It's only when the total CSF WBC is high that we need to look carefully at the differential, in which case the predominant cell subtype can help clue us in to the underlying diagnosis.

Neutrophils: A predominance (>50%) of neutrophils points toward an acute bacterial infection of the CNS (bacterial meningitis or encephalitis), especially in the setting of a markedly elevated total CSF WBC count (>1,000 cells/μL). Neutrophilic predominance is also seen in the first 24 hours of some viral CNS infections.

Lymphocytes: When you see more than 50% lymphocytes in the CSF, think viruses, fungi, and tuberculosis. Lymphocytic predominance may also be seen in CNS malignancies, including leptomeningeal metastasis. Rarely, we see lymphocytic predominance early in the course of bacterial meningitis.

Eosinophils: Eosinophilic predominance (>50%) is very rarely seen. When there are a significant number of eosinophils in the CSF (>~10%), the most common causes are parasitic infections of the CNS, such as cysticercosis or schistosomiasis. Other diseases to consider include tuberculosis, rocky mountain spotted fever, some fungal infections (eg, coccidioidomycosis), lymphoma, and obstructive hydrocephalus.

Monocytes: Generally not helpful.

How to Interpret the Cerebrospinal Fluid White Blood Cell Count on a Traumatic Tap

Any bleeding into the CSF—from either a subarachnoid hemorrhage or a traumatic tap—may cause an elevation in the CSF WBC count; after all, the blood that leaks into the CSF contains WBCs as well as RBCs. In the case of a subarachnoid hemorrhage, the elevated WBC count is usually not the primary concern, for obvious reasons. But how can you interpret an elevated CSF WBC count in a patient who undergoes a traumatic tap?

Suppose Camilla, a 20-year-old college student, comes to the emergency department with 1 day of headache, fever, neck stiffness, and confusion. She gets an LP to rule out meningitis. Here are her cell counts (from the first tube drawn):

WBC: 22 cells/μL

RBC: 18,000 cells/μL

The first tube appears grossly bloody, but the blood completely clears by the fourth tube—this was a traumatic tap. But her CSF WBC count appears to be abnormally elevated, albeit not markedly so. How many of these WBCs are due to the bleeding from the traumatic tap versus a possible CNS infection? *In a patient with a normal serum WBC count, you can estimate that a traumatic tap will increase the CSF WBC count by 1 WBC/ μL for every 1,000 RBCs/μL that leak into the CSF.* So, in Camilla's case, we can subtract 18 (18,000/1,000 = 18) from the CSF WBC count to obtain a "corrected" value of 4 WBC/μL (22 – 18 = 4). Her corrected CSF WBC count is acceptably within normal.

If the patient's serum WBC count is abnormally elevated (>11,000 WBC/μL), it stands to reason that more WBCs will leak into the CSF in the same volume of blood. The opposite is true in cases of leukopenia (<4,000 WBC/μL). Therefore we recommend *not* using the above simplified correction method when your patient has an abnormal serum WBC count. Instead, plug the CSF and serum cell counts into an online calculator that adjusts for the serum WBC count.

Glucose

Glucose is normally transported from the blood into the CSF and serves as the main fuel for the CNS. So, unlike RBCs and WBCs, we expect to find glucose in the CSF. How much?

For a patient with a normal blood glucose, the normal range for the CSF glucose is 40 to 80 mg/dL. However, the CSF glucose rises and falls with the blood glucose. For this reason, it's important to compare the glucose in the CSF to the glucose in the serum; a CSF to serum glucose ratio of 0.5 to 0.8 is generally considered normal. Consider both the measured value and the CSF/blood glucose ratio when interpreting this test.

An abnormally low CSF glucose (<40 mg/dL or CSF/blood glucose ratio <0.5) is a classic sign of bacterial meningitis. Imagine the bacteria eating the glucose to help you remember this (the degree to which this actually happens is unclear). However, a low CSF glucose by itself is not diagnostic of a bacterial infection; both fungal and tubercular CNS disease may also produce a low CSF glucose. The lower the CSF glucose, the higher the specificity for bacterial meningitis. Patients with viral meningitis typically present with a normal CSF glucose.

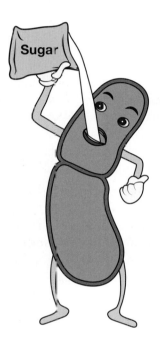

Figure 10.6 Imagining bacteria (such as this gram-negative rod) eating the sugar in the CSF may help you remember the association of bacterial meningitis with a low CSF glucose. CSF, cerebrospinal fluid.

The only noninfectious causes of a low CSF glucose are those that produce inflammation sufficiently severe to prevent the transport of glucose from the blood to the CSF. Examples include severe subarachnoid hemorrhage, CNS malignancies, and neurosarcoidosis.

Hyperglycemia is the only cause of an abnormally high CSF glucose (>80 mg/dL). The blood/CSF glucose ratio tends to remain normal in such patients.

Protein

The blood-CSF barrier allows very little protein to cross into the CSF. Most of this protein is made up of albumin, the most abundant protein in the blood. The normal range for the CSF protein is 15 to 60 mg/dL; in neonates, up to 170 mg/dL may be normal.

An abnormally low CSF protein is uncommon and has a very limited differential diagnosis. Either there is a low protein level in the blood (most commonly hypoalbuminemia) or there is a CSF leak leading to rapid production of CSF (which does not innately contain protein and therefore dilutes out the protein).

An abnormally high CSF protein is a nonspecific finding that tells us "something is not right" in the CNS. It results from two main mechanisms:

- The disruption of the blood-CSF barrier (leading to protein leakage into the CSF)

- The production of proteins within the CSF by inflammatory cells or foreign antigens

Therefore, any CNS infection or disease resulting in significant inflammation may elevate the CSF protein. Common culprits include bacterial or fungal meningitis, CNS malignancy, subarachnoid hemorrhage, autoimmune diseases such as multiple sclerosis or Guillain-Barré syndrome, and even some medications (nonsteroidal anti-inflammatory drugs [NSAIDs] in particular can cause an aseptic meningitis with high CSF protein).

The CSF protein may be either normal or slightly elevated (<150 mg/dL) in viral meningitis. The notable exception to this is West Nile virus, which can mimic bacterial meningitis and cause a profoundly elevated (up to 900 mg/dL) CSF protein level.

How to Interpret the Cerebrospinal Fluid Protein on a Traumatic Tap

When blood leaks into the CSF, it takes both WBCs and protein with it. You already know how to interpret the CSF WBC count in this context; what about the CSF protein? In the setting of a traumatic tap (or subarachnoid hemorrhage, in which case a CSF protein analysis is clearly not your main concern), the *CSF protein increases by 1 mg/dL for every 1,000 RBCs/μL*. Suppose Camilla, our young patient with possible meningitis from the box on page 142, undergoes a traumatic tap with the following results:

CSF protein: 75 mg/dL

CSF RBCs: 18,000 cells/μL

Her CSF protein appears to be mildly elevated (>60 mg/dL). How much of this protein is due to the bleeding from the traumatic tap versus a possible CNS infection? Based on the numbers indicated, we can subtract 18 mg/dL (18,000/1,000 = 18) from the CSF protein to obtain a "corrected" value of 57 mg/dL (75 – 18 = 57). Her corrected CSF protein is normal. This makes bacterial meningitis less likely (remember that viral meningitis can produce a normal CSF protein).

Sometimes it can be helpful to look for specific proteins called *oligoclonal bands* in the CSF. "Oligo" means "a few," and the term *oligoclonal bands* refers to limited groups of antibodies that show up as bands on a gel strip during a testing process called immunofixation. These are classically associated with multiple sclerosis. We will discuss their clinical utility further in Chapter 21.

Central Nervous System Infections: Putting It Together

You've now learned all of the basic tests that we routinely send on the CSF. Along the way, you may have noticed our emphasis on differentiating among types of CNS infections. Our basic CSF studies provide quick results that, taken together, may point us toward a particular type of pathogen so that we can adjust our management appropriately (eg, start empiric antibiotics before cultures and other test results are back). Here's a helpful summary table:

Remember that these are patterns, not absolute rules. Rather than relying solely on any one single value, look at all of your CSF findings together when deciding on the likelihood of a particular type of CNS infection.

Table 10.1 CSF Patterns in CNS Infections

CNS Infection	Total WBC	Predominant Cell	Opening Pressure	Glucose	Protein
Normal	0-5/µL	N/A	70-200 mm H$_2$O	40-80 mg/dL	15-60 mg/dL
Bacterial	↑ or ↑↑	Neutrophils	↑	↓	↑ or ↑↑
Viral	↑	Lymphocytes	Normal	Normal	Normal or ↑
Fungal	↑	Lymphocytes	↑	↓	↑

CNS, central nervous system; CSF, cerebrospinal fluid; WBC, white blood cell.

Lactate

Although the cell counts, opening pressure, glucose, and protein are helpful in distinguishing bacterial from viral meningitis, there can be considerable overlap. For example, imagine a patient with headache, fever, and photophobia, whose labs show a mildly elevated CSF protein, low-normal CSF glucose, and a CSF WBC count of 150 with a slight neutrophilic predominance. These results could be consistent with either a viral or bacterial meningitis. You would like a tool to further inform this distinction—and you want the answer quickly.

CSF lactate has emerged as a way to differentiate bacterial from viral meningitis. Like the serum lactate (see Chapter 9), a CSF lactate level can be obtained very quickly.

A CSF lactate less than 35 mg/dL makes bacterial meningitis much less likely.

We recommend using this test to help rule out bacterial meningitis when you have low to moderate suspicion.

Gram Stain and Bacterial Cultures

The definitive—and most specific—method for determining whether a patient has bacterial meningitis or encephalitis is to perform a Gram stain and bacterial culture. Both of these tests should ideally be done prior to the administration of any antibiotics, which significantly decreases their sensitivity. However, you absolutely should *not* wait for the results to initiate antibiotic treatment if you have any suspicion for a bacterial infection of the CNS—just get the tests drawn first if at all possible.

The Gram stain gives us results within minutes to hours and tells us *if* bacteria are present. It is much more specific than it is sensitive: a positive test makes a bacterial infection very likely, but a negative test (the absence of any Gram-staining organisms) does not rule out a bacterial infection. The bacterial cultures take longer—it may take several days for some organisms to grow. However, unlike the Gram stain, bacterial cultures can identify the specific organism and give you information about antibiotic susceptibilities. If you have any suspicion at all for bacterial meningitis or encephalitis, obtaining a CSF Gram stain and bacterial cultures is mandatory.

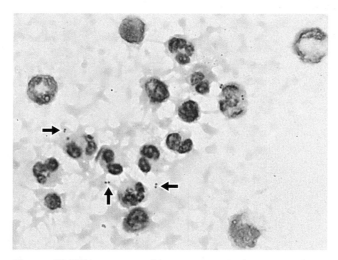

Figure 10.7 The arrows point to gram-negative coccobacilli—meningococci—in the CSF. CSF, cerebrospinal fluid. (Reprinted from Engleberg NC, DiRita VJ, Dermody TS. *Schaechter's Mechanisms of Microbial Disease*. 5th ed. Wolters Kluwer Health; 2013.)

There are many other stains besides Gram stain used to test for various CNS pathogens. Examples include the *acid-fast bacillus stain for tuberculosis* and the *India ink stain for cryptococcal meningitis*. Similarly, there are many cultures besides bacterial cultures that may be indicated in certain clinical scenarios, especially in immunosuppressed patients or in those with disease-specific risk factors. Here we have focused on the widely applicable Gram stain and bacterial cultures that are indicated in *everyone* with possible bacterial meningitis or encephalitis. We will review additional tests for specific pathogens in Chapter 14.

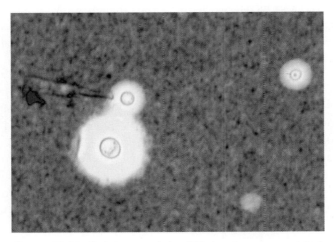

Figure 10.8 India ink prep of the CSF showing encapsulated cryptococcal yeast. CSF, cerebrospinal fluid. (Reprinted from Cornelissen CN, Hobbs MM. *Lippincott Illustrated Reviews: Microbiology*. 4th ed. Wolters Kluwer; 2020.)

Molecular Testing

If you are performing an LP, you will almost always order the basic panel that includes a cell count and differential, glucose, and protein, possibly with a lactate tossed in. If infection is on your differential diagnosis, and it usually is, you will add a Gram stain and culture. Not that many years ago, that was about all we had. Today, a host of CSF molecular tests are available to aid in the evaluation of meningitis and encephalitis. These are generally not ordered routinely, but can be especially useful when a Gram stain and culture are negative, when there is a history of prior antibiotic use, or when a viral pathogen is suspected.

One molecular test that has been around seemingly forever is the cryptococcal antigen. This test is highly sensitive and specific for cryptococcal meningitis. Results usually come back in an hour or so, much faster than culture.

For bacterial meningitis, while Gram stain and culture remain the gold standard, nucleic acid amplification tests (NAATs), such as PCR, are increasingly being employed. They can be ordered singly or more commonly as a panel targeting common pathogens such as *Streptococcus pneumoniae* and *Neisseria meningitidis*. False negatives are rare, but false positives can occur.

Molecular testing is now the standard of care when a viral CNS infection is suspected. These tests, too, can be ordered singly or as a panel. The single tests—for example, against HSV, Epstein-Barr virus, and/or varicella-zoster virus, as guided by pretest probability—are generally preferred over multiplex NAATs (see discussion in Chapter 14, page 201), which are less sensitive for herpes virus infection. NAAT is also available for West Nile virus, although a CSF viremia is only present early in the disease, so if you don't run the test early you may get a false negative; antibody testing of the serum and CSF is still the standard of care.

Cytology

Although several of the CSF tests we have discussed are useful in cases of suspected CNS malignancy—including WBCs and lymphocytes (high), glucose (low), and protein (high)— none are specific for either primary CNS malignancy or leptomeningeal metastasis. CSF cytology offers an array of tests that examine individual cells and cell markers that are specific indicators of CNS malignancies such as CNS lymphoma, meningioma, or CNS leukemia. These tests tend to require relatively large volumes of CSF (sometimes as much as 15 mL) and are expensive. CSF cytology is indicated only when you have suspicion for malignancy involving the CNS.

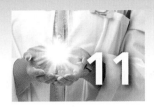

11 Pleural Fluid

We all have blood in our vessels and cerebrospinal fluid (CSF) in our subarachnoid space, but most of us do not walk around with a significant amount of fluid in or around our lungs.* A pleural effusion is an accumulation of fluid between the pleura, the two layers that line the lungs. Regardless of the underlying cause, the potential symptoms range from none to mild cough or chest discomfort to life-threatening respiratory failure.

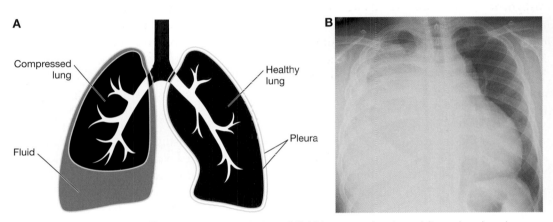

Figure 11.1 A. A pleural effusion is an accumulation of fluid between the visceral (inner layer) and parietal (outer layer) pleura. (Courtesy Pikovit/Shutterstock.) B. Chest x-ray of a patient with a huge right-sided pleural effusion. Only pleural effusions of at least 300 to 500 mL will reliably show up on chest x-ray. (From Lee EY. *Pediatric Radiology: Practical Imaging Evaluation of Infants and Children.* Wolters Kluwer; 2018.)

A pleural effusion presents a unique diagnostic opportunity for the clinician. Because pleural fluid sits outside the lung parenchyma, it can be easily accessed, thereby allowing us to make a more accurate diagnosis than would otherwise be possible.

The procedure for sampling a pleural effusion is called a *thoracentesis*. A thoracentesis can be therapeutic, diagnostic, or both.

- A *therapeutic* thoracentesis entails removing a large volume of fluid (sometimes more than 1 L) in order to alleviate associated symptoms.

- Our focus will be on the *diagnostic* thoracentesis, during which a small volume of pleural fluid is sampled to be analyzed.

---

*A tiny volume of pleural fluid—up to about 10 mL—is considered normal. This thin liquid film helps decrease the friction between the lungs and the chest wall.

Indications for a Thoracentesis

Any new pleural effusion should prompt consideration of performing a thoracentesis. The only situations in which a new pleural effusion should *not* be sampled are when:

1. The diagnosis is already obvious. An example would be a patient with clear clinical evidence of a heart failure exacerbation presenting with moderate symmetric bilateral pleural effusions.

2. The pleural effusion is very small. About 50 mL is required for a sufficient diagnostic yield. If the distance from the pleural fluid line to the chest wall on a recumbent chest x-ray is less than 1 cm, there probably isn't enough pleural fluid to sample. Additionally, in the case of a very small effusion, the risk of causing a *pneumothorax* with a thoracentesis increases significantly.

 ## *Contraindications to Thoracentesis*

Just as with a lumbar puncture, do not perform a thoracentesis through infected skin because of the risk of spreading the infection into the pleural space ("seeding"). Many clinicians will also avoid performing a thoracentesis on a patient with a severe coagulopathy, although the data to support this practice are a bit fuzzy. There are no hard-and-fast thresholds regarding such blood clotting parameters as the prothrombin time–international normalized ratio (PT-INR), activated partial thromboplastin time (aPTT), or platelet count (see Chapter 20), or when to correct a coagulopathy with blood products before thoracentesis. Weigh the urgency of the thoracentesis against the risk of bleeding (and please don't forget to include your patient in the conversation!).

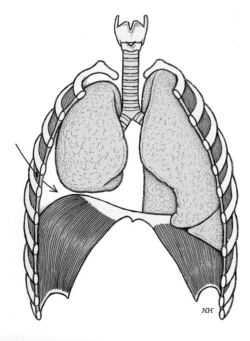

Figure 11.2 An illustration of a right-sided basal pneumothorax after a thoracentesis (site of the arrow). (Adapted from Neil O. Hardy, Westpoint, CT.)

How a Thoracentesis Is Done

Most clinicians now use ultrasound guidance to confirm the location of the pleural effusion and identify the optimal spot in the chest (one of the intercostal spaces) for needle insertion. Correct anatomic placement of the needle is extremely important. It should be placed over the superior aspect of the rib to avoid the neurovascular bundle that runs below the inferior portion of the rib. A catheter is threaded over the needle once it is in the pleural space, and at least 50 mL of fluid is then drained. An experienced operator can typically perform a diagnostic thoracentesis in about 15 minutes.

 ## *Types of Pleural Effusions*

We use pleural fluid studies to differentiate between two basic categories of pleural effusion: *transudative* and *exudative*. By making this distinction we can begin to narrow the differential diagnosis.

Transudative Effusions

Transudative effusions are caused by abnormal pressures across the pleura—the fluid is literally pushed (positive pressure) or sucked (negative pressure) into the pleural space. The underlying problem here is typically *not* with the lungs or pleura themselves. Think of processes that cause generalized fluid overload and edema when you think of transudative effusions: *heart failure, hepatic cirrhosis with large volume ascites,* and *renal failure* (particularly nephrotic syndrome and obstructive uropathy). *Atelectasis*, the collapse of alveoli (usually from taking shallow breaths in the setting of prolonged immobility or a rib fracture), may sometimes cause a transudative effusion due to increased intrapleural negative pressure.

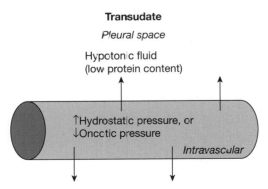

Figure 11.3 Transudates are caused by pressure imbalances.

Exudative Effusions

Structural problems with the pleura or lungs may cause leakage of fluid into the pleural space (with or without associated impaired lymphatic drainage, ie, trapped fluid). The result is an exudative effusion. Because anything that causes inflammation of the lungs or pleura can cause an exudative effusion, the differential diagnosis here is very broad. If you can remember the main causes of transudative effusions, simply remember the causes of exudative effusions as "everything else." Common examples include:

- Pulmonary infection (eg, bacterial or viral pneumonia, tuberculosis)

- Acute respiratory distress syndrome (ARDS; often in the setting of pancreatitis)

- Connective tissue disease (eg, lupus or rheumatoid pleuritis)

- Pulmonary embolism

- Malignancy involving the lungs or pleura

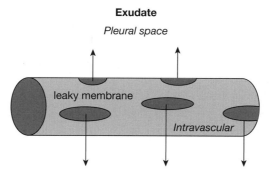

Figure 11.4 Exudates are caused by abnormal, "leaky" pleura.

Light's criteria give us a straightforward way to identify whether an effusion is transudative or exudative using just two pleural fluid studies: the *protein* and *lactate dehydrogenase (LDH)*. If one or more of Light's criteria are fulfilled, we consider the effusion *exudative*:

1. Ratio of pleural fluid protein to serum protein is greater than 0.5.
2. Ratio of pleural fluid LDH to serum LDH is greater than 0.6.
3. Pleural fluid LDH is greater than two-thirds the lab's upper limit of normal for serum LDH (the upper limit of normal varies by lab).

Light's criteria are more sensitive than they are specific— in other words, with these criteria you will not miss many exudates but you may occasionally mischaracterize a transudative effusion as exudative.

Characterization of a pleural effusion as transudative or exudative is fundamental to its interpretation and should almost always come before any other analysis.

An Alternative to Light's Criteria: The Three Test Rule

Instead of using Light's criteria, some pulmonologists are now using the "Three Test Rule," a set of criteria that require only pleural fluid analysis and spare the patient a blood draw. The effusion is considered exudative if one or more of the criteria are met:

1. Pleural fluid LDH is greater than two-thirds the laboratory's upper limit of normal for serum LDH

2. Pleural fluid protein is greater than 3.0 g/dL

3. Pleural fluid cholesterol is greater than 55 mg/dL

Sensitivity and specificity are very similar to those for Light's criteria.

 ## Testing the Pleural Fluid

Gross Appearance and Color

The gross appearance of pleural fluid can give us clues about what our subsequent tests may show and even about the underlying diagnosis.

Transudates are typically translucent and appear pale yellow ("straw colored"). Pleural fluid that is opaque or any other color is very likely an exudate. We've included a few high-yield fluid characteristics with associated diagnoses in Table 11.1. Remember that these are associations, not strict one-to-one relationships (ie, you should still send your basic fluid studies even if the appearance of the fluid points toward a particular diagnosis).

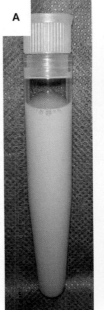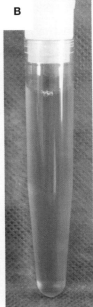

Figure 11.5 The opaque whitish-yellow pleural fluid on the left (A) could represent pus (empyema) or a lipid effusion. The translucent yellow fluid on the right (B) is most likely transudative. (Courtesy of Sabine Semrau, Department of Radiation Oncology, Universitätsklinikum Erlangen.)

Table 11.1 Pleural Fluid Characteristics and Associated Etiologies

Color or Characteristic	Association
Translucent yellow	Transudate • Heart failure • Cirrhosis with ascites • Renal disease (nephrotic syndrome, ipsilateral urinary obstruction) • Atelectasis
Red (fresh blood) or brown (old blood)	Malignancy Pulmonary infarction Trauma Asbestosis Postpericardiotomy syndrome
White or milky	Chylothorax (lymphatic fluid)[a] Cholesterol effusion[a] Empyema
Black	Fungal infection (eg, aspergillosis)
Dark green	Biliopleural fistula (biliothorax)
Color of tube feeds or catheter contents	Feeding tube or catheter has infiltrated pleural space
Viscous	Mesothelioma Empyema
Debris particles	Rheumatoid pleurisy
Food particles	Esophageal rupture
"Anchovy paste"	Ruptured amebic liver abscess
Foul odor	Anaerobic empyema
Ammonia odor	Urinothorax

[a]Both chylothorax and cholesterol effusions look milky due to their high lipid content. Chylothorax consists of lymph, which is very high in triglycerides, and is often due to a mechanical insult such as trauma, recent surgery, or lymphatic obstruction. A cholesterol effusion looks similar ("pseudochylothorax") but contains cholesterol crystals and usually forms as a result of chronic inflammation, most commonly in rheumatoid pleurisy and tuberculosis.

Recognizing a Traumatic Thoracentesis

Let's say your thoracentesis yields red fluid. How do you know if your patient has a bloody pleural effusion or if a vessel was nicked during the procedure (traumatic aspiration)?

Blood that has been sitting in the pleural space for more than a few hours does not clot well, whereas fresh blood from a traumatic aspiration clots within a few minutes. Changing color or appearance over seconds to minutes as the fluid drains implies self-limited bleeding at or near the entry site and is another sign of a traumatic aspiration.

If a postprocedure chest x-ray shows a larger effusion than before the procedure, by far the most likely explanation is a traumatic hemothorax.

Cell Count and Differential

Think of this as a complete blood count (CBC) that is run on the pleural fluid. The results include total red blood cells (RBCs) and total white blood cells with differential (neutrophils, lymphocytes, and eosinophils). You should almost always order this test if you are going to the trouble of performing a diagnostic thoracentesis. Although the results tend to be nonspecific—you are unlikely to make the final diagnosis based solely on the cell counts—they may be helpful in pointing you in the right direction.

Remember that any significant amount of pleural fluid (>~10 mL) is inherently abnormal, so there are no well-established normal ranges for cell counts. We do not categorize any cell count as "normal" or "abnormal." Instead, we consider the range in which it falls and correlate this with the most likely diagnoses. Here's what we mean:

White Blood Cell Count: A total white blood cell count of more than 50,000 cells/μL is highly suggestive of a *complicated parapneumonic effusion*. The term *parapneumonic* means accompanying a pneumonia. The term *complicated* here means that the pleural space has actually been invaded by microorganisms (most commonly bacteria) and is not just reacting to a nearby infection. When a complicated parapneumonic effusion presents as frank pus, we call it an *empyema*. The treatment of any complicated parapneumonic effusion includes both antibiotics and prompt drainage.

The effusion is more likely to be transudative—and very unlikely to be due to an inflammatory or infectious process—if the white blood cell count is less than 1,000 cells/μL.

"Intermediate" white blood cell counts between 1,000 and 50,000 cells/μL are seen in a broad range of inflammatory, infectious, and malignant diseases. Acute processes such as bacterial pneumonia (*without* bacteria having infiltrated the pleural space, ie, an *uncomplicated* parapneumonic effusion) tend to produce a white blood cell count more than 10,000 cells/μL. Chronic processes such as malignancy and tuberculosis tend to produce a white blood count less than 5,000 cells/μL.

Neutrophils: Remember that neutrophils are early "first responder" white blood cells. As such, neutrophilic predominance (>50%) indicates either acute or ongoing pleural injury (in contrast to old or resolving pleural injury). Common causes of neutrophilic predominance include pneumonia and recent pulmonary infarction (eg, due to trauma or pulmonary embolism). Although most malignant effusions demonstrate lymphocytic predominance, neutrophilic predominance is occasionally seen.

Lymphocytes: Lymphocytic predominance (>50%) is very common and has a wide differential diagnosis. Common causes include malignancy, tuberculosis, and autoimmune diseases such as sarcoidosis and chronic rheumatoid pleurisy.

Eosinophils: Eosinophilic predominance (>50%) is almost unheard of. Instead, we refer to "pleural fluid eosinophilia," which is defined as more than 10% eosinophils. We see pleural fluid eosinophilia in parasitic lung diseases, chronic eosinophilic pneumonia (this one shouldn't be too difficult to remember), pneumothorax, hemothorax, pleural drug reactions,* and asbestosis.

Red Blood Cell Count: It is common for almost any type of pleural effusion to contain up to several thousand RBCs—even some transudative effusions may contain more than 10,000 RBCs/μL. Because it takes only about 5,000 RBCs/μL to produce a red ("blood-tinged") discoloration, grossly bloody pleural fluid is not a very specific finding (don't forget to rule out traumatic aspiration, as discussed in the box "Recognizing a Traumatic Thoracentesis"). However, an RBC count of more than 100,000 RBCs/μL (expect this fluid to appear dark red) is far less common and is typically seen only in malignancy, trauma (with resulting hemothorax), and pulmonary infarction.

You can divide the pleural fluid RBC count by 100,000 to obtain an estimation of the pleural fluid hematocrit (eg, 2,000,000 RBCs/μL in the pleural fluid divided by 100,000 = 20% hematocrit). A hemothorax is diagnosed when the pleural fluid hematocrit is 50% or more. With patients who present with a hemothorax, you need to include aortic and myocardial rupture in your differential diagnosis.

Protein

A protein level should be part of any pleural fluid analysis. Not only does the protein help you determine whether the fluid is transudative or exudative (see Light's criteria on page 152), but the range in which the value falls may help further narrow the differential diagnosis:

- Most transudates have a protein level of less than 3.0 g/dL.

- The pleural fluid protein is almost always greater than 4.0 g/dL in tuberculosis.

- A pleural fluid protein of greater than 7.0 g/dL is concerning for a monoclonal gammopathy such as multiple myeloma or Waldenström macroglobulinemia.

When Light's Criteria Lie: Using the Protein and Albumin Gradients

Consider Frances, a 62-year-old woman, who is being treated in the hospital for a heart failure exacerbation with aggressive intravenous diuretic therapy. She has a moderate right-sided pleural effusion that has improved only slightly with diuresis. A diagnostic and

---

*The list of potential offenders is long, but some drugs used in psychiatry and neurology, for example, fluoxetine and valproic acid, are often implicated.

therapeutic thoracentesis is performed that, surprisingly, shows mild elevations in both the LDH (>0.6 × serum LDH) and protein (>0.5 × serum protein). She appears to have an exudative effusion based on Light's criteria, yet your clinical suspicion is high that her pleural effusion is due to heart failure (transudative).

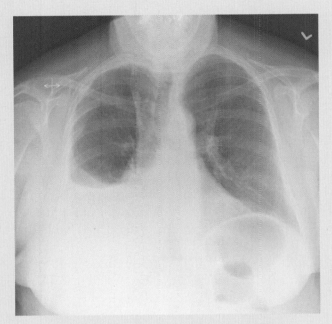

Figure 11.6 Could Frances' right-sided pleural effusion be due to heart failure or perhaps a superimposed pneumonia? (From Smith WL, Farrell TA. *Radiology 101: Basics and Fundamentals of Imaging*. 4th ed. Wolters Kluwer Health; 2014.)

Is it possible that Light's criteria could be misleading us here? Yes! It turns out that diuretics can cause an increase in several commonly measured pleural fluid components, including both the protein and LDH. The mechanism is presumably forced diffusion of water out of the pleural fluid, increasing the concentration of its various solutes. The result is a "pseudoexudate": a transudative effusion that appears to be exudative based on the protein and/or LDH.

How can we tell if we are dealing with a real exudate or a pseudoexudate? First of all, consider the degree of elevation in the protein and/or LDH: extremely high values (eg, a protein of 6 g/dL or an LDH of 1,000 IU/L) are almost certainly indicative of a true exudative effusion. Second, studies have shown that diuretic use has only a minimal effect on two additional parameters, both of which can be used to help identify pseudoexudates:

1. Serum to pleural fluid protein gradient = serum protein − pleural fluid protein

2. Serum to pleural fluid albumin gradient = serum albumin − pleural fluid albumin

In the setting of active diuresis, a serum to pleural fluid protein gradient of greater than 3.1 g/dL and/or a serum to pleural fluid albumin gradient of greater than 1.2 g/dL is suggestive of a transudate (pseudoexudate). We suggest that you calculate these values in addition to—not instead of—Light's criteria in patients undergoing diuresis when the pleural fluid protein and/or LDH is mildly elevated. As always, do not rely on just one value or calculation in isolation to make your diagnosis. Take all of your numbers together and, of course, consider the clinical context.

Lactate Dehydrogenase

LDH is an enzyme present in all tissues that plays an important role in anaerobic metabolism. When cells are damaged, LDH is released. The concentration of LDH, therefore, correlates with the degree of tissue damage. So when we measure pleural fluid LDH, we are in effect measuring the extent and severity of pleural injury (see Chapter 20 for further discussion of serum LDH).

As is the case with most pleural fluid studies, there is no clearly defined "normal" or "abnormal" pleural fluid LDH. As a point of reference, the upper limit of normal for *serum* LDH is about 200 IU/L in most labs, so we expect the pleural fluid LDH of a transudate to be less than about 130 IU/L ($\frac{2}{3} \times 200 = 134$).

Plug the pleural fluid LDH (along with the protein) into Light's criteria to determine whether the effusion is transudative or exudative. If you find that you are dealing with a transudate, the LDH must be low and can help you no further. On the other hand, the LDH can range widely in the case of an exudative effusion. In many illnesses (the data are most robust in pulmonary malignancy), increasing pleural fluid LDH over time corresponds to worsening or treatment-resistant disease. Trending the pleural fluid LDH over time can help inform prognosis and indicate the potential need for adjustment or escalation of treatment.

When you're dealing with just a single isolated measurement, here's how the LDH range can help you narrow your differential diagnosis:

- Pleural fluid LDH more than 1,000 IU/L is most commonly seen in empyema and rheumatoid pleurisy, and less often in malignancy and tuberculosis. Paragonimiasis, a rare parasitic infection of the lungs caused by eating raw crayfish (more common in Asia and Africa than in North America), can also cause a pleural fluid LDH more than 1,000 IU/L.

- *Pneumocystis jirovecii* pneumonia ("PJP"), a fungal lung infection common in immunocompromised patients, characteristically produces a pleural fluid LDH that is higher than the serum LDH (pleural fluid-serum ratio >1.0).

Many exudative effusions have both an elevated LDH and protein. If, however, you see a high pleural fluid LDH (>0.6 × serum LDH) accompanied by a relatively *low* pleural fluid protein (<0.5 × serum protein), consider a parapneumonic effusion (especially PJP), malignancy, or urinothorax (a rare condition in which there is retroperitoneal leakage of urine into the pleural space).

Glucose

In the absence of pleural damage, glucose freely diffuses from the blood through the pleura into the pleural space. As a result, we expect pleural fluid glucose to be the same or similar to the blood glucose in all transudates. Even many exudates contain a glucose level similar to that in the blood. We recommend you consider a "normal" pleural fluid glucose to be at least $0.5 \times$ serum glucose; in patients who are not hyperglycemic, this usually comes out to be approximately 60 mg/dL or more.

Pleural fluid glucose drops when (1) severe pleural damage blocks diffusion of glucose across the pleura, or (2) metabolically active infectious, neoplastic, or inflammatory cells in the pleural space "eat up" (ie, utilize) glucose. The worse the pleural damage, or the more numerous the unwelcome metabolically active cells or organisms, the lower the pleural fluid glucose.

- A "moderately low" pleural fluid glucose—usually in the range of 30 to 50 mg/dL (depending on the blood glucose)—suggests lupus pleuritis, tuberculosis, esophageal rupture, or malignancy. In the case of malignancy, the lower the glucose, the higher the tumor burden.

- Glucose can be even lower—around 0 to 30 mg/dL—in rheumatoid pleurisy and in a complicated parapneumonic effusion. A pleural fluid glucose of 0 to 10 mg/dL is almost always due to either empyema or rheumatoid pleurisy.

A pleural fluid glucose that is significantly *higher* than the blood glucose is rare and has a short differential diagnosis limited to two very specific clinical scenarios:

1. A catheter (eg, central line) has been misplaced in the pleural space and glucose-rich fluid (eg, tube feeds, dextrose solution) is being infused through it.

2. A patient on peritoneal dialysis has developed a pleural effusion due to upward migration of the glucose-rich peritoneal dialysate into the pleural space.

pH

The tiny amount of normal pleural fluid has a slightly higher concentration of bicarbonate than the blood, giving it a pH of about 7.60 (recall that the normal pH of arterial blood is ~7.40). An abnormally high pleural fluid pH (>~7.7) is extremely unusual and unlikely to be diagnostically helpful (it is occasionally seen in *Proteus* infections). On the other hand, an abnormally low pleural fluid pH is found in many diseases and is a sign of either pleural acid production from bacteria or damaged cells, or of trapped hydrogen ions from scarring, inflammation, or tumor. In general, the more the pleural fluid pH drops below 7.30, the higher the clinical concern for severe, acute, or life-threatening diseases.

Here's how various pH ranges correlate with diagnosis:

- Most transudative effusions have a pH of 7.40 to 7.55.

- Most exudative effusions have a pH of 7.30 to 7.45.

- A pH less than 7.30 ("pleural fluid acidosis") is most commonly caused by empyema, tuberculosis, malignancy (in which the low pleural fluid pH correlates with poorer prognosis), and connective tissue diseases (particularly rheumatoid pleurisy).

- A parapneumonic effusion with a pH less than 7.20 indicates a severe infection (possibly empyema) that needs to be drained.

- A pH less than 6.0 is highly concerning for esophageal rupture.

Think of the pleural fluid LDH, glucose, and pH all in one "bucket"; they all tend to correlate. Specifically, a low pH almost always corresponds to a low glucose and a high LDH. If you see a pleural fluid pH less than 7.30 with a normal glucose and normal/low LDH, consider repeat testing—one or more of the results may have been a lab error.

Additional Pleural Fluid Tests: Homing in on the Diagnosis

The pleural fluid tests we have discussed so far are indicated for almost all pleural effusions. They give us a sense of the category of disease we are dealing with (transudate or exudate, acute or chronic, severe or non-severe), and this is vital information. Do not skip these tests. However, except in cases of extreme results (eg, an undetectably low glucose or a pH <6.0), these tests tend not to be very specific. Once you have used your basic labs to lay the diagnostic foundation—establishing a reasonable differential diagnosis in the process— it's often time to get more granular.

The tests in Table 11.2 help to rule in or rule out specific diagnoses. Because they answer very specific questions (eg, "Is this a cholesterol effusion?"), they aren't always indicated.

Finally, don't forget to send a *Gram stain and bacterial culture* on pleural fluid when you are concerned about the possibility of a complicated parapneumonic effusion. These tests can definitively identify bacteria in the pleural space and can direct subsequent therapy. If feasible, send both of these tests prior to the administration of any empiric antibiotics in order to increase their sensitivity. Remember that the Gram stain gives results within minutes to hours and tells us *if* bacteria are present (and whether they are gram-negative or gram-positive), whereas bacterial cultures take up to several days and tell us *which* bacteria are present. Both tests are far more specific than they are sensitive: a negative Gram stain and/or bacterial culture does *not* rule out a complicated parapneumonic effusion.

You are now familiar with the vast majority of common tests ordered on pleural fluid. As is the case with CSF analysis, there are many other pleural fluid tests that apply only to very specific clinical scenarios. Examples include viral, fungal, and mycobacterial cultures; polymerase chain reaction (PCR) tests; and antigen and antibody tests. We will address many of these specific tests in Chapter 14.

Table 11.2 Tests of the Pleural Fluid Beyond the Ordinary

Pleural Fluid Study	Relevant Physiology/ Mechanism	When to Order	Interpretation
Cholesterol	Released from degenerating pleural cell membranes in chronic inflammation	Concern for cholesterol effusion (eg, milky effusion, possible RA or TB)	>250 mg/dL diagnoses a cholesterol effusion
Triglycerides (TG)	Mechanical trapping of TG-rich lymphatic fluid (chyle) in the pleural space	Concern for chylothorax (eg, milky effusion, trauma, known malignancy)	If >110 mg/dL, chylothorax is very likely. If <50 mg/dL, chylothorax is excluded.
Amylase	Produced by pancreas (pancreatic amylase) and salivary glands (salivary amylase)	Concern for pancreatic effusion or esophageal rupture	1. Pleural amylase > serum amylase suggests pancreatic or esophageal effusion[a] 2. Send pancreatic and salivary isoenzymes to differentiate
Creatinine	Cleared by the kidneys. Concentration is higher in the urine than in the serum	Transudative effusion concerning for urinothorax (eg, in urinary obstruction)	Pleural fluid creatinine > serum creatinine diagnoses urinothorax
Adenosine deaminase (ADA)	Enzyme involved in proliferation and differentiation of T lymphocytes (highly active in TB)	Differentiate TB from malignant effusion	If >40 U/L, TB is much more likely than malignancy
Cytology	Malignant cells often appear atypical	Concern for malignancy	1. Positive cytology establishes the diagnosis of malignancy 2. Negative cytology does *not* rule out malignancy (~60% sensitivity). Consider repeat thoracentesis if suspicion is high

[a]Whereas an elevated pleural pancreatic amylase is highly specific for a pancreatic effusion, an elevated pleural salivary amylase can be found in both esophageal rupture and in malignant effusions. Know your clinical context!
RA, rheumatoid arthritis; TB, tuberculosis

Pleural Fluid Tests That Are Unlikely to Be Helpful

1. *N-Terminal pro–Brain Natriuretic Peptide (NT-proBNP)*

   Elevated NT-proBNP in the blood is a helpful marker of heart failure (see Chapter 15). We suggest sending a *blood* NT-proBNP if you are concerned about a possible cardiac pleural effusion. Because blood NT-proBNP correlates very well with pleural fluid NT-proBNP, the added value of the pleural fluid NT-proBNP is minimal. Additionally, pleural fluid NT-proBNP can be falsely elevated in critically ill patients.

2. *Procalcitonin*

   Blood procalcitonin may have some utility in the evaluation and management of pneumonia (see Chapter 14), but current data are not convincing that pleural fluid procalcitonin adds any value in differentiating a parapneumonic effusion from other exudates. We do not suggest ordering a pleural fluid procalcitonin level.

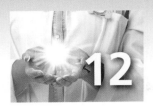

12 Peritoneal (Ascitic) Fluid

The peritoneum is the multilayered lining of the abdominal cavity that serves to protect and support the vital organs within it ("intraperitoneal" organs), including the spleen, liver, stomach, and most parts of the small and large intestines. The ovaries are also an intraperitoneal organ.

The outer *parietal* peritoneum forms part of the abdominal wall (think of this layer as a big burlap sack), and the inner *visceral* peritoneum lines each organ (think of this layer as a shrink wrap). The potential space between these two layers is the *peritoneal cavity*. Like the pleural space, the peritoneal cavity does not normally contain a significant amount of fluid.* Any peritoneal fluid that accumulates is called *ascites* and is, by definition, abnormal.

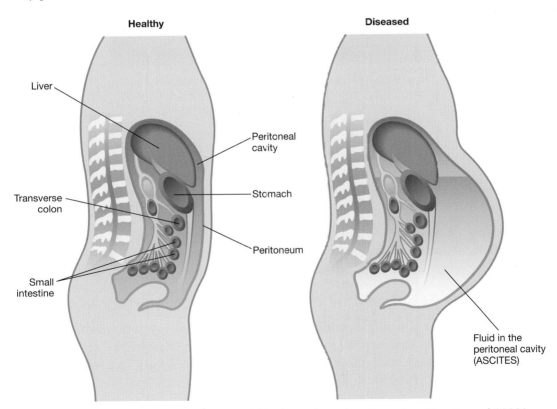

Figure 12.1 We call fluid that accumulates within the peritoneal cavity *ascites*. (Courtesy rob9000/ Shutterstock.)

---

*A small volume—about 50 to 75 mL—of peritoneal fluid serves as lubrication between the abdominal wall and the visceral organs.

Any disease that can cause generalized volume overload can cause ascites. Examples include hepatic cirrhosis (by far the most common cause of ascites), heart failure, and renal failure, the same diseases that can cause transudative pleural effusions. Ascites may also develop from disease of any organ inside or adjacent to the peritoneum (including the peritoneum itself). Examples include malignancy (most commonly ovarian cancer), infection (eg, tuberculous or fungal peritonitis), and pancreatitis.

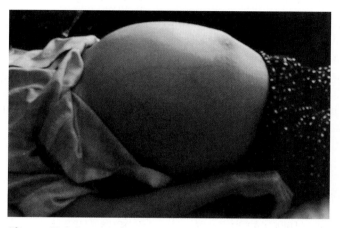

Figure 12.2 Large-volume "tense" ascites, as depicted here, can be extremely uncomfortable. (From Sun T. *Parasitic Disorders: Pathology, Diagnosis, and Management.* 2nd ed. Lippincott Williams & Wilkins; 1999; Figure 44.12)

- Ascites can become infected by bacteria at any time (fungal infection can occur but is much less common). *Spontaneous bacterial peritonitis (SBP)* occurs when preexisting ascites becomes infected without any obvious source; this is by far the most common form of bacterial peritonitis.

- We diagnose *secondary bacterial peritonitis* when there is a precipitating source of intra-abdominal infection or inflammation such as a bowel perforation or appendicitis. Surgical intervention is often necessary.

We can't know for sure whether ascitic fluid is infected without sampling it directly.

The procedure for sampling ascitic fluid is called a *paracentesis*. Like a thoracentesis, a paracentesis can be *therapeutic*, where a large volume of ascites is drained for symptom control; *diagnostic*, where ascites is drained for analysis; or both. We will focus on the diagnostic paracentesis and ascitic fluid testing.

Indications for Paracentesis

Perform a diagnostic paracentesis when you need to answer one or both of these questions:

1. What is the cause of the ascites?

2. Is the ascites infected (and, if so, why and with what organism)?

With this in mind, there are two major indications for a paracentesis:

1. *Any new-onset ascites*

Even when the cause appears obvious (eg, a patient with a recent diagnosis of cirrhosis with portal hypertension), a paracentesis should still be performed to definitively rule out other etiologies and, perhaps more importantly, ensure that the fluid is not infected.

2. *Significant clinical changes in a patient with preexisting ascites*

Examples include new fever, altered mental status, leukocytosis, and renal failure. Many clinicians consider hospital admission—regardless of the reason for admission—enough of a "clinical change" to necessitate a paracentesis in patients with ascites.

The bottom line is that the threshold for performing a diagnostic paracentesis is actually quite low. Even though this is an invasive procedure, it is a very powerful diagnostic tool, is typically quick and easy, and the risk of complications is low.

Contraindications to Paracentesis

There are no *absolute* contraindications to paracentesis. Even the *relative* contraindications—times when you should consider delaying paracentesis or correcting risk factors for complications—are few.

Paracentesis is generally safe in patients with an elevated prothrombin time (PT)/international normalized ratio (INR) or low platelet count (these are both very common in patients with cirrhosis due to liver dysfunction). The bleeding risk is very low, especially when the paracentesis is done under ultrasound guidance, and the minimal benefits of pretreating with blood products are far outweighed by the risks in most circumstances. Patients with either *disseminated intravascular coagulation (DIC)* or *primary hyperfibrinolysis* are the exceptions to this rule. In the former case, transfuse platelets with or without fresh frozen plasma before performing a paracentesis. In the latter case, aminocaproic acid or tranexamic acid should be given to reduce bleeding risk.

A paracentesis should not be done "blind," that is, without ultrasound guidance, in any patient with severe bowel distension (eg, due to ileus or mechanical bowel obstruction) because of the increased risk of bowel perforation. Ultrasound guidance lowers this risk substantially.

Finally, do not perform a paracentesis through infected tissue or surgical scars. In the former case, you risk seeding the peritoneal space with infection. In the latter case, the bowel may be tethered to the abdominal wall underneath and the risk of bowel perforation with paracentesis is increased.

 ## *How a Paracentesis Is Done*

With the patient in the supine position, a pocket of ascites is identified with a bedside ultrasound. The most common site—and generally considered the safest—is the left lateral lower quadrant, where the abdominal wall is thin, bowel loops are rarely in the way, and abdominal wall collateral vessels are usually absent. Either with or without continued ultrasound guidance, the peritoneum is punctured with a needle and a catheter threaded over it for fluid removal.

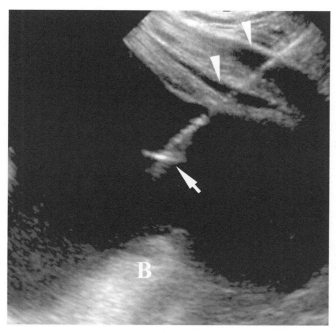

Figure 12.3 Paracentesis performed under ultrasound guidance. The needle (arrow) has passed through the skin and peritoneum (arrowheads) into the ascitic fluid (black). The bowel (B) is safely avoided. (From Penny SM. *Introduction to Sonography and Patient Care.* 2nd ed. Wolters Kluwer; 2021.)

The "Bread-and-Butter" Ascitic Fluid Studies

The following tests are indicated whenever a diagnostic paracentesis is performed, regardless of the suspected etiology. They provide invaluable information about the underlying cause of ascites and the likelihood of infection. Often they are all you need to make an accurate diagnosis.

- Gross appearance

- Albumin (with calculation of the serum-to-ascites albumin gradient, or SAAG)

- Cell count and differential

- Total protein

- Gram stain and bacterial cultures

Gross Appearance

This is free information. The appearance of the ascitic fluid will rarely if ever give you the diagnosis outright, but it can help inform your differential diagnosis before your labs come back. Although ascites due to cirrhosis is usually translucent yellow or clear, it can also be bloody or milky, so do not use the gross appearance to rule out cirrhosis as the cause of the ascites. You can use the following general associations to help guide your clinical thinking:

Table 12.1 Gross Appearance of Ascitic Fluid and Likely Causes

Color or Characteristic	Associated Diagnoses
Translucent yellow or colorless	Cirrhosis
Red or bloody	Traumatic paracentesis Bleeding from previous tap Malignancy (particularly HCC[a]) Cirrhosis
Cloudy or opaque	Infection (any cause)
Milky	Malignancy Lymphatic injury (eg, from surgery) Infection (tuberculosis, filariasis) Cirrhosis
Dark brown ($\uparrow\uparrow$ bilirubin)	Gallbladder rupture Perforated duodenal ulcer

[a]About half of ascites due to hepatocellular carcinoma (HCC) is bloody.

The Serum-to-Ascites Albumin Gradient: Is Portal Hypertension Present?

By far the most common cause of ascites is portal hypertension, defined as abnormally high pressures within the portal venous system running from the gastrointestinal (GI) tract and spleen to the liver. Thus, it makes sense to start your ascitic fluid analysis by asking the question, "Is this ascites due to portal hypertension?"

In the United States, cirrhosis is by far the most common cause of both portal hypertension and ascites. Other common causes of portal hypertension with resulting ascites include schistosomiasis (a parasitic infection that is much more common outside the United States, especially in the developing world), Budd-Chiari syndrome (obstruction of the hepatic vein by invasive cancer or thrombus), and chronic right-sided heart failure (systemic venous blood backs up from the right side of the heart → inferior vena cava → liver → portal system).

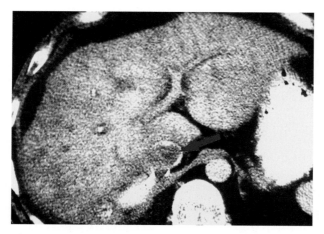

Figure 12.4 This patient with an invasive right adrenal carcinoma has a large associated occlusive inferior vena cava thrombus (red arrow) with resulting Budd-Chiari syndrome, a rare but devastating cause of liver failure and ascites. (From Brant WE, Helms CA. *Fundamentals of Diagnostic Radiology*. 4th ed. Lippincott Williams & Wilkins; 2012.)

Portal hypertension ultimately leads to ascites by causing increased circulatory hydrostatic pressures. The fluid that spills out into the peritoneum is thin and watery and has a very low albumin content compared to the blood. By quantitatively comparing the serum albumin and ascitic fluid albumin, we can identify whether portal hypertension is the underlying cause of the ascites:

$$SAAG = \text{serum albumin} - \text{ascites albumin}$$

1. *SAAG of 1.1 g/dL or more* is consistent with portal hypertension.

   a. Cirrhosis
   b. Right-sided heart failure
   c. Schistosomiasis
   d. Budd-Chiari syndrome

2. *SAAG less than 1.1 g/dL* is consistent with *something else* (eg, infection, malignancy).

If at all possible, the serum albumin should be checked on the same day as the paracentesis.

Think of portal hypertensive or "high SAAG" ascites as analogous to a transudative pleural effusion. Just as we use pleural fluid protein and lactate dehydrogenase (LDH) to identify pleural transudates versus exudates, we use ascitic fluid albumin to identify ascites that is "high SAAG" (portal hypertension) versus "low SAAG" (not portal hypertension).

Cell Count and Differential: Is the Ascites Infected?

The ascitic fluid cell count and differential includes the total white blood cell (WBC) count with differential (neutrophils, lymphocytes, and eosinophils) and the total red blood cell (RBC) count. It can tell you whether the ascites is infected well before bacterial cultures come back. In this way, the cell count and differential often dictate important management decisions—for example, whether to start potentially life-saving antibiotics. Do not forget to send this important test with every paracentesis.

White Blood Cell Count and Differential: Neutrophils, lymphocytes, and eosinophils are typically reported as percentages of the total WBC count rather than as absolute numbers. In order to calculate the absolute number of any of these cell types, multiply the percentage (as a decimal—eg, use 0.45 for 45%) by the total WBC count.

- An absolute neutrophil (polymorphonuclear [PMN]) count of 250 cells/μL or more is both sensitive and specific for bacterial peritonitis (either spontaneous or secondary) and is almost always an indication to start empiric antibiotics. *This is the highest yield test in this chapter.*

- A total WBC count of greater than 10,000 cells/μL—regardless of the differential—should prompt suspicion for possible secondary peritonitis (eg, bowel perforation, intra-abdominal abscess).

- A total WBC count of greater than 250 cells/μL with lymphocytic predominance (>50% lymphocytes) suggests peritonitis due to tuberculosis (TB) or malignancy.

Peritoneal Dialysis–Related Peritonitis

Peritoneal dialysis works by producing iatrogenic ascites: dialysate fluid is intermittently infused into and drained from the peritoneal cavity in order to filter out waste products. This form of dialysis has several advantages, not the least of which is that it can be done at home. On the other hand, peritonitis is common in these patients, due either to contamination of the dialysate or of the dialysis catheter itself. We call this form of peritonitis "peritoneal dialysis–related peritonitis"; it is its own category of peritonitis, separate from both spontaneous and secondary bacterial peritonitis. Patients may develop nonspecific symptoms such as abdominal discomfort, fever, and confusion, or they may be asymptomatic. Cloudy peritoneal fluid should raise your level of suspicion.

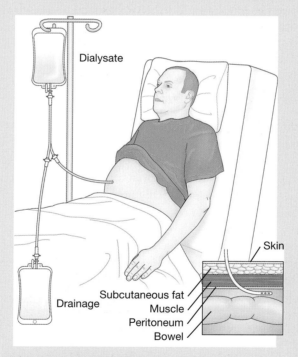

Figure 12.5 Peritoneal dialysis. On average, each patient undergoing peritoneal dialysis experiences one episode of peritonitis every 2 to 3 years. (From Hinkle JL, Cheever KH. *Brunner & Suddarth's Textbook of Medical-Surgical Nursing.* 14th ed. Wolters Kluwer; 2018.)

How do you interpret a peritoneal fluid cell count and differential in a patient on peritoneal dialysis in whom you are concerned for peritonitis? Normal peritoneal fluid in a patient on peritoneal dialysis contains no more than 8 WBCs/mm^3. *If the WBC count is more than 100 cells/mm^3, or is more than 8 cells/mm^3 with greater than 50% neutrophils, the patient likely has peritonitis and should be treated accordingly.* Do not forget to send a Gram stain and bacterial cultures.

Correcting the White Blood Cell Count and Neutrophil Count When the Ascites Is Bloody

Blood that spills into the peritoneal cavity—either due to a traumatic paracentesis or to internal bleeding—contains both RBCs and WBCs (including neutrophils). When interpreting the cell count and differential, you need to know how many WBCs, including neutrophils, are present because of bleeding rather than inflammation or infection of the ascites. *Subtract 1 neutrophil for every 250 RBCs; subtract 1 WBC for every 750 RBCs.* These "corrected" numbers tell you what the neutrophil and WBC counts would be in the absence of bleeding, and therefore are the best numbers on which to base your management decisions.

Here's an example of a cell count and differential from a bloody paracentesis sample:

RBC: 25,000 cells/mm^3

WBC: 500 cells/mm^3

Neutrophils: 60%

You now need to do three quick calculations:

1. Calculate the corrected WBC count: Subtracting 1 WBC for every 750 RBCs yields a corrected WBC count of 467 cells/mm^3 (500 − 25,000/750 = 467).

2. Calculate the uncorrected neutrophil count: Multiplying the total uncorrected WBC count by 60% yields an uncorrected neutrophil count of 300 cells/mm^3 (500 × 0.6 = 300). The neutrophil count is more than 250 cells/mm^3—should we start antibiotics? Not so fast.

3. Calculate the corrected neutrophil count: Subtracting 1 neutrophil for every 250 RBCs yields a corrected neutrophil count of 200 cells/mm^3 (300 − 25,000/250 = 200).

Note that this method can result in a corrected neutrophil count that is negative. This phenomenon is related to the rapid lysis of neutrophils that are present in bloody ascites. Treat a negative neutrophil count as 0.

Red Blood Cell Count: We refer to any ascitic fluid with 10,000 RBCs/μL or more as *hemorrhagic ascites.* This is the number of RBCs required to cause ascites to appear grossly pink or "blood tinged." Hemorrhagic ascites is found most commonly with malignancy (particularly hepatocellular carcinoma), traumatic aspirations (the blood should clear as you aspirate more fluid), and cirrhosis. Except in cases of traumatic aspirations, hemorrhagic ascites is associated with high rates of bacterial peritonitis and an overall poor prognosis.

Total Protein Concentration

In the past, the ascitic fluid total protein was used to characterize ascites as transudative versus exudative, as is still done with pleural effusions. It turns out that the SAAG is a much more useful and reliable way to characterize ascites (ie, in terms of the presence or absence of portal hypertension). However, the ascitic fluid total protein remains useful for a few specific reasons:

- It can help to differentiate cardiac ascites from uncomplicated cirrhotic ascites, both of which have a SAAG of 1.1 g/dL or more. The total protein is reliably 2.5 g/dL or more in cardiac ascites and less than 2.5 g/dL in uncomplicated cirrhotic ascites.

- It can help to determine if the patient has a high risk of developing SBP. Any ascitic fluid with a total protein less than 1 g/dL likely has very low levels of protective immunoglobulins and complement (both are proteins), and as such is predisposed to SBP. Consider prophylactic antibiotics for these patients.

- It can help to identify ascites due to nephrotic syndrome (with resulting hypoalbuminemia). In these patients, the SAAG will be less than 1.1 g/dL and the protein will be less than 2.5 g/dL. This combination of a low SAAG and a low protein is unusual and strongly supports nephrotic syndrome in the right clinical context.

Table 12.2 Common Causes of Ascites Categorized by SAAG and Protein

Cause of Ascites	SAAG (g/dL)	Protein (g/dL)
Cirrhosis	≥1.1	<2.5
Right-sided heart failure	≥1.1	≥2.5
Nephrotic syndrome	<1.1	<2.5
Most other causes	<1.1	≥2.5

SAAG, serum-to-ascites albumin gradient.

Gram Stain and Bacterial Cultures

You should almost always send these tests with a diagnostic paracentesis. If at all possible, send the Gram stain and bacterial cultures before administering any empiric antibiotics, which significantly reduces the sensitivity of these tests.

Remember that the Gram stain gives us results within minutes to hours and tells us *if* bacteria are present (and whether they are gram-negative or gram-positive), whereas bacterial cultures take up to several days and tell us *which* bacteria are present. Even if the neutrophil count has already confirmed bacterial peritonitis, the Gram stain and cultures allow you to target your antibiotic therapy to the relevant pathogen(s).

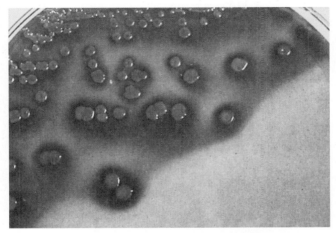

Figure 12.6 The two most common causes of spontaneous bacterial peritonitis are *Escherichia coli* and *Klebsiella*, both lactose-fermenting gram-negative rods that produce purple colonies on MacConkey agar, as depicted. (From Procop GW, Koneman EW. *Koneman's Color Atlas and Textbook of Diagnostic Microbiology*. 7th ed. Lippincott Williams & Wilkins; 2016.)

Ascitic fluid bacterial cultures showing growth of multiple organisms (a "polymicrobial" infection) should raise suspicion for secondary bacterial peritonitis. Finally, don't forget that the Gram stain and bacterial cultures are both far more specific than they are sensitive—do not use these tests alone to rule *out* bacterial peritonitis.

Glucose and Lactate Dehydrogenase (LDH): Identifying Secondary Bacterial Peritonitis Due to Bowel Perforation

Bowel perforation is a surgical emergency. Unfortunately, signs, symptoms, and even the ascitic fluid neutrophil count cannot reliably distinguish patients with bowel perforation from those with SBP. Luckily, we can use three ascitic fluid tests to identify those who may have bowel perforation: the total protein, glucose, and LDH. Send an ascitic fluid *glucose* and *LDH* in addition to your bread-and-butter tests if you have any clinical concern for bowel perforation (eg, a patient with presumed SBP who has not responded appropriately to antibiotics).

Patients who meet two of the following three criteria are likely to have a bowel perforation and require urgent follow-up (eg, imaging and/or surgery):

1. Total ascitic protein more than 1 g/dL

2. Ascitic glucose less than 50 mg/dL

3. Ascitic LDH more than the upper limit of normal for serum LDH

These criteria are more sensitive than specific. The most common alternative diagnosis in patients who meet at least two criteria is malignancy (particularly peritoneal carcinomatosis).

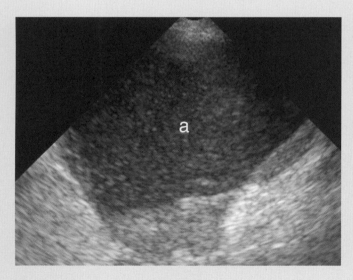

Figure 12.7 The dense white specks in this patient's ascites (a) represent debris particles that have spilled out from the bowel due to perforation. Early diagnosis is crucial—this is a surgical emergency. (From Brant WE, Helms CA. *Fundamentals of Diagnostic Radiology.* 4th ed. Lippincott Williams & Wilkins; 2012.)

In general, lower ascitic glucose tends to correlate with higher ascitic LDH; both indicate more severe or extensive local inflammation or infection. The utility of ascitic fluid glucose and LDH in narrowing your differential diagnosis is otherwise quite limited.

Additional Ascitic Fluid Studies

The tests in Table 12.3 are indicated in specific clinical scenarios.

Table 12.3 Ascitic Fluid Tests to Order in Specific Clinical Scenarios

Ascitic Fluid Study	Relevant Physiology/ Mechanism	When to Order	Interpretation
Amylase	Enzyme produced by the pancreas	Concern for pancreatic ascites[a]	Ascitic > serum amylase *or* ascitic amylase >1,000 IU/L suggests pancreatic ascites
Bilirubin	Concentration is high in the bowel, bile ducts, and gallbladder	Brown ascites	Ascitic > serum bilirubin suggests perforation of bowel or biliary tree
Triglycerides (TG)	Concentration is high in lymph; surrogate for lymphatic injury or obstruction	Milky ascites	Ascitic TG >200 mg/dL suggests: • Malignancy • Lymphatic anomaly or injury • Cirrhosis • Tuberculosis or filariasis (more so outside the United States)
Cytology	Malignant cells often appear atypical	Concern for malignant ascites	1. Positive cytology establishes the diagnosis of malignancy 2. Negative cytology does *not* rule out malignancy (~65% sensitivity)

[a]Leakage of pancreatic secretions, usually due to pancreatic duct injury in the setting of chronic or acute pancreatitis.

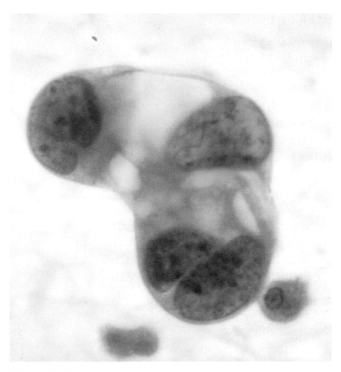

Figure 12.8 Ascitic fluid cytology demonstrating metastatic ovarian adenocarcinoma. Cytology is almost always positive in patients with peritoneal carcinomatosis; sensitivity is far lower in the absence of direct peritoneal involvement (eg, in tumors isolated to the liver such as hepatocellular carcinoma or lymphoma). (From Rubin E, Farber JL. *Pathology*. 3rd ed. Lippincott Williams & Wilkins; 1999.)

Ascitic Fluid Studies That Are Generally Unhelpful

Tuberculosis: adenosine deaminase and mycobacterial smear
The enzyme *adenosine deaminase (ADA)* is important in the proliferation and differentiation of T lymphocytes, which play a major role in the immune response to TB. ADA is often helpful in the diagnosis of pulmonary TB, and an ascitic fluid ADA activity level greater than 40 IU/L is suggestive of tuberculous peritonitis (lymphoma in particular may cause false positives). However, the big problem with the ascitic fluid ADA is that it is only about 30% sensitive for detecting TB in the setting of cirrhosis, by far the most common cause of ascites in the United States. *We recommend sending an ascitic fluid ADA only if you are suspicious for tuberculous peritonitis in a patient without cirrhosis.*

The sensitivity of an ascitic fluid *mycobacterial smear* is even worse—approaching 0% (!)—even in the absence of cirrhosis, so there really isn't any situation in which you should bother sending this test.

If you are suspicious for tuberculous peritonitis, send *mycobacterial cultures*. Ultimately, a peritoneal biopsy is often required to definitively make this diagnosis. See Chapter 14 for further discussion on testing for TB.

Infection: pH and Lactate

When these tests are run on the blood or on other body fluids (eg, pleural fluid), they can be helpful for the detection of infection or tissue hypoperfusion. Unfortunately, neither ascitic fluid pH nor ascitic fluid lactate seems to add any information that is helpful for management (eg, neither is sensitive nor specific for ascitic fluid infection).

Malignancy: Fibronectin, Cholesterol, Carcinoembryonic Antigen, and Cancer Antigen 125

Ascitic fluid fibronectin and cholesterol are "humoral tests of malignancy" that are usually elevated in cases of malignant ascites, including in the setting of peritoneal carcinomatosis. Unfortunately they are also elevated in a wide range of other conditions such as cardiac ascites, pancreatic ascites, and tuberculous ascites. The poor specificity of both ascitic fluid fibronectin and ascitic fluid cholesterol limits their clinical value.

Poor sensitivity and specificity make ascitic fluid *carcinoembryonic antigen* (CEA; a GI tumor marker) and *ascitic fluid cancer antigen 125* (CA 125; an ovarian cancer marker) unhelpful in either diagnosing or ruling out malignant ascites.

 # 13 Synovial Fluid

Most of our joints contain synovial fluid, a highly viscous solution that serves mainly as lubrication to prevent friction between articular surfaces. Synovial fluid is a mixture of hyaluronic acid (this is the lubricant) and small molecules filtered in from the plasma (eg, glucose, electrolytes). You'll find synovial fluid inside any mobile joint: the shoulders, elbows, wrists, hips, knees, ankles, and even the fingers and toes. There isn't a lot of synovial fluid in normal, healthy joints. The knee, for example, contains about 1 to 3.5 mL of fluid. Inflammation increases the volume of fluid, producing a joint effusion.

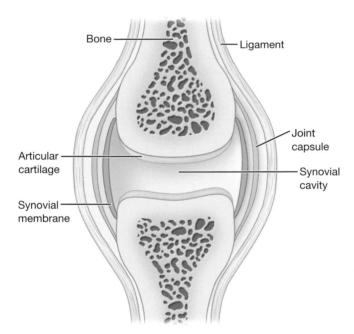

Figure 13.1 A typical synovial joint. The synovial membrane, the inner layer of the joint capsule, produces synovial fluid that lubricates and nourishes the joint. The other joints—termed "solid" joints—consist only of fibrocartilage that provides stabilization but does not allow for much movement at all. Examples include the joints between the bones of the skull and those between the vertebral bodies. In these cases, there is no joint cavity. Don't try to stick a needle into a solid joint. (From Anderson MK, Barnum M. *Foundations of Athletic Training: Prevention, Assessment, and Management*. 6th ed. Wolters Kluwer; 2017.)

Just like all the other fluids we have reviewed (cerebrospinal, pleural, peritoneal), synovial fluid sits inside its own special sequestered space, in this case the joint capsule. Although blood tests may sometimes give us clues as to what may be going on inside a joint, only by directly sampling the synovial fluid can we really know for sure. The process of sampling synovial fluid is called *arthrocentesis*.

Indications for Arthrocentesis

Any *new joint swelling or effusion*—especially when symptoms are acute, monoarticular, and/or severe—should prompt consideration of an arthrocentesis. Why? An arthrocentesis gives you a lot of valuable diagnostic information that you can't otherwise obtain even from advanced imaging studies such as computed tomography (CT) or magnetic resonance imaging (MRI). Perhaps most importantly, an arthrocentesis is the only way to rule out an acute bacterial infection of the joint (septic arthritis), a diagnosis you can't afford to miss.

An arthrocentesis may not be necessary when the diagnosis is already clear. For example, a patient with known rheumatoid arthritis presenting with symmetrical joint pain and swelling similar to past flares may be able to be treated empirically. The same approach could apply to a patient with known gout presenting with recurrent pain and swelling of the first metatarsophalangeal joint. But remember not to anchor: don't just automatically assume that your patient's new joint swelling is due to their known arthritic disease without solid evidence. For example, patients with rheumatoid arthritis are susceptible to joint infections with staphylococci. When in doubt, tap the joint.

Contraindications to Arthrocentesis

Do not perform an arthrocentesis through infected skin or soft tissue (eg, cellulitis) because of the risk of seeding the joint space with infection. In general, arthrocentesis is safe in patients with a coagulopathy (if, for example, they have an elevated prothrombin time [PT]/ international normalized ratio [INR] or partial thromboplastin time [PTT], thrombocytopenia, or are on treatment with blood thinners). The risk of iatrogenic hemarthrosis is extremely low.

How an Arthrocentesis Is Performed

The specifics vary depending on the joint, but the basics remain the same: the skin is sterilized and (usually) numbed, then—with or without ultrasound guidance—a needle is introduced into the joint cavity and a sample of synovial fluid is aspirated. Ideally at least 1 mL of fluid is obtained for analysis, but even a single drop is better than nothing since microscopic examination is still possible.

Synovial Fluid Studies

There are only a few studies routinely ordered:

- Appearance (no tests necessary—just look)
- Cell count and differential
- Microscopic analysis for crystals
- Gram stain and bacterial culture

Appearance

Normal synovial fluid is clear (or faint yellow), transparent, and viscous.

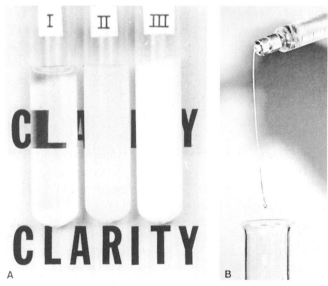

Figure 13.2 A. Tube I contains normal, transparent synovial fluid. The opaque synovial fluid in tubes II and III is abnormal. B. Normal synovial fluid is viscous enough that we expect it to form a "string" at least approximately 4 cm long when dangled from the tip of a syringe or pinched between two fingers. (From William J. Koopman, Larry W. *Moreland, Arthritis and Allied Conditions A Textbook of Rheumatology*. 15th ed. Lippincott Williams & Wilkins; 2005.)

Synovial fluid that is opaque, thin, or any color but clear or faint yellow is abnormal:

- White or dark/deep yellow discoloration indicates inflammation, whereas red or dark brown discoloration indicates bleeding (ie, hemarthrosis).

- Thin synovial fluid suggests inflammation, which causes the accumulation of enzymes that break down the proteins responsible for maintaining the fluid's normal viscosity. As inflammation becomes more severe (ie, in purulent effusions), the fluid may become thick and viscous again due to the sheer density of the inflammatory cells themselves.

None of the above findings are very sensitive. In other words, normal-appearing synovial fluid (*lack* of any of the above abnormal findings) does not rule out underlying pathology. Use the gross appearance of the synovial fluid as a clue rather than an answer. You'll need to do more studies to establish a diagnosis.

Cell Count and Differential

Normal synovial fluid contains very few cells—it is effectively "acellular." So instead of considering normal ranges for cell counts (white blood cells [WBCs] and red blood cells [RBCs]), we consider ranges of values that correlate with different diseases. Use the ranges mentioned in the following as a guide, not as a strict set of absolute rules—there are many exceptions.

- WBC less than 2,000 cells/mm^3 indicates a *noninflammatory effusion*, consistent with osteoarthritis, avascular necrosis, or joint trauma.

- WBC between 2,000 and 50,000 cells/mm^3 indicates an *inflammatory effusion*. Your differential diagnosis here is very broad. In general, expect a WBC count on the lower end of this range in systemic lupus erythematosus, scleroderma, sarcoidosis, and the seronegative spondyloarthropathies. Rheumatoid arthritis, gout, pseudogout, and miscellaneous infectious causes of arthritis (Lyme disease, gonorrhea, fungal, or mycobacterial) can produce WBC counts anywhere in this wide range.

- WBC more than 50,000 cells/mm^3 indicates *septic arthritis* until proven otherwise. A patient with such a high synovial fluid WBC count likely needs empiric antibiotics until both a Gram stain and bacterial culture come back with a more definitive answer. Note that the cutoff of 50,000 cells/mm^3 is more specific than it is sensitive; do not rule *out* septic arthritis if the WBC count is less than 50,000 cells/mm^3.

- Most noninflammatory and chronic inflammatory effusions demonstrate lymphocytic predominance. As the percentage of neutrophils increases, the likelihood of acute inflammatory arthritis (eg, an acute flare of gout, pseudogout, or rheumatoid arthritis) or septic arthritis increases. Synovial fluid with more than 50,000 WBCs/mm^3 and more than 75% neutrophils is highly concerning for septic arthritis.

The RBC count is usually not necessary to diagnose hemarthrosis; the synovial fluid appears pink, red, or dark brown upon aspiration. Expect an effusion that looks like this to contain at least 2,000 RBCs/mm³. You can differentiate true hemarthrosis from a traumatic tap in two ways: first, true hemarthrosis will be uniformly bloody as fluid is aspirated, whereas a traumatic tap may at first appear clear then become bloody (as blood spills into the joint space from the blood vessel that was nicked). Second, true hemarthrosis will typically not clot after aspiration, whereas a traumatic tap will.

Microscopic Analysis for Crystals

Gout and pseudogout—the "crystalline arthropathies"—are common and treatable. Diagnosis by synovial fluid microscopy is quick, easy, and cheap. For these reasons, you should almost always order a crystal analysis after a diagnostic arthrocentesis, even if your suspicion for gout or pseudogout is low. Many labs perform microscopic crystal analysis on all synovial fluid samples regardless of whether this test is ordered.

Crystal analysis involves examining a sample of synovial fluid under a microscope using polarized light. Both gout crystals (monosodium urate, or MSU) and pseudogout crystals (calcium pyrophosphate dihydrate, or CPPD) are *birefringent*, meaning that they appear in two different colors depending on their orientation relative to the direction of polarization of light. This concept is much easier to understand using pictures:

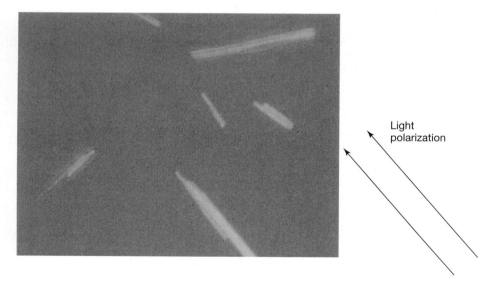

Light polarization

Figure 13.3 Gout: Monosodium urate crystals look like *needles*. They are *negatively birefringent*, meaning that they appear yellow when their long axis is parallel to the direction of polarization of light and blue when their long axis is perpendicular to the direction of polarization of light. (From Iannotti JP, Williams GR. *Disorders of the Shoulder: Diagnosis and Management: Shoulder Reconstruction*. 3rd ed. Wolters Kluwer Health; 2014.)

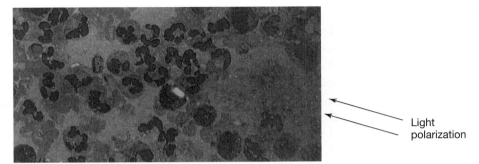

Light polarization

Figure 13.4 Pseudogout: Calcium pyrophosphate dihydrate crystals are *rhomboid*. They are *positively birefringent*, meaning that they appear blue when their long axis is parallel to the direction of polarization of light and yellow when their long axis is perpendicular to the direction of polarization of light. (From McClatchey KD. *Clinical Laboratory Medicine*. 2nd ed. Lippincott Williams & Wilkins; 2002.)

The sensitivity of crystal analysis depends on who is doing it (the nice way of saying this is that it is "operator dependent"). In general, MSU crystals are easier to detect than CPPD crystals, but both can be missed. The overall sensitivity of polarized microscopy for gout, for example, is about 85%. So there will be some cases of both gout and pseudogout in which no crystals will be seen. The specificity for both gout and pseudogout is quite good.

When Crystals Aren't the Whole Story

Consider a patient with a history of pseudogout who presents with a red, hot, and swollen knee. You perform an arthrocentesis that yields dark yellow, opaque synovial fluid with a WBC count of 30,000/mm³ (85% neutrophils). CPPD crystals are noted to be present. Can you be confident that this inflammatory effusion is due to an acute pseudogout flare?

Not necessarily. You may see crystals in the synovial fluid of any patient with a history of gout or pseudogout *even in the absence of an acute flare*. In other words, whereas crystals indicate the presence of a crystalline arthropathy, they do not necessarily indicate the presence of an acute flare. If many of the crystals are *intracellular*—that is, found inside inflammatory cells such as neutrophils or macrophages—the likelihood that the patient is having an acute flare of gout or pseudogout is much higher.

Suppose many CPPD crystals are found inside neutrophils. Along with the elevated synovial fluid WBC count, this finding confirms an acute pseudogout flare. But can you be confident that the patient does not also have an infection of the joint? After all, many causes of arthritis—including gout and pseudogout—increase the risk of septic arthritis of affected joints. Your next steps depend heavily on your supporting clinical and laboratory data. If your patient is infected (eg, bacteremic), immunosuppressed, has a recent history of intravenous (IV) drug use, and/or the synovial fluid demonstrates an extremely high WBC count (see page 181), do not let a few crystals knock septic arthritis off your differential.

Occasionally, other types of crystals may be found in the synovial fluid. Perhaps the most important example is *basic calcium phosphate (BCP; also called hydroxyapatite)*, which tends to form in large joints already affected by osteoarthritis, chronic CPPD arthritis, or prior traumatic injuries. BCP often does not cause any symptoms, but its presence can be associated with "Milwaukee shoulder syndrome," a form of chronic, destructive shoulder arthritis that can cause recurrent noninflammatory effusions and often affects the periarticular structures of the rotator cuff. BCP crystals are not visible on polarized microscopy; a special stain called alizarin Red S is required for proper visualization, and even then both sensitivity and specificity are not great.

Other crystals that may be seen include calcium oxalate (seen mainly in dialysis patients) and cholesterol (seen in chronic inflammation). In most cases, their presence is unlikely to change management—just know that these crystals exist.

Gram Stain and Bacterial Cultures

The Gram stain gives us results within minutes to hours and tells us *if* bacteria are present (and whether they are gram negative or gram positive), whereas bacterial cultures take up to several days and tell us *which* bacteria are present. Positive bacterial cultures are the gold standard for the diagnosis of septic arthritis.

False negatives are extremely common on a synovial fluid Gram stain—this test is only 30% to 50% sensitive. The sensitivity of synovial fluid bacterial cultures is much better, about 80% to 85%, but it decreases significantly if you give antibiotics before aspirating the joint. For this reason, if at all possible, arthrocentesis should be performed before administering antibiotics.

Tests for Other Infectious Diseases

If you are concerned about Lyme arthritis, send a blood sample for a Lyme enzyme-linked immunosorbent assay (ELISA) with reflex Western blot; we expect any patient with Lyme arthritis to have positive serologies (see Chapter 14 on diagnosis of Lyme disease). A synovial fluid sample can be sent for a polymerase chain reaction (PCR) test for *Borrelia burgdorferi* (about 70% sensitive). It is unhelpful to send synovial fluid for Lyme ELISA and/or Western blot.

Send fungal or mycobacterial (tuberculosis) cultures if you are suspicious for fungal or mycobacterial arthritis, respectively. These cultures are likely to take at least a few days to grow. In the case of mycobacterial arthritis, diagnosis often requires synovial biopsy.

If you suspect gonococcal arthritis, send synovial fluid cultures and alert the laboratory to your suspicion so that appropriate culture modifications can be made. Even with these modifications, however, synovial fluid cultures are not sensitive for gonococcal arthritis. In the appropriate clinical context (eg, a sexually active patient with tenosynovitis, oligoarticular large joint arthritis, and characteristic gonococcal skin lesions), gonococcal arthritis can be diagnosed with a positive nucleic acid amplification test (NAAT) run on any sample, including urine, blood, mucosa (eg, skin lesions), or synovial fluid. Although the synovial fluid gonococcal NAAT has very good accuracy and is more sensitive than synovial fluid cultures, it is not universally available.

Diagnosis of the abovementioned diseases often involves additional tests of multiple compartments including the blood, urine, skin, and sometimes even the cerebrospinal fluid (CSF). We review these tests in Chapter 14.

Cytology

Occasionally, a tumor may invade the joint space (eg, osteosarcoma, bony or synovial metastases). In these cases, a tissue biopsy is typically required for diagnosis. Nevertheless, if you suspect an underlying malignancy, send the synovial fluid for cytology, or simply inform the lab of your concern; microscopy is routinely performed as part of synovial fluid analysis anyway. Cells with characteristic atypical morphologies indicate malignancy.

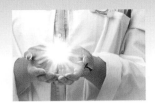

Bonus Chapter: A Few Words About Notation

In today's world, where the electronic medical record (EMR) has eclipsed the handwritten note, the recording and storage of lab results happen automatically. However, there will undoubtedly be times when it is more convenient to jot down the results with paper and pen, perhaps to facilitate a quick handoff or because the EMR is not working. For these situations, it is good to know that there are simple ways that have stood the test of time for recording lab results. The most common are used to record the complete blood count (CBC), basic metabolic panel (BMP), liver function tests, and blood gases. Here they are—and remember that you will not be judged by your artistic ability but by the clarity with which you express the numbers:

CBC

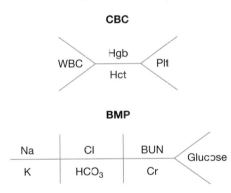

WBC ⟩ Hgb / Hct ⟨ Plt

BMP

Na | Cl | BUN ⟩ Glucose
K | HCO₃ | Cr

Liver Function Tests and Calcium

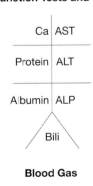

Ca | AST

Protein | ALT

Albumin | ALP

Bili

Blood Gas

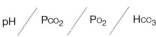

pH / Pco_2 / Po_2 / Hco_3

Section 3
Other Tests You Need to Know

 What This Section Is All About

In this section you will learn:

- When to order and how to interpret many important tests we have not yet discussed.
- For each of these tests:
  - What is the purpose of the test?
  - What is the proper clinical context in which to order the test?
  - How do you interpret the results? What are the strengths and limitations of the test?

In Section 2 you encountered many of the most commonly ordered lab tests. But, of course, you have not met *all* of the lab tests you need to know. In this section, we will focus on many of these additional tests, some of which are frequently used, some not so much but which stand out as critical for establishing diagnoses you don't want to miss.

We have grouped these lab tests by organ system because that's how we traditionally tend to think about these things, recognizing that boundaries are fuzzy and there is considerable overlap among these categories. Don't worry, though—we will point out the full utility of each test as we discuss it.

We have also grouped tests that are frequently ordered together and that share a common clinical context. Thus, you will see headings such as Sexually Transmitted Infections, Autoimmune and Metabolic Liver Disease, and Hemolysis to name just a few.

Finally, in a few of the chapters we will introduce you to basic testing concepts that tend to come up frequently within a specific field. One example is the chapter on Infectious Diseases: Principles of Testing, which will cover topics such as cultures, antigen tests, polymerase chain reaction (PCR) tests, and serologies (antibody tests).

Sometimes we will express our own personal opinion about why and when to order these tests, as well as when not to, but we will make it clear that it is just our opinion, and you can take it or leave it at your discretion as you learn more.

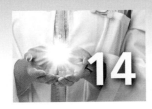# 14 Infectious Diseases

PRINCIPLES OF TESTING

 ## Methods of Testing

We will review four fundamental techniques:

- Cultures
- Immunologic assays for antibodies (serologic tests) and antigens
- Nucleic acid amplification tests (NAATs)
- Tissue biopsy with microscopy

Cultures

Cultures are the traditional gold-standard method for detecting infectious pathogens. The concept is simple: take a sample from the patient (eg, blood, urine, stool, cerebrospinal fluid [CSF], pleural fluid, peritoneal fluid) and place it in conditions conducive to the growth of the target pathogen(s). Then, wait—sometimes days, sometimes longer—to see if anything grows.

Cultures are very specific—the growth of a particular organism can be confirmed visually, and additional tests can help determine the precise organism and its susceptibility to various antimicrobials.

Sensitivity, however, may be limited depending on how fastidious the organism is, the extent of the infection, previous treatment, the immunologic status of the patient, and the nature of the sample source. It is important that *cultures be ordered and drawn prior to the administration of antimicrobials whenever possible*, since antibiotics significantly reduce the culture sensitivity.

The most frequently ordered cultures are optimized for the detection of common bacterial pathogens. At your institution, these default cultures may be called "routine cultures," "bacterial cultures," or simply "cultures." Understand that these cultures are not designed to pick up many fungal, parasitic, viral, or atypical bacterial infections; if any of these are suspected, specialized cultures (usually involving the use of special growth media) or other diagnostic tests may be needed. Examples of such difficult-to-culture bacteria include *Haemophilus* and *Legionella*. All viruses as well as many fungi and parasites fall into this category as well. On the other hand, some organisms, such as *Staphylococcus aureus*, usually grow very quickly (usually within 1-2 days) in routine cultures.

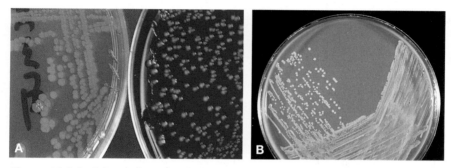

Figure 14.1 A. *Salmonella* spp. growing on MacConkey (left) and blood (right) agars. B. *Haemophilus influenzae* growing on chocolate agar. "Agar" is the general term for the gelatinous media used to culture many common microorganisms (mostly bacteria). Routine cultures typically employ multiple agars, each optimized for the growth of different common pathogens. When clinically significant organisms are found to be growing, the addition of different antibiotics to different areas of the plate can help determine the organism's antibiotic susceptibility (eg, if the organism does not grow where ampicillin was added, it must be susceptible to ampicillin). (From Procop GW, Church DL, Hall GS, et al. *Koneman's Color Atlas and Textbook of Diagnostic Microbiology.* 7th ed. Wolters Kluwer; 2017.)

An organism that is difficult or slow to grow in cultures is termed *fastidious.* Knowing an organism's fastidiousness can greatly impact clinical management: for example, because *S. aureus* grows rapidly, many experts opt to discontinue empiric coverage for methicillin-resistant *Staphylococcus aureus* (MRSA) if blood and sputum cultures remain negative after 2 to 3 days. Mycobacteria, on the other hand, grow very slowly, so cultures must be monitored for several weeks.

Colonizers and Contaminants: Finding an organism does not necessarily mean that you have found the cause of your patient's disease. Even when we are healthy, we are crawling with microorganisms. In fact, many of these little residents—such as the bacteria found in the gut microbiome—play an important role in maintaining our health. We refer to these benign organisms as *colonizers*, many of which are commonly found in the oropharynx, nose, gastrointestinal (GI) tract, urinary tract, and skin.

When a sample is drawn from one of these compartments, typical colonizers are often easily recognized by the lab technician and either discounted or labeled appropriately (eg, as "normal respiratory flora"). Sometimes, however, a colonizer in one patient may represent a pathogen in another. This is particularly relevant in the case of urine cultures, when the finding of bacteriuria may represent asymptomatic bacteriuria or a urinary infection. Treatment may or may not be indicated based on the clinical context (eg, the presence or absence of associated symptoms, comorbidities, or upcoming planned urologic procedures).

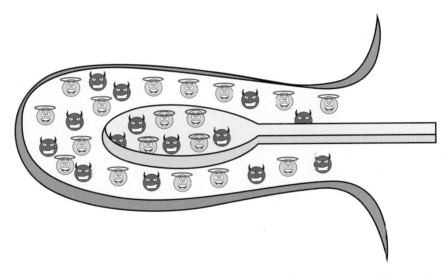

Figure 14.2 When performing cultures of a non-sterile compartment, it is critical to differentiate colonizers from disease-causing pathogens. This isn't always easy—microorganisms do not always declare themselves as good or evil.

Some body compartments—such as the blood and CSF—are normally sterile, meaning that the presence of any microorganisms is abnormal and should be considered evidence of infection until proven otherwise.

Occasionally, organisms from a non-sterile outside source, such as the skin, may make their way into a sample. When this happens, we refer to these organisms as *contaminants*. Contamination is especially common during the collection of blood cultures. Skin colonizers such as *Staphylococcus epidermidis* may make their way into the sample after improper or insufficient skin disinfection prior to venipuncture.

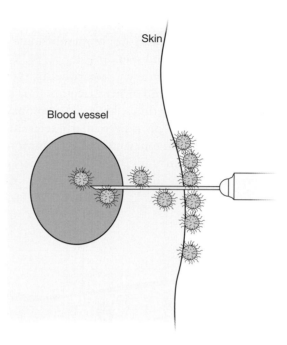

Figure 14.3 Improper skin disinfection can allow colonizers from the skin to make their way onto a needle tip. They may contaminate the sample and lead to positive blood cultures when bacteremia is not present.

How can we know if a given organism is a contaminant? Sometimes the identity of the organism itself is enough: *Propionibacterium acnes*, for example, a common skin colonizer, is a very rare cause of bacteremia. If found on blood cultures, *P. acnes* is almost certainly a contaminant. *S. aureus* and *Candida* species, on the other hand, should never be considered contaminants if found on blood cultures.

Some organisms, such as coagulase-negative *staphylococci* (CoNS), may cause bacteremia or represent contaminants. In these cases, clinical context must be weighed heavily. Blood cultures growing CoNS in a patient with high fevers and an indwelling medical device, for example, are concerning for true CoNS bacteremia; the same result in an otherwise healthy patient may not be. Additionally, consider how many of your cultures are growing the organism in question—if multiple blood cultures drawn from different sites are growing CoNS, contamination is far less likely than if just one of several is growing CoNS. It is usually helpful to repeat cultures in cases of uncertainty.

Blood Cultures: When you order a routine blood culture, a blood sample is drawn and separated into anaerobic and aerobic bottles that facilitate the growth of anaerobic and aerobic organisms, respectively. At least approximately 8 to 10 mL of blood is required per bottle. The growth media are optimized to detect the most common bloodstream infections, including most bacteria as well as some yeast and fungi (eg, *Candida* and *Aspergillus* species). Sensitivity varies greatly by organism, site of infection, and sample volume, and ranges from less than 50% to greater than 90%. In order to optimize sensitivity, it is important to *draw at least two blood cultures from different sites* (ideally on different sides of the body) whenever blood cultures are indicated.

Urine Cultures: To minimize the risk of contamination, a urine sample for culture should ideally be obtained via a midstream clean catch (for how to do this, see Chapter 8). A result of at least 10^5 colony-forming units (CFU)/mL is widely considered to be a positive result indicative of true bacteriuria. Among patients whose picture is otherwise convincing for urinary tract infection (UTI)—particularly female patients (for reasons that are unclear)—results as low as 10^2 CFU/mL may be consistent with a UTI.

What Is a Colony-Forming Unit and How Does the Lab Measure It?

A *colony* is a bunch of microorganisms—in most cases bacteria—growing together in what appears to be a large, amorphous agglomeration (see Figure 14.1A). The term *CFU* is simply a fancy way of referring to a single bacterium that can reproduce and give rise to an entire colony of similar bacteria. How does the lab go from a lump of bacteria on an agar plate to determining how many CFUs are present? The answer is simple: serial dilutions. A sample of the colony is suspended and then put through serial dilutions, each of which is plated. At some point, one of the plates will produce a limited and countable number of bacterial colonies. Multiply the number of colonies by the dilution factor and you get the total CFUs.

By far the most common indication for urine culture is a suspected UTI. *It is generally unwise to send urine cultures in patients without signs or symptoms of a UTI unless the finding of asymptomatic bacteriuria would change management.* General indications for screening and potential treatment of asymptomatic bacteriuria include pregnancy, planned urologic procedures, and recent renal transplantation.

Sputum Cultures: Sputum cultures are rarely needed in patients with *upper* respiratory infections, such as patients with typical symptoms of a cold. But they are an important part of the workup of suspected *lower* respiratory tract infections. Because the respiratory tract—especially the upper respiratory tract, including the oropharynx—contains many normal colonizers, the finding of one or more organisms on sputum culture does not necessarily mean that there is a respiratory infection or, if an infection is present, that the cultured organism is the cause. The sample should be collected from as low in the respiratory tree as possible.

The diagnostic yield of a sputum culture depends heavily on how it is obtained:

- *Expectorated sputum*: Patients rinse their mouth (ideally they do not eat or drink for 1-2 hours beforehand), then attempt to cough up sputum into a sample cup, which is then submitted for culture. Convenience and noninvasiveness make this the most popular method for obtaining sputum cultures. However, many patients—even those with pneumonia—are unable to produce significant sputum this way. A respiratory therapist can use procedures like nebulizers, suction, and manual percussion for assistance. Even when sputum can be obtained, sample quality is highly variable. Often, the sample may consist largely of oropharyngeal secretions (with many contaminants) rather than sputum from the lower respiratory tract. Some laboratories use the squamous epithelial count (SEC) to assess specimen quality and may reject specimens with more than a set number of squamous cells (10 per low-power field is a common cutoff).* Estimates of the overall sensitivity of expectorated sputum cultures for bacterial pneumonia vary significantly, but it is likely not higher than 75% even under optimal conditions. However, the finding of a pathogenic species such as *Streptococcus pneumoniae* or *Haemophilus influenzae* is highly specific.

- *Bronchoscopic specimens:* Consider bronchoscopic sampling in patients with possible pneumonia—primarily those who are very sick—in whom expectorated sputum either cannot be obtained or has been unrevealing. A bronchoscopy bypasses the dense oropharyngeal flora and allows for direct sampling of the lower respiratory tract via lavage and brushing. Sensitivity varies significantly by technique, operator, and organism, but is overall widely considered to be better than that of expectorated sputum.

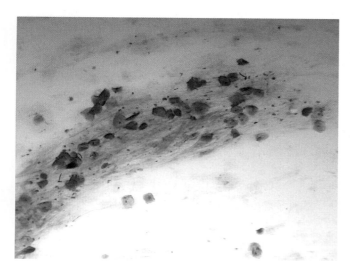

Figure 14.4 Gram-stained sputum sample showing many squamous epithelial cells; cultures of this sample probably will not be helpful. (Image provided by Dr. Robert Fader.)

---

*A high SEC indicates that the specimen is contaminated with saliva (the upper respiratory tract, unlike the bronchi, is lined with squamous epithelial cells).

- *Deep endotracheal specimens:* A sputum sample taken from the distal end of the endotracheal tube should be obtained from patients who are intubated.

Positive sputum culture results are typically reported semiquantitatively, either using words such as "rare, few, moderate, abundant" or using numbers such as "1+, 2+, 3+, 4+." Whether or not a result represents a true positive—that is, represents a likely etiologic pathogen—depends on the organism, with most requiring at least moderate or 3+ growth to be considered pathogenic. Some organisms, even when growing abundantly on sputum cultures, are highly unlikely to represent true pulmonary pathogens; examples include Coagulase-negative Staphylococci (CoNS) and *Candida* species.

Other Cultures: Any body fluid sample can be cultured when infection is suspected— examples include the CSF, pleural fluid, peritoneal fluid, synovial fluid, stool, and superficial or deep wounds (eg, ulcers, abscesses). If you culture the GI tract or the skin (especially superficial wounds), expect to find colonizers. The other compartments mentioned should normally be sterile.

Immunologic Methods: Antigen and Antibody Testing

Antigen and antibody testing represent two sides of the same coin: an antigen test looks for some component or marker of the pathogen(s) of interest (eg, hepatitis B surface antigen), whereas antibody testing looks for signs of an immune response to that component or marker (eg, hepatitis B surface antibody). Antigen and antibody tests can often produce results faster than cultures and usually require less involved specimen handling and manipulation.

The finding of a given antigen can often be taken as evidence of active infection with the organism of interest—examples include hepatitis B surface antigen, *S. pneumoniae* urinary antigen, COVID-19 antigen, and many others. Sensitivity and specificity vary significantly by pathogen and specimen source.

Antibodies, on the other hand, do not necessarily indicate active or recent infection. The appearance of a given antibody must necessarily occur *after* that of its corresponding antigen, and may indicate that an infection is recent (eg, hepatitis B core immunoglobulin [Ig]M; see Chapter 17), remote (eg, hepatitis B core IgG), or cleared, or that the host is immune (eg, hepatitis B surface antibody). This may seem confusing, but it is actually a good thing! By understanding the timing of a given antibody's appearance and its antigen specificity, we can learn much more about the patient's disease state than just whether or not they are actively infected. Importantly, however, the lag time between antigen and antibody appearance means that antibody testing may miss cases of active infection early in the disease course. We discuss antibody testing, including the basic antibody classes, in more depth in Chapter 22.

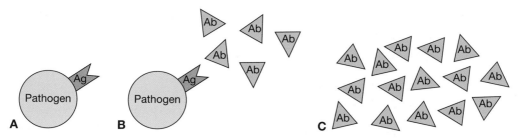

Figure 14.5 A simple schematic of a theoretical pathogen with a single surface antigen and corresponding antibody. Early in the disease course (A), the antigen is detectable but neutralizing antibodies have not yet formed. Later on (B), antibodies develop and may for a time be able to be detected along with the antigen. As the immune response kicks into full gear, antibody titers rise dramatically and bind the antigen sufficiently to neutralize the pathogen; at this point, antibodies but *not* antigen may be detectable (C). Not all organisms follow this exact pattern—we give this example to demonstrate why antigen positivity usually correlates with active infection, whereas antibody positivity may have multiple interpretations.

There are many laboratory methods for antigen and antibody detection. Two of the most common are the enzyme-linked immunosorbent assay (ELISA) and Western blot tests.

Enzyme-Linked Immunosorbent Assay: ELISA is used quite frequently to test for specific infections, but can be used to test for almost any antigen or antibody you want. For example, when screening for autoimmune disorders, the target isn't an antigen on the surface of an infectious organism but rather an antibody, specifically an autoantibody.

You will not have to run an ELISA yourself; you only have to order it and your lab will run the test for you. Here's how an ELISA works:

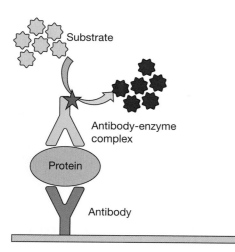

Figure 14.6 Cartoon schematic of a typical "sandwich" enzyme-linked immunosorbent assay. The amount of color change (see the following discussion) corresponds to the concentration of the target protein in the patient sample.

1. Make an antibody ("A") that binds to the protein of interest ("P"). In the case of infectious diseases, P is usually an antigen on the surface of the pathogen. Fix the antibody A to a plate.

2. Add the patient sample (usually blood). If the patient has P, it will bind to A and also become fixed to the plate.

3. Take more of A and link it to an enzyme ("E"), making "AE." Add AE to the plate. If there is P on the plate, AE will bind to it. All this binding will make a sandwich: A-P-AE.*

4. Add a substance ("substrate") that gets turned a nice bright color by the enzyme (E). The more bright color you see when you add the substrate, the more AE must be fixed to the plate, and the more P must be in the patient's sample.

Bottom line: more color change = more protein (antigen or antibody) of interest.

ELISA testing tends to be sensitive but not very specific. False positives are not at all uncommon. Therefore, a positive ELISA test is often followed up by a more specific test, the Western blot.

Western Blot: The *Western blot test* is generally run as a confirmatory test when the ELISA is positive. It is similar to an ELISA but involves an extra initial step where the patient's sample is subjected to electrophoresis, which separates out proteins of interest by size and charge. Ultimately, like with an ELISA, enzyme-linked antibodies and a substrate (the thing that changes colors in the presence of the enzyme) are both added. Western blot tends to be more specific but less sensitive than ELISA. Results of a Western blot are usually qualitative (eg, positive or negative), whereas those of an ELISA are typically quantitative.

Nucleic Acid Amplification Test

NAAT involves combining a patient sample with synthetic cellular machinery that replicates (ie, amplifies) a genetic sequence specific to a given organism if it is present in the sample.

---

*This is called a "sandwich ELISA." There are other variations of ELISA that work slightly differently, but the basic principles remain the same.

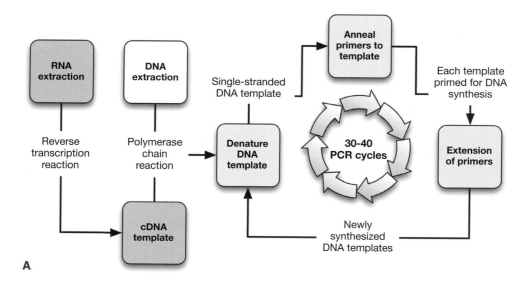

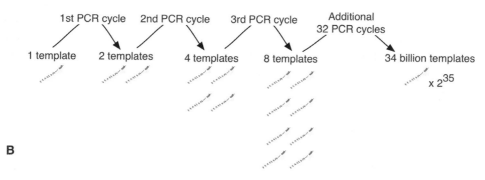

Figure 14.7 The most common type of NAAT is called PCR (in clinical practice, the terms NAAT and PCR are generally used interchangeably), in which genetic amplification is accomplished through the use of primers (small fragments of single-stranded DNA) and construction enzymes called DNA polymerases; cycles of DNA strand separation (allowing for primer binding) and replication are achieved through repeated temperature changes (A). Amplification occurs exponentially, so it only takes 30 to 40 PCR cycles to make billions of copies of a given genetic sequence (B), enough to then be detected by methods such as gel electrophoresis. cDNA, complementary DNA; NAAT, nucleic acid amplification test; PCR, polymerase chain reaction. (From Attilio Orazi A, Foucar K, Knowles D, Weiss LM, *Knowles Neoplastic Hematopathology*. 3rd ed. Lippincott Williams & Wilkins; 2013.)

The sensitivity and specificity of NAAT vary, of course, by organism and specimen source, but overall both tend to be excellent. High accuracy, combined with relatively low cost and short turnaround time, makes NAAT quite popular. It has replaced more traditional methods like culture or immunologic testing as a first-line test for many infectious diseases. We will point out when and where NAAT, rather than other methods, is best utilized as initial and/or follow-up testing in specific clinical scenarios.

Multiplex Assays

With multiplex testing, a single specimen can be tested for numerous pathogens simultaneously. Two widely used panels are the GI panel and the respiratory pathogen panel; each tests for many of the most common infectious organisms that may be present. The specific organisms that are included in these panels vary from lab to lab. Results are often available within just a few hours. The diagnostic yield is impressive; for example, the accuracy of multiplex testing of stool samples for bacterial pathogens may even exceed that of stool cultures. However, these assays cannot distinguish between actual infection and colonization, and you still need cultures to assess antibiotic sensitivity and resistance.

Biopsy: When Tissue Is the Issue

The details involved in direct tissue examination—that is, biopsy with microscopic examination—fall outside the scope of this book. Biopsy is typically reserved for cases when the diagnosis cannot be made noninvasively and/or when the patient is very sick and a prompt definitive diagnosis is urgently needed. When performed, biopsy tends to be quite specific but—depending on the organism and tissue—may not be as sensitive as one would wish. Once tissue is obtained, many of the abovementioned techniques may be used to aid in diagnosis.

 ## *The Source of the Infection*

Where we test—or which body fluid(s) we choose to test—matters. Thinking practically about the localization of any given infection makes this point obvious. For example, most patients with a UTI have evidence of bacteria in the urine but less commonly in the blood, and almost never in other compartments like the respiratory tract or CSF. Colloquially, we refer to the organ or organ system in which an infection originates as the *infectious source*. The source may or may not be apparent based on the patient's clinical presentation, and the infection may or may not have spread to other compartments.

When deciding which organ(s) or body compartment(s) to test, take into account both those that are most likely to be affected *and* those that, if affected, would prompt a change in management.

Urine *and* blood cultures may make sense in an older adult patient with multiple comorbidities who is febrile with evidence of UTI on urinalysis, both because of the reasonable likelihood of blood culture positivity and the potential effect of blood culture results on the choice, intensity, and duration of antibiotic. On the other hand, a young otherwise healthy patient with similar signs and symptoms might not need blood cultures because of the very low likelihood of blood culture positivity and the high likelihood of clinical improvement with a short course of antibiotics.

Source Unknown

In many instances, you may suspect that your patient has an infection but there is no clear source. This is a particularly common scenario in the inpatient setting.

Suppose a patient is hospitalized for a small bowel obstruction that resolves with medical management, but a few days after admission develops new fevers without any clear localizing symptoms (eg, cough that might indicate a respiratory origin, or dysuria from a UTI).

One common approach is to initiate a relatively broad infectious workup consisting of noninvasive tests for common infections: blood cultures, urinalysis, urine cultures, and sometimes sputum cultures and/or rapid influenza and COVID-19 tests; a chest x-ray is often added if there is any consideration of pneumonia. This approach can be helpful in identifying common community- and hospital-acquired infections, and it is very often a reasonable first step. But it is also insensitive. Far from ruling out infection categorically, this basic workup may miss many pathogens (most nonbacterial and many bacterial pathogens) and does not test at all for infections of several organ systems such as the central nervous system (CNS; meningitis) or GI tract (colitis). When the initial workup proves unrevealing and infection remains a serious consideration, additional testing (eg, imaging of the abdomen and pelvis, tests for specific pathogens such as *Clostridium difficile*, repeat cultures, or immunologic tests) may be warranted.

COMMON RESPIRATORY PATHOGENS

Most patients who present with a typical *upper* respiratory infection do not require testing. They have a self-limited viral illness that, annoying as it may be, will usually resolve in a matter of days or a couple of weeks. But there are other circumstances where laboratory testing for respiratory pathogens can be important, in particular when you suspect the possibility of strep throat, flu, respiratory syncytial virus (RSV), pertussis, bacterial pneumonia, or COVID-19.

 ## *Pharyngitis*

Is it *strep throat* or not? Most of the time (but not all of the time—more later), that's the only question you need to answer for your patients who present with a sore throat.

Strep Throat

The Centor criteria are widely used to determine the likelihood of strep and guide your choice of additional laboratory testing and treatment:

There are various opinions on how to apply these criteria, but the most common approach, and one we like, is to

- empirically treat anyone with a score of 4 or more with an antibiotic

- test anyone with a score of 2 or 3 for strep, and let the results guide your decision to treat

- neither test nor treat anyone with a score of 0 or 1 (ie, assume they have a viral infection)

Table 14.1 Centor Criteria for Strep Throat

Criterion	Answer	Points
Age	3-14 yr[a]	+1
	15-44 yr	0
	>44 yr	−1
Swollen tonsils, or tonsillar exudate	No	0
	Yes	+1
Tender or swollen anterior cervical lymph nodes	No	0
	Yes	+1
Temp > 100.4 °F	No	0
	Yes	+1
Cough	No	+1
	Yes	0

[a]Strep is rare in children under the age of 3.

When testing is called for, the initial test should be a *rapid strep test*. Although throat culture remains the gold standard, the rapid antigen tests found in most offices are reasonably sensitive (60%-95%) and very specific (>95%). In adults who have a positive test, treatment can be instituted right away. In adults with a negative rapid strep test, you should follow up with a culture only if your clinical suspicion for strep remains high. All children, however, should have a culture done following a negative rapid test.

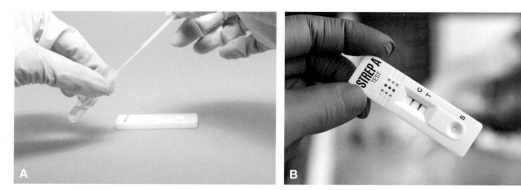

Figure 14.8 How to do a rapid strep test. The sample, obtained from the back of the throat, is placed in the testing fluid and stirred. (A) Several drops of the fluid are then deposited in the well of the test cartridge and allowed to migrate up along the strip. If streptococcal antigens are present in the sample, they will interact with antibodies impregnated in the strip to form a visible line. (B) Results are ready in minutes; the above test is positive. (Courtesy UNIKYLUCKK/Shutterstock and angellodeco/ Shutterstock.)

A sample for a *throat culture* should be taken by swabbing the posterior pharynx, both tonsillar regions, and any area that looks inflamed; try to avoid the cheeks and tongue. The swab is then placed in transport media and sent to the lab where it will be cultured.

Other Causes of Pharyngitis

Fusobacterium is an anaerobic bacterium that is increasingly being recognized as a cause of pharyngitis. Patients tend to be quite ill and will not respond to the oral antibiotics used to treat strep throat. The most feared complication is Lemierre syndrome, septic thrombophlebitis of the internal jugular vein. You will need to alert the lab if you suspect this infection, because it requires special aerobic cultures to grow.

You also need to consider *chlamydial* and *gonococcal pharyngitis* in sexually active adolescents and adults. Testing for sexually transmitted infections (STIs) is discussed later in this chapter.

Viral etiologies you need to think about and do not want to miss include *COVID-19* (page 216), *infectious mononucleosis* (page 209), and *HIV infection* (page 229).

Influenza

During the flu season, there is often no need to test for flu; the diagnosis can be made with a high degree of accuracy by recognizing the typical symptoms (eg, acute-onset fever, myalgias, and cough) in a patient when the prevalence of the disease in the community is high. Testing for flu is warranted when:

- Patients present with flu-like symptoms when it is early or late in flu season; flu is then just one among several other diagnoses that must be considered.

- Because of age, underlying comorbidities, or immunocompromise, your patient is at risk for complications of flu *and the diagnosis would alter management* (if you are going to start treatment for the flu anyway, ask yourself why you are running the test).

- The respiratory illness is sufficiently severe to merit hospitalization.

Almost all clinics can run in-office *rapid antigen tests* on oropharyngeal or nasopharyngeal (preferred) specimens, often in concert with COVID-19 testing. Results are available within minutes. These tests are highly specific but not very sensitive. To achieve close to 100% sensitivity, you need a *polymerase chain reaction (PCR)*, the results of which take more time to come back. One approach in the outpatient setting is to start with a rapid antigen test and, if it is negative and you still have a high suspicion for flu, order a PCR.

 ## Respiratory Syncytial Virus

Largely but not exclusively a disease of children, RSV is a lower respiratory tract infection for which testing is only indicated when it will affect management. Most otherwise healthy patients will recover with supportive care alone. Those whose illness is sufficiently severe to require hospitalization and those who are immunocompromised should have the diagnosis confirmed by laboratory testing, because antiviral medications, intravenous immunoglobulin (IVIG), and/or corticosteroids may be indicated.

PCR testing of a nasal wash or nasopharyngeal swab is the most sensitive test but is not universally available. Rapid antigen testing can be used alone or in conjunction with PCR; it has a sensitivity of approximately 80% and specificity of more than 95%. False negatives can occur in patients already receiving prophylaxis with the antiviral drug palivizumab.

 ## Pertussis

This illness is most common among infants, but can affect older children and adults as well. Early antibiotic treatment can shorten the duration of the illness and prevent spread, so you don't want to miss this diagnosis. Tip-offs that pertussis may be present include the following:

- A paroxysmal, severe cough
- The characteristic inspiratory whoop
- Post-tussive vomiting
- An absent or low fever

None of these symptoms are sufficiently specific to obviate the need for testing. The test of choice is a *PCR* for *Bordetella pertussis* on a sample taken from the posterior nasopharynx. A specimen for *culture* is often sent at the same time. Culture results take longer to come back than PCR results—3 to 7 days versus 1 to 2 days. PCR is also more sensitive; it can detect much smaller viral loads than culture. Unlike cultures, PCR is not affected by prior antibiotic therapy. If only one of the two tests is positive—for example, a positive PCR and a negative culture—you should assume the patient has pertussis. Both PCR testing and cultures have false negatives if run 4 or more weeks *after* the onset of symptoms; at that point, if you want to confirm that your patient has had pertussis, you would need to order *serology* to look for antibodies against *Bordetella*. Rapid antigen testing is not available.

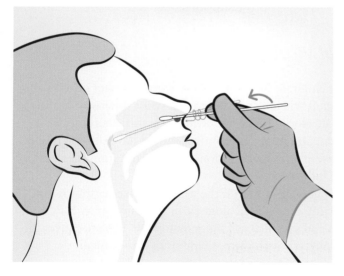

Figure 14.9 Obtaining a specimen from the posterior nasopharynx in a patient with an upper respiratory infection. (Courtesy ketpixel/Shutterstock.)

What Kind of Swab Should I Use?

For best results when testing for either flu or pertussis, use a flocked swab when available (they almost always are). Flocked swabs have many short, thin absorbent nylon fibers that can trap the specimens in the outermost layer of the swab where they are most accessible for testing. Detection rates are higher with flocked swabs than traditional fiber swabs.

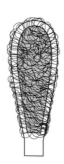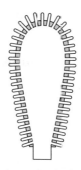

Figure 14.10 Comparison of non-flocked (traditional nylon; left) and flocked (right) swabs.

 ## *Bacterial Pneumonia*

The diagnosis of bacterial pneumonia primarily involves a careful history, physical exam, and—often—a chest x-ray. In many patients, primarily in otherwise healthy outpatients, no lab testing is needed at all, and empiric antibiotic therapy is recommended as the first step in management. However, laboratory testing is appropriate for patients who are sufficiently ill to require hospitalization as well as for those who acquire pneumonia while in the hospital.

When a laboratory evaluation is called for, testing includes, at the very least:

- Sputum Gram stain and culture

- Complete blood count (CBC) with differential

Additional tests depend on how sick the patient is and the clinical history. These tests may include the following:

- Blood culture in patients with severe pneumonia

- *Legionella* and pneumococcal testing (see later)

- Flu testing (see earlier)

- Tuberculosis (TB) testing (see page 217)

- Testing for opportunistic infections in immunocompromised patients (eg, molecular tests, fungal cultures, and testing for *Pneumocystis jirovecii*)

Pneumococcal Pneumonia

S. pneumoniae (pneumococcus) is the leading bacterial cause of community-acquired pneumonia. A Gram stain and culture of a good sputum sample (see page 195 for details on sputum sampling) will allow you to diagnose a majority of cases of pneumococcal pneumonia. Some cases, however, can be missed, especially if antibiotics have already been started.

Pneumococcal pneumonia is one of the respiratory infections for which we have a *urine antigen test*. A test for pneumococcal urinary antigen is about 70% sensitive and, unlike a sputum analysis, remains highly sensitive even if empiric antibiotic therapy has already been started. Send a pneumococcal urine antigen test along with sputum gram stain and cultures when laboratory testing for pneumonia is indicated.

Legionnaires' Disease

Legionnaires' disease, caused by *Legionella* species, typically presents as pneumonia. The patient's symptoms, physical exam, and/or chest x-ray cannot reliably distinguish it from other causes of pneumonia. However, suggestive features include high fevers, GI or neurologic symptoms, or certain high-risk exposures (eg, to a possible contaminated water supply or, more directly, to a local outbreak). Often the diagnosis is not suspected until the patient fails to respond to a β-lactam antibiotic.

Available testing for legionella infection includes a *urinary antigen test, sputum PCR,* and *sputum culture* (but the organism requires a special medium to grow so you must tell the lab that this is what you are looking for). The urine antigen test has the quickest turnaround time, on the order of 1 to at most 3 days. Sensitivity is around 75%, limited largely by the test's ability to detect only one serotype of the organism. Specificity is nearly 100%.

Even in patients with a positive urinary antigen, a sputum analysis should be obtained to identify the specific species as an epidemiologic aid in determining the source of the infection and thereby helping to control local outbreaks of the disease. Sputum PCR has a high specificity (83%) and may have a higher sensitivity (90%) than sputum culture (very variable depending on multiple factors such as sputum yield and culture techniques, with numbers running the gamut from 20% to 80%).

Procalcitonin

Bacterial infections can induce the synthesis of procalcitonin in tissues throughout the body, a process normally limited to the thyroid. Procalcitonin has been touted as a way to help distinguish bacterial pneumonia from other causes of respiratory symptoms including nonbacterial pneumonia. One advantage it offers is the short turnaround time to get a result, usually within 1 to 2 hours. There is evidence that employing it as a guide may reduce the use of antibiotics in patients with suspected pneumonia without increasing adverse outcomes. All of this may sound good, but:

- Procalcitonin is not as accurate in distinguishing bacterial pneumonia from viral pneumonia as we would like (sensitivity is ~55% and specificity is ~76%).

- Many other conditions—some medications, toxins, severe stressors such as burns, trauma, pancreatitis, fungal infections, and inflammatory and autoimmune disorders—can also cause an elevated procalcitonin.

- It is expensive.

So what is the bottom line regarding when and in whom to order a procalcitonin? Although it shows some promise, procalcitonin is not currently recommended as a guide for starting empiric therapy; in almost all cases of suspected bacterial pneumonia you will want to start empiric therapy anyway and wait for the other more definitive tests to come back. Procalcitonin may be useful for determining when hospitalized patients or patients with community-acquired pneumonia who have taken several days of an antibiotic can stop their medication; a declining procalcitonin below 0.25 ng/mL is usually used as a cutoff.

Procalcitonin remains a controversial topic, so rather than go it alone you should check with how the infectious disease specialists at your particular institution view it and what their experience has been.

Using Multiplex Polymerase Chain Reaction Testing for Respiratory Pathogens

As we already discussed on page 201, panels are available to screen for a wide array of respiratory pathogens, including many of those we've discussed in this chapter. These panels are increasingly being used, particularly in hospital settings, and especially for patients who are severely ill or immunocompromised where a precise diagnosis is likely to impact management. The test is run on a sample obtained via a nasopharyngeal swab. One potential pitfall is the incidental detection of colonizers—that is, organisms that are present but are not causing the patient's illness. These panels can also be extremely expensive. Exactly how and when to use these panels remains controversial.

EPSTEIN-BARR VIRUS

Infectious mononucleosis (IM) typically presents with pharyngitis, cervical (often posterior cervical) adenopathy, fever, and marked fatigue. The most specific symptom is splenomegaly (palatal petechiae are a close second), but it is present in fewer than 10% of patients at presentation. Although treatment for IM is purely supportive (specific antiviral therapy has no clear clinical benefit), diagnosis is important: patients who test positive should be counseled to temporarily avoid contact sports because of the associated risk of splenic rupture. Further, you can spare your patient unnecessary, potentially harmful antibiotics if you find that their upper respiratory infection is due to Epstein-Barr virus (EBV).

 Heterophile Antibodies

The initial test for IM is to look for *heterophile antibodies*. These are low-affinity IgM antibodies that bind to the red blood cells of species other than humans. They appear to play no role in the pathogenesis of IM; rather, they are just a by-product of the generalized B-cell activation induced by the virus. Heterophile antibody tests can be run rapidly. The most popular, the *monospot* test, has a sensitivity of about 85% and specificity of nearly 100%.* Heterophile antibodies are not usually present in children 4 years of age and younger, so diagnosis in this population should be done via serologic testing.

 ## Serologic Testing

Heterophile antibody assays can be negative during the first week of the illness. Although it is usually not necessary to confirm the diagnosis that quickly, when there is urgency—for example, in athletes who need to know if it is safe to play—you can order a *viral capsid antigen (VCA) IgM* that rises very quickly after infection. VCA IgM has very good specificity for acute IM and may catch early infections that are missed by heterophile testing (excellent sensitivity).

EBV VCA IgM is usually ordered as part of an EBV antibody profile, which also includes an *EBV VCA IgG* and *Epstein-Barr nuclear antigen (EBNA) IgG*. The VCA IgG is also elevated early in the disease and persists for the lifetime of the patient. EBNA rises much later, about 3 to 4 months after the onset of the illness, and also persists over the course of a lifetime. Therefore, a positive EBNA early in the course of a patient's illness indicates prior exposure to EBV but NOT acute IM. Most of the US population will have been exposed to EBV by early adulthood and—particularly in those who were infected early in life—will have had only mild disease or no symptoms at all and will therefore not know they were previously infected; the EBNA can confirm that they did in fact have IM at some point in the past.

Some EBV panels also include IgG to what is called the early antigen (EA). *EA IgG* comes in two varieties—anti-D and anti-R. Anti-D is consistent with recent infection and vanishes with recovery. It does not appear to add much to the information provided by the VCA IgM. Anti-R is only seen in a minority of patients, is of no real clinical utility, and is not always included in the laboratory analysis.

PCR testing, although available, has not been validated for the diagnosis of IM and is not Food and Drug Administration (FDA) approved for this purpose.

What about the role of persistent EBV infection in causing chronic fatigue? This is a controversial topic. The virus does persist in B cells for the lifetime of the patient and, as mentioned earlier, once individuals have had IM, immunologic evidence of infection persists as well. However, no clear-cut causal connection has been established with chronic fatigue syndrome (now renamed systemic exercise intolerance disease). Reactivation of latent EBV can occur, albeit not commonly, in settings of immunosuppression or whenever there is any stress—such as another infection—to the immune system.

There is a rare lymphoproliferative disorder called chronic active EBV infection, mostly seen in immunocompromised individuals, that is characterized by persistent EBV viremia, cytopenias, and a clonal lymphoid or natural killer (NK) cell population.

---

*But not exactly 100%; false positives occasionally occur with lymphoma, leukemia, malaria, and other viral infections such as cytomegalovirus (CMV).

Table 14.2 Epstein-Barr Virus Antibody Profiles

Status	VCA IgM	VCA IgG	EBNA IgG
No exposure	Negative	Negative	Negative
Acute infection	Positive	Positive	Negative
Past infection	Negative	Positive	Positive
Reactivation	Positive	Positive	Positive

IgG, immunoglobulin G; IgM, immunoglobulin M; EBNA, Epstein-Barr nuclear antigen; VCA, viral capsid antigen.

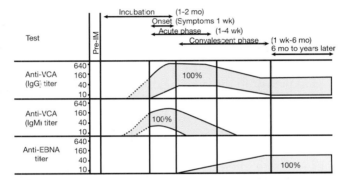

Figure 14.11 How the various antibody titers rise and fall during a typical course of IM. EBNA, Epstein-Barr nuclear antigen; IgG, immunoglobulin G; IgM, immunoglobulin M; IM, infectious mononucleosis; VCA, viral capsid antigen. (Adapted with permission from Henle G, Henle L. Horowitz CA. Epstein-Barr virus specific diagnostic tests in infectious mononucleosis. *Hum Pathol.* 1974;5:551.)

Patients with IM can be quite sick, and it is often appropriate to draw a CBC in these patients as part of the initial workup. The report may come back with several abnormalities. The white blood cell count is typically elevated (rarely above 20.000/µL) with more than 50% lymphocytes. Many—more than 10% of the lymphocytes—may be described as *atypical lymphocytes*. These cells have abundant cytoplasm, are larger than normal lymphocytes and are often oddly shaped (see Figure 14.12).* The presence of more than 10% atypical lymphocytes has a sensitivity of approximately 75% and a specificity of approximately 92% for IM; if there are more than 20% atypical lymphocytes, the specificity rises to 98%. Atypical lymphocytes are therefore associated in most people's minds with IM, but the specificity is not 100%, and they can also be seen in a host of other acute viral illnesses, such as viral hepatitis, HIV infection, and various childhood illnesses such as measles, mumps, and rubella (MMR).

---

*For those of you who wish to know, these atypical lymphocytes are activated cytotoxic T cells.

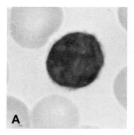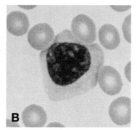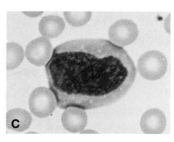

Figure 14.12 A. A normal, typical lymphocyte. B and C. Atypical lymphocytes in a patient with infectious mononucleosis; note the copious cytoplasm and odd shapes compared to the normal cell. (From Greer JP, Arber DA, Glader B, et al. *Wintrobe's Clinical Hematology*. 13th ed. Lippincott Williams & Wilkins; 2014.)

Patients may also have mild thrombocytopenia. Other findings, such as hemolytic anemia, can be seen with severe disease.

More common—and present in the large majority of patients at some point in the course of their illness—are *elevated liver transaminases*. These can get quite high but typically return to baseline as the disease resolves. This finding is so common that you should suspect another diagnosis if the patient's liver panel is normal.

CYTOMEGALOVIRUS

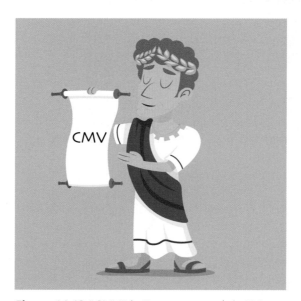

Figure 14.13 "CMV" in Roman numerals is 905. This useless fact, something we couldn't help noticing and that has gone unremarked in the medical literature, has no clinical significance. (Courtesy Meilun/Shutterstock.)

Most of us are infected with CMV at some point in our lives, but few of us know it. In immunocompetent patients, CMV infection typically presents without symptoms or as a self-limited EBV-like mononucleosis syndrome ("heterophile negative mononucleosis"). Laboratory testing may help confirm the diagnosis in such cases but rarely changes management.

Immunocompromised patients, on the other hand, are much more likely to develop organ- or life-threatening disease due to CMV. Prompt diagnosis can mean the difference between life (with the initiation of appropriate antiviral therapy) and death. Even among such patients, however, it is important to remember that CMV infection may occur in the absence of associated clinically significant disease.

CMV *disease* is only diagnosed when the patient is both infected with CMV (eg, PCR and/or serology is positive) *and* has an otherwise unexplained clinical illness that can be reasonably attributed to CMV.

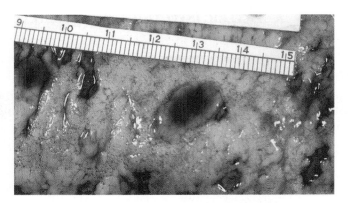

Figure 14.14 The ulcerated colon of a patient who required a bowel resection for cytomegalovirus colitis. Prompt diagnosis is paramount. (From Riddell R, Jain D. *Lewin, Weinstein and Riddell's Gastrointestinal Pathology and Its Clinical Implications.* 2nd ed. Wolters Kluwer Health; 2014.)

 ## *Polymerase Chain Reaction*

NAAT by PCR allows for the detection and quantification of CMV DNA in a sample (eg, blood, stool, CSF, tissue biopsy). Many assays are available, all of which tend to have excellent sensitivity and specificity. In general, if invasive or disseminated CMV is suspected, both the blood and a sample from the affected compartment (eg, bronchoalveolar lavage in pneumonitis or stool in colitis) should be sent for CMV PCR. However, many patients without actual CMV disease, especially if immunocompromised, may shed CMV from various sites, including the lungs, GI tract, and the CNS (detected in the CSF). Therefore, a positive PCR from one of these compartments does not necessarily indicate active infection.

The best way to confirm active infection is tissue biopsy (see section "Microscopy With Staining").

Most assays can detect a viral load as low as less than 100 units/mL and as high as more than 10,000,000 units/mL. There is no widely established consensus on what viral load should universally be considered clinically significant—the clinical picture, then, is all the more important in making the diagnosis of CMV disease. If the viral load is low and the clinical picture is uncertain, trending the viral load over time may help determine if CMV disease is in the process of developing or worsening.

 ## Antigen Testing

CMV antigen testing involves detection of a viral protein called *pp65* by immunofluorescence.

Specimen handling can be challenging and involved, and sensitivity can be very poor in patients with baseline neutropenia. Because of these limitations, PCR is by far the more popular test.

 ## Antibody Testing

IgM antibodies usually become detectable within 2 weeks of the onset of symptoms, followed by IgG antibodies about a week later. IgM antibodies subsequently wane over a few months, whereas IgG antibodies tend to persist for life. Here's what all this means for the interpretation of CMV antibody testing:

- The presence of IgM antibodies makes CMV infection within the past few months very likely. However, a single measurement of CMV IgM antibodies cannot reliably distinguish between acute (within 1-2 weeks) and recent (within a few months) infection.

- The absence of IgM antibodies does not rule out acute CMV infection, especially if symptoms have been present for less than 2 weeks.

- The presence of IgG antibodies indicates past CMV exposure; it does *not* distinguish among those with active, asymptomatic, or resolved disease.

- IgG antibody titers that increase by at least 4-fold over at least 2 weeks indicate likely acute CMV infection.

Serology is commonly used to diagnose CMV disease in immunocompetent patients. PCR is the preferred method in those who are immunocompromised, at least in part because it provides rapid and reliable results that do not require repeat sample acquisition. Additionally, those who are immunocompromised may have impaired antibody production, theoretically reducing the sensitivity of serologic testing.

There are a few specific clinical scenarios in which CMV serology is particularly helpful. Because CMV is known to persist in a latent state inside host monocytes after initial infection, those with IgG positivity—and therefore evidence of past exposure—are at risk for future reactivation, especially if they are immunocompromised, and may warrant monitoring as a result. CMV serologic status is also commonly assessed in potential organ transplant recipients and donors. A patient who is seronegative (ie, CMV IgG negative) is at risk for acquisition of CMV disease from an organ donor who is seropositive.

 ## Viral Culture

Culture media containing human fibroblasts can be used to grow CMV from blood, CSF, or any other infected source. CMV can usually be detected within 2 to 3 days. Sensitivity, however, tends to be poor, particularly for blood samples. Overall, given the availability of better tests such as PCR, viral cultures are not commonly performed.

 ## Microscopy with Staining

When noninvasive methods are unrevealing and/or when tissue biopsy is feasible (or obtained for other reasons), microscopy with staining can be used to identify the intracellular inclusions characteristic of CMV-infected tissues. This is the gold-standard test for the diagnosis of tissue-invasive CMV.

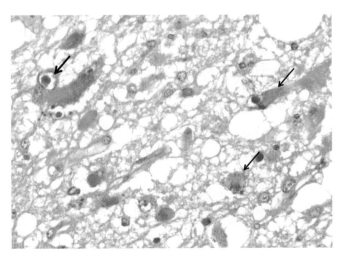

Figure 14.15 Both intranuclear inclusions (thick arrow, top left) and intracytoplasmic inclusions (thin arrows) may be seen in cytomegalovirus-infected tissues. (From Murat G. *Neuropathologic Evaluation: From Pathologic Features to Diagnosis*. Wolters Kluwer Health/Lippincott Williams & Wilkins; 2013.)

COVID-19

There are three types of tests for the SARS-CoV-2 virus that causes COVID-19. Two (real-time polymerase chain reaction [RT-PCR] and rapid antigen testing) are widely used and important, and one (anti-SARS-CoV-2 antibodies) should be used only in rare circumstances.

 ## *Real-Time Polymerase Chain Reaction*

This test detects viral RNA and is extremely sensitive, able to detect as few as hundreds or even just tens of viral particles. It is considered the gold standard for testing patients with suspected acute infection. The test sample should be obtained with a nasopharyngeal swab (some labs will run the test on saliva). Sensitivity and specificity for SARS-CoV-2 infection are said to approach 100%, but one must then ask—compared to what? There is no other useful meaningful standard. The main drawback to PCR testing is that it can detect RNA fragments as well as intact virus, and therefore mistakenly indicate that infection is ongoing when actually the body is just shedding viral remnants. PCR may remain positive for weeks to months after the clinical resolution of infection.

 ## *Rapid Antigen Testing*

This test for viral proteins is the one that people perform at home (a point-of-care test). You have almost certainly seen the test cards and have watched the sample move along the surface where it interacts at one line with test antibodies and another with a control. These types of assays are referred to as *lateral flow assays*. It takes only a few minutes to get a result. Like the PCR, the sample should be obtained via a nasopharyngeal swab (again, some tests can be run on saliva).

Rapid antigen testing is not nearly as sensitive as PCR, requiring millions of virus particles to turn positive. It is therefore not of much use in asymptomatic patients—for example, at the very onset of infection—when the viral load is small. Because of its convenience, its main role is in diagnosing infection in symptomatic patients. Rapid tests turn positive within several days of the onset of symptoms. Sensitivity ranges widely—from 30% to 90%—in symptomatic patients depending upon the test (and there are many of them), the timing, the presence or absence of symptoms, and the dominant circulating variant. However, the lower sensitivity compared to PCR testing may actually be a boon, because it will report a positive result only when there is a high viral load, sufficiently high to make the infection contagious to others. Specificity is above 90%, but of course this means that there are occasional false positives.

Anti-SARS-CoV-2 Antibodies

There are almost no reasons to order this test. Antibody titers start to rise approximately 1 to 2 weeks after infection, so it is of no use in diagnosing acute infection. Titers do not correlate well with immune protection. The only value of this test is to confirm prior infection or vaccination, but as of this writing virtually everyone has had the disease at least once and/or been vaccinated.

TUBERCULOSIS

Although TB is uncommon in the United States—where there are an estimated 9,000 cases per year—approximately 10 million people per year are diagnosed with TB worldwide, and 1.4 million people die of the disease. It has been estimated that as many as 1.7 *billion* people worldwide may actually harbor latent TB, of whom 5% to 10% will go on to develop active disease at some point during their lifetimes.

 ## Screening for Latent Tuberculosis

Generalized screening of the population as a whole is not recommended. Screening for TB should be directed toward patients at high risk for TB. These include:

- Anyone who has been in contact with someone who has tested positive for TB or likely has TB
- All infants, children, and adolescents exposed to an adult with latent or active TB
- Health care workers who care for patients who are at high risk for TB
- Employees and residents of homeless shelters, nursing homes, and correctional facilities
- People who have been medically underserved
- Anyone with a history of drug or alcohol abuse
- Patients with HIV, diabetes mellitus, silicosis, chronic renal failure, malignancy, leukemia, body weight less than 90% of ideal, or who have had a gastrectomy or jejunoileal bypass
- Patients on immunosuppressive therapy
- Recent immigrants (within the previous 5 years) from (or frequent travelers to) a country with a high rate of TB

There are two types of tests that are used to screen for latent TB: *tuberculin skin test (TST)* and *interferon gamma release assays (IGRAs)* of the blood. Neither tests directly for *Mycobacterium tuberculosis.* Rather, they look for evidence of cellular immunity to the organism that would indicate the patient has had a prior infection. Although their specificity and sensitivity differ somewhat, they have been shown to be equally effective at preventing future cases of active TB. Neither test, however, is able to rule out TB with 100% accuracy, even when used together. And, importantly, neither can distinguish latent TB from active TB.

Tuberculin Skin Test

This test, properly called the Mantoux tuberculin test, involves intradermal injection of a collection of tuberculin antigens referred to as *purified protein derivative (PPD).** Many clinicians simply refer to this test as "a PPD."

The test is administered as follows:

- Draw up 0.1 mL (5 tuberculin units) of tuberculin into a 27-gauge syringe (colloquially known as a TB syringe); make sure the solution has not expired!

- Clean a small area of the patient's volar forearm with an alcohol swab.

- Enter at a 15° angle (yes, that is nearly parallel to the arm), creating a small intradermal bubble (if there is no bubble, you have not done the injection properly).

- If there is a small spot of blood after you withdraw the needle, you can gently remove it with a gauze pad or cotton ball without affecting the result.

- Wait 48 to 72 hours and have the patient return so the test result can be ascertained. Do not wait longer—20% of positive tests will be negative if read after 72 hours.

- If there is a wheal, measure the largest diameter in millimeters. Measure the induration, not the extent of any erythema. It is the diameter of induration that matters.

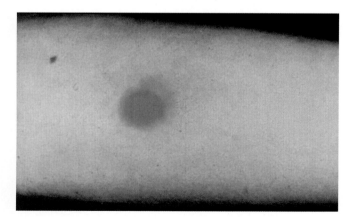

Figure 14.16 A positive PPD test. (From Onofrey BE, Leonid S, Holdeman NR. *Ocular Therapeutics Handbook: A Clinical Manual.* 4th ed. Wolters Kluwer; 2020.)

---

*PPD is actually a bunch of molecules—the majority of which are proteins—collected from culture media of *M. tuberculosis.*

A wheal is a sign of a positive reaction, but how big a wheal? That depends on why you are doing the test and who your patient is:

Table 14.3 What Qualifies as a Positive PPD

Size of Wheal Considered Positive	Patients in Whom This Is Positive
Any reaction	Patients with HIV with close contact with a contagious person
≥5 mm	Patients with HIV, close contacts of contagious persons, immunosuppressed patients, patients with fibrotic changes on chest x-ray consistent with old TB
≥10 mm	Patients at high risk of reactivation (see discussion earlier; this includes health care workers), children under the age of 4, residents of high-risk settings, persons born abroad from regions with a high incidence of TB
≥15 mm	Anyone over the age of 4 with a low likelihood of TB (not falling into any of the above categories)

PPD, purified protein derivative; TB, tuberculosis.

Interferon Gamma Release Assays

These are blood tests. Blood is drawn up into several separate tubes usually in a kit supplied by your lab.

There are two of these tests currently available in the United States:

1. *QuantiFERON-TB Gold Plus* uses ELISA technology to measure the level of interferon that is produced when the patient's blood is exposed to mycobacterial antigens.

2. The *T-SPOT.TB* works under the same principle, but measures the number of interferon-secreting cells when exposed to mycobacterial antigens.

Results of either are reported as positive, negative, or indeterminate/invalid (ie, uninterpretable). An indeterminate/invalid result may occur in the setting of high-dose steroid use, advanced HIV, or sometimes pregnancy. Indeterminate/invalid tests should be repeated.

Which Test Should I Order?

In most settings, either the TST or an IGRA is fine—you can ask your patients which they would prefer. As mentioned earlier, the two tests are equivalent in terms of reducing reactivation of TB (up to 90% compared to those who are not tested and treated).

Interferon testing offers the advantage that the patient does not have to return for a second visit. It is therefore a good choice in patients who may not be able to return to have their skin test read. It is also more specific than the TST, which does not distinguish between

M. tuberculosis and atypical mycobacterial antigens. The TST may also be positive in patients who have been vaccinated with *Bacillus Calmette-Guérin* (BCG),* whereas interferon testing is not affected by prior BCG vaccination.

However, the TST has advantages as well: it is less expensive and does not require a laboratory to run the test.

So how do you decide? In most instances, shared decision-making with your patient is the way to go.

With either method, if you are testing someone with a history of close contact with someone who has TB and get a negative result, a second test should be done 8 to 10 weeks later. This is recommended because early after exposure the TST and interferon tests may still be negative.

People traveling to areas where TB is endemic should be tested both before (to get a baseline) and 8 to 10 weeks after returning from their trip.

When the Tuberculin Skin Test and Interferon Gamma Release Assay Disagree

What should you do if you get both tests, either together or serially, and one comes back positive and one negative? Do you just go ahead and treat for latent TB—knowing that the commonly used medications carry potential side effects—or do you just follow your patient clinically?

Suppose the PPD comes back positive in a patient at low risk who is from a region with a very low prevalence of TB. It is then reasonable to check an IGRA, primarily to rule out a nontuberculous mycobacterial infection. Let's say the IGRA now comes back negative. Although the risk of TB is low in this situation, it is not zero; patients with discordant results have a higher risk of TB than those in whom both tests are negative.

For all patients who are tested for TB, but especially for those with discordant results, there are online calculators that can help you determine the chances that your patient has latent TB that will one day reactivate; these take into account risk factors such as age, exposure, immigration history, and BCG vaccination history. But these will not give you a yes or no answer, only a percent probability that can be helpful in deciding your next steps.

Two-Step Testing: Boosted Tuberculin Skin Test

After many years—exactly how long varies from person to person—immune reactivity to TB can wane. Therefore, the Centers for Disease Control and Prevention (CDC) recommends two-step TST in patients who have not been tested in years. Two-step testing is also recommended as baseline screening for those who have never been tested before, for those without documentation of prior testing, for health care workers, and for other persons who require periodic testing such as nursing home residents.

---

*BCG is an attenuated strain of *Mycobacterium bovis* often given in regions with high rates of TB to reduce the risk of TB in children.

How does two-step testing work to increase the sensitivity of TST? In patients with a remote TB exposure whose immunity has waned, the first TST is not sufficient to generate a positive test, but it is able to reawaken the body's memory of the prior TB infection. The second TST, done 1 to 3 weeks later on the opposite forearm, functions as a booster, and—with their immunologic memory rejuvenated—will elicit a positive response.

 ## Testing Patients Who May Have Active Tuberculosis

When you have a patient who by history and exam may have active TB—the appropriate term now is *tuberculosis disease*—you will need to order a chest x-ray and *sputum for an acid-fast bacillus (AFB) smear and culture.** A positive TST or IGRA indicates a likely history of TB infection but is neither sensitive nor specific for the diagnosis of active disease.

The *AFB smear* is a simple procedure with a quick turnaround time. By acid fast, we mean that once the bacteria have been stained with dye, they do not decolorize when an acid solution is applied; under the light microscope, they will hold the dye and appear red or pink. This traditional staining technique has poor sensitivity. However, sensitivity increases when multiple specimens are collected. Therefore, we advise repeating sputum collection for AFB smears 3 times with at least 8 hours between samples.

Many labs today use a fluorochrome dye and, when available, light-emitting diode (LED) microscopy, a technique that further increases sensitivity compared to traditional staining and light microscopy. None of these techniques, however, can distinguish *M. tuberculosis* from other acid-fast organisms.

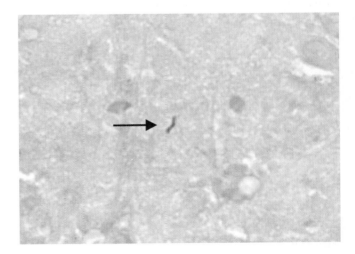

Figure 14.17 The arrow points to an acid-fast mycobacterium. (From Torbenson MS. *Biopsy Interpretation of the Liver.* 4th ed. Wolters Kluwer; 2022.)

---

*In patients with extrapulmonary TB, you will want to obtain samples from any other infected region(s) as well as the sputum; the more sites you sample, the higher the yield.

How to Collect a Sputum Sample for an Acid-Fast Bacillus Smear

Obtaining a good sputum sample is key to making the diagnosis of active TB. You should collect at least 3 mL of sputum (although most labs will accept 2 mL). Testing is best done first thing in the morning. After rinsing out the mouth, patients should be instructed to take a deep breath, hold it for 5 seconds, repeat the deep breath, and then cough forcibly. The sputum that accumulates in the mouth is then spat into a collecting cup.

A *sputum culture* is essential in any patient with suspected active TB. It is typically required to pin down the diagnosis and is the only test that can reliably determine drug susceptibility.

Sputum culture is both more specific and more sensitive than the AFB smear for active TB. Whereas the AFB stain will be positive only when there are at least 10,000 bacteria/mL, culture can detect as few as 10 bacteria/mL. However, TB takes up to several weeks to grow in cultures.

NAAT can confirm the diagnosis of active TB far more rapidly than cultures—within 1 to 3 days—but is less sensitive than cultures. Some believe that it may soon replace the AFB smear as an initial rapid test. Some but not all NAAT assays can identify the organism's pattern of drug resistance.

FUNGAL DISEASES

Invasive fungal disease typically demands an aggressive diagnostic workup, whereas a minor or superficial fungal infection does not.

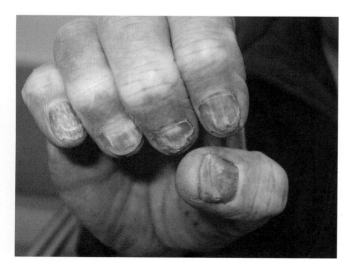

Figure 14.18 Diagnosis of nail fungus, or *onychomycosis*, typically requires only a history and physical. If you are uncertain of the diagnosis, nail clippings can be sent to the lab for analysis. (From Stedman TL. *Stedman's Medical Dictionary*. 28th ed. Lippincott Williams & Wilkins; 2006.)

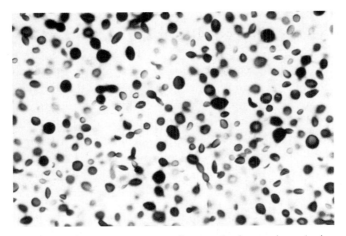

Figure 14.19 *Cryptococcus neoformans* in the cerebrospinal fluid of a patient with cryptococcal meningitis. When cryptococcal infection is a possibility, aggressive and timely laboratory testing must be pursued. (From Cornelissen CN, Hobbs MM. *Lippincott Illustrated Reviews: Microbiology*. 4th ed. Wolters Kluwer; 2020.)

Invasive fungal infections are much more common in patients who are severely immunocompromised. Immunocompromised patients also tend to have a significantly higher organism burden, meaning that in the setting of any given fungal infection, they tend to be infected with a higher number of organisms than those who are immunocompetent. Taken together, these two facts mean that the yield of fungal tests tends to be higher in immunocompromised patients.

Here we emphasize some of the most widely used tests for fungal diseases, many of which can detect multiple different species of fungus.

Fungal Cultures

Although some fungi grow in standard bacterial culture media, many require modified media. Sabouraud agar, which contains peptones (short protein chains) that allow many fungi to grow, is a common choice. If you suspect a fungal infection, communicate your suspicions to the laboratory (eg, as a comment on the order for cultures) in case media modifications are needed.

Fungal cultures allow for antimicrobial susceptibility testing once a given organism is identified. Their sensitivity depends on the organism and specimen source. Because many fungi grow slowly, fungal cultures may take weeks to turn positive.

Given the limited sensitivity and long turnaround time of fungal cultures, additional testing (discussed on the next several pages) is usually indicated in the meantime.

Fungal Wet Mount: KOH and Saline Prep

Fungal wet mount entails microscopic examination of a specimen (eg, a skin scraping or body fluid) suspended in a solution of either potassium hydroxide (KOH, a procedure aptly termed a *KOH prep*) or saline. Often, a substance called calcofluor white is added; it binds to components of fungal cell walls and produces a fluorescent glow, improving visualization.

The most common indications for a wet mount include suspected superficial fungal infections of the skin, hair/scalp, nails, or mucous membranes. Examples include dermatophyte infections (eg, tinea cruris or ringworm) and candidal vaginitis. In cases of minor or superficial infections, a wet mount alone is usually sufficient to make a diagnosis in the setting of a compatible history and physical.

The biggest advantage of a wet mount is its rapid turnaround time—you can do this yourself in the office (see page 238). Sensitivity varies significantly by specimen source and organism, but overall is poor enough that, most of the time, you should not consider a negative wet mount to be definitive evidence that a patient does not have a fungal infection, especially if your clinical suspicion is high. When positive, wet mount allows for visualization of the basic morphology of any fungi that are present, which is usually sufficient to identify the culprit organism. Wet mount is not quite as specific as fungal cultures; occasional false positives may result from misinterpretation of calcofluor dye binding patterns (eg, binding to blood vessels in the sample).

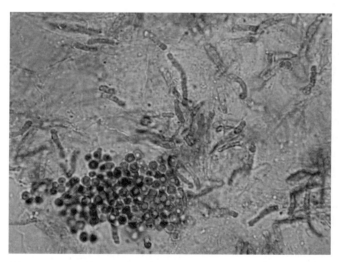

Figure 14.20 Classic "spaghetti and meatballs" appearance of *Malassezia* species (the cause of tinea versicolor) on a KOH prep. (From Goroll A, Mulley AG. *Primary Care Medicine: Office Evaluation and Management of the Adult Patient*. 8th ed. Wolters Kluwer; 2021.)

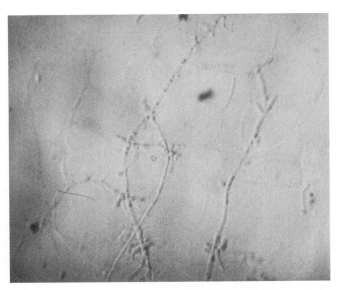

Figure 14.21 A KOH prep showing branching hyphae typical of *Candida* species. (From Fleisher GR, Ludwig S, Baskin MN. *Atlas of Pediatric Emergency Medicine*. Lippincott Williams & Wilkins; 2004.)

 ## β-ᴅ-*Glucan*

1,3-β-ᴅ-glucan (BG) is a cell wall component shared by many fungi, including *Aspergillus* species, *Candida* species, and *P. jirovecii*, all of which can be detected by this test. Zygomycetes such as *Mucor* and *Rhizopus* species (causes of mucormycosis) and *Cryptococcus* species must be diagnosed by other means—they lack BG in their cell wall. Experts differ on whether or not a serum BG should be part of the workup of all patients with suspected invasive fungal disease. It is probably most helpful in patients who are severely immunocompromised.

BG is detected by spectrophotometry, a method that identifies a given compound's characteristic pattern of absorption or emission of light over a particular range of wavelengths. Ultimately, the output of the assay is an *optical density* of light, which can then be mathematically converted to a BG concentration.

Results greater than 80 pg/mL are considered positive and are highly suggestive of fungal infection. Estimates of specificity range from 75% to 95% depending on the organism and source of infection. Specificity tends to increase as BG concentration increases above 80 pg/L. *Positive* and *specific* here mean that the patient likely has a fungal infection, but identification of which fungal infection requires additional testing. Sending a BG alone tends not to be sufficient for the workup of invasive fungal disease; fungal cultures, wet mount, and organism-specific testing (discussed on the next few pages) should be sent along with it.

Occasional false positives may occur in patients infected with *Pseudomonas aeruginosa* (a bacterium, not a fungus), because this organism contains a protein similar to the BG found in many fungi. Otherwise, most false positives are due to iatrogenic causes such as the introduction of cellulose fibers found in certain hemodialysis membranes or some surgical gauzes, or the recent administration of IVIG or even albumin.

Results less than 60 pg/mL are considered negative. Estimates of the sensitivity of various BG assays range from 55% to 95% depending on the population, organism, and infectious source. In the case of suspected invasive aspergillosis, BG is believed to be significantly more sensitive than galactomannan (see Table 14.4). Overall, a negative BG should generally decrease your suspicion for a fungal infection, but should not rule out the possibility entirely if the pretest probability is high.

Results between 60 and 80 pg/mL are regarded as indeterminate and generally should not drastically alter your suspicion (ie, posttest probability) for fungal infection.

 ## *Organism-Specific Testing*

When added to one or more of the abovementioned tests, organism-specific tests tend to improve diagnostic sensitivity and specificity. Table 14.4 highlights the pros and cons of some of the most important organism-specific tests.

Table 14.4 Organism-Specific Testing

Organism	Test	Key Points
Aspergillus spp.	Galactomannan antigen (serum or BAL)—component of *Aspergillus* cell wall	Predictive value for invasive disease depends heavily on the clinical situation: for example, positive predictive value is excellent in a bone marrow transplant recipient, but fairly poor in an otherwise healthy patient.
	PCR (serum)	Sensitivity ~85%, specificity ~75%: both improve when multiple specimens are sent.
Pneumocystis jirovecii	PCR (BAL, induced sputum, or lung tissue)	High sensitivity and specificity
	Microscopy with staining (eg, GMS, Wright-Giemsa)	Sensitivity may exceed 95% on BAL.
	Culture	This organism cannot be cultured.

Table 14.4 Organism-Specific Testing (*continued*)

Organism	Test	Key Points
Candida spp.[a]	Culture	Grows on bacterial and standard fungal media
	PCR	Not routinely used
	T2Candida assay (serum)—novel DNA amplification and detection technique	Rapid and highly sensitive but expensive and not universally available
Cryptococcus spp.	Antigen (serum or CSF)	High sensitivity and specificity Sensitivity for cryptococcal pneumonia is nearly 100% in those with AIDS but drops to 60%-70% in those with other immunocompromising conditions.
	Culture	Requires special media to optimize sensitivity
	Microscopy with staining—India Ink	Rapid turnaround time but poor sensitivity
	PCR	Can be done alone or as part of a multiplex panel Rapid turnaround time High sensitivity and specificity in patients with AIDS; accuracy not well established in other populations
Histoplasma capsulatum	Antigen (serum, urine, or BAL)	High specificity (other endemic mycoses may cause occasional false positives) BAL is sensitive for pulmonary histoplasmosis; otherwise the sensitivity of this test is not very good.
	Antibody	Titers rise 2-4 wk from symptom onset and may persist for years. Does not distinguish chronic vs resolved infection
	PCR	Not routinely used

(continued)

Table 14.4 Organism-Specific Testing (*continued*)

Organism	Test	Key Points
Blastomyces spp.	Antigen (serum or urine)	High sensitivity but specificity <80%
	Antibody	Not routinely used
	PCR	Not routinely used
Coccidioides spp.	Antibody	Two-step testing: ELISA → confirmatory immunodiffusion Antibodies do ***not*** persist after resolution of infection; positive result indicates active or recent infection.
	Antigen (serum, urine, or CSF)	Sensitivity and specificity are not well established but specificity is likely >90%. Consider sending along with antibody testing in severely immunocompromised patients.
	PCR	Not routinely used

BAL, bronchoalveolar lavage; CSF, cerebrospinal fluid; ELISA, enzyme-linked immunosorbent assay; GMS, Gomori methenamine silver; PCR, polymerase chain reaction.
[a]Beware: *Candida* is a common colonizer of the gastrointestinal/genitourinary tracts, skin, and oral mucosa.

What About Noninvasive Aspergillosis?

Noninvasive aspergillosis may present as an *aspergilloma* (a fungus ball typically found in a lung cavity that was previously formed by an unrelated disease such as TB or emphysema; diagnosis may often be made radiographically) or as *allergic bronchopulmonary aspergillosis (ABPA)*, a form of hypersensitivity to *Aspergillus* seen in immunocompetent patients with asthma. In ABPA, asthma-like and constitutional symptoms are common. Laboratory diagnosis entails checking *total serum IgE* (a result >1,000 ng/mL supports the diagnosis of ABPA), the *serum eosinophil count* (a result >500/mm³ supports the diagnosis), and several tests for *Aspergillus*-specific hypersensitivity:

- *Aspergillus antigen skin testing*: the antigen is injected subcutaneously—significant inflammation at the site of injection 48 to 72 hours later is considered a positive result.

- *Serum precipitating antibodies to Aspergillus*

- *Serum anti-Aspergillus IgE and IgG antibodies*

Diagnostic criteria are complex; overall, a definitive diagnosis of ABPA requires that several of the abovementioned tests are positive. Note that galactomannan is not on the list of tests—it is not helpful in the diagnosis of ABPA.

HUMAN IMMUNODEFICIENCY VIRUS

There are two main reasons to send HIV testing:

1. Diagnosis: rule out acute or chronic infection in a patient with compatible symptoms (eg, acute retroviral syndrome, which can include unexplained constitutional symptoms, lymphadenopathy, pharyngitis, mucocutaneous ulcers, rash, diarrhea).

2. Screening: precise recommendations vary by organization.

   • The CDC recommends screening *all* individuals between ages 13 and 64 at least once, regardless of the presence or absence of risk factors.

   • Those with risk factors (eg, recent HIV exposure, intravenous [IV] drug use, high-risk sexual activity) should be tested at least yearly, and as often as every 3 to 6 months.

   • HIV testing is recommended for pregnant women during each pregnancy (ideally during the first trimester).

Your overall threshold for sending HIV testing should be low. Acute HIV infection has many mimics, such as infectious mononucleosis or even a typical viral upper respiratory infection. Chronic infection can easily go unnoticed as patients may remain asymptomatic for years until developing a potentially deadly opportunistic infection, such as *Pneumocystis jirovecii* pneumonia (PJP). Additionally, making the diagnosis of HIV early drastically alters its clinical trajectory. Available treatments (antiretroviral therapy [ART]) are extremely effective in driving down the viral load, driving up the CD4 cell count, and preventing disease complications.

The two essential tests for diagnosis are the fourth-generation antigen/antibody immunoassay and HIV RNA (viral load).

 ## Fourth-Generation Combination Antigen/Antibody Immunoassay

The combined antigen/antibody immunoassay is the initial test of choice regardless of the presence or absence of symptoms or suspected disease chronicity. This test is "combined" in that it detects both the *p24 antigen* (a protein that forms the capsid around the viral RNA) and antibodies to *p24*, *gp 41*, and *gp 120* (the latter two antigens are components of the viral envelope that facilitate entry into the host cell). Results are reported as positive or negative.

Sensitivity and specificity are excellent, with one very important caveat: p24 antigen does not become detectable until about 2 to 3 weeks after exposure, and the antibodies take 3 weeks to 3 months to become detectable. This means that *the fourth-generation immunoassay will occasionally miss acute HIV infection, especially if exposure occurred less than 2 weeks prior to testing.* For this reason, if acute infection is suspected, HIV RNA testing (discussed next) should be sent along with the combination immunoassay. When acute infection is not a concern, a negative combination immunoassay reliably rules out HIV.

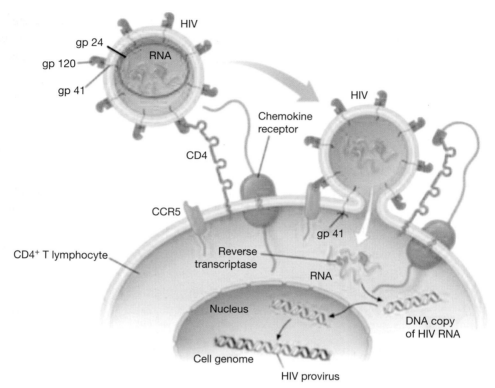

Figure 14.22 Diagram of the structure of the HIV virion as it infects a CD4 cell. The fourth-generation HIV immunoassay detects the p24 antigen (here labeled "gp 24") and antibodies to p24, gp 41, and gp 120. Earlier generations of this test are not as sensitive because they detect the antibodies only (not the p24 antigen). (From Pawlina W, Ross MH. *Histology: A Text and Atlas.* 8th ed. Wolters Kluwer; 2018.)

Some institutions may label the combination immunoassay test "HIV-1/2 screen," which refers to the fact that the target antigen and antibodies are found in infection with both subtypes of HIV, HIV-1 and HIV-2, which are otherwise clinically indistinguishable but have different drug resistance patterns. A positive immunoassay result reflexes to an *HIV-1/HIV-2 differentiation assay*, which allows for tailoring of treatment to HIV-1 or HIV-2. A positive antigen/antibody test followed by a *negative* HIV-1/HIV-2 differentiation assay is considered overall an indeterminate result and should be followed by an HIV RNA test.

 ## RNA (Viral Load) Testing

Because the overall sensitivity and specificity of the combination immunoassay is excellent, additional testing is often not required. There are, however, a few situations in which NAAT (also just called nucleic acid testing, or NAT) for HIV RNA should be sent:

- *Suspected acute infection*: Because HIV viremia can be detected as early as 5 days after exposure, NAAT can occasionally detect early infection that is missed by immunoassay. However, even

NAAT may miss cases of acute HIV in patients with extremely recent exposure (anywhere from 5 to 15 days prior). If both the combination immunoassay and HIV RNA are negative in such a patient and clinical suspicion for HIV remains, testing should be repeated 1 to 2 weeks later.

- *Positive combination immunoassay with a negative HIV-1/HIV-2 differentiation assay*: This result is considered "indeterminate" and may be the result of isolated p24 antigen positivity (which would not trigger a positive differentiation assay). In this scenario, a positive HIV RNA test confirms (presumably acute) infection. A negative HIV RNA test rules out infection in the vast majority of cases; some clinicians choose to repeat a fourth-generation screen in a few months.

- *Disease and treatment monitoring*: Periodic monitoring of the viral load (along with CD4 count) should be performed in patients with confirmed HIV to track the disease course and help determine the treatment response.

- Other clinical scenarios in which HIV RNA testing is recommended include suspected neonatal HIV infection and HIV screening of donor blood.

Many HIV RNA tests can detect a viral load as low as 20 copies/mL. Patients with acute HIV infection typically have a viral load more than 100,000 copies/mL. A weakly positive result (eg, <2,000 copies/mL) may warrant repeat testing to rule out a false positive; consider consultation with an infectious disease specialist in this scenario.

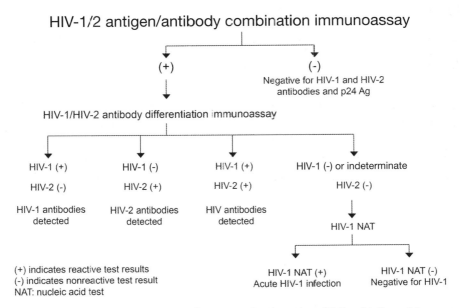

Figure 14.23 Suggested algorithm for HIV testing based on CDC guidelines. Many consider those with suspected acute infection to be an exception because the combination immunoassay alone cannot reliably rule out HIV in these patients; adding on a NAT test up front may increase sensitivity in these individuals. (Courtesy Centers for Disease Control and Prevention [CDC].)

Other Laboratory Features Associated With Human Immunodeficiency Virus

The following lab results are seen in some but not all patients with HIV:

- Cytopenias, most commonly leukopenia with lymphopenia; less commonly mild anemia and/or thrombocytopenia

- Occasional atypical lymphocytes on blood smear or a false-positive heterophile antibody test. Taken together with symptoms such as sore throat and lymphadenopathy, this may lead to mistaking acute HIV infection for IM. Repeat testing (both the heterophile test and HIV antigen/antibody) may be helpful if your suspicion for HIV is high.

- Elevated liver enzymes (usually mild elevations in aspartate aminotransferase [AST] or alanine aminotransferase [ALT]); it is unclear to what extent these findings, when present, may represent a direct effect of the HIV virus versus comorbid conditions or antiretroviral medication toxicity.

 Once the Diagnosis Is Made

In addition to checking an HIV RNA viral load, several tests are recommended in any patient newly diagnosed with HIV:

1. **CD4 helper T-cell count by flow cytometry**

   The CD4 count correlates with the patient's degree of susceptibility to opportunistic infections and helps to determine if any infectious prophylaxis is indicated. The CD4 count should subsequently be followed periodically along with viral load to monitor disease course and treatment response.

   - A normal CD4 count for an otherwise healthy person is at least 800 cells/μL. AIDS is diagnosed at a CD4 count less than 200 cells/μL, at which point prophylaxis for *P. jirovecii* is indicated.

   - The absolute CD4 count can be misleadingly high in a patient with leukocytosis or misleadingly low in a patient with leukopenia. In these scenarios, the CD4 *percentage* can be helpful; we expect the CD4 percentage to change significantly along with the absolute CD4 count if patients have had a true change in their HIV-related immunologic status. For example, a patient with HIV who develops leukopenia while on an antibiotic may have a drop in the absolute CD4 count that corresponds to the drop in total white blood cell count. If the CD4 percentage remains stable compared to previously, it is unlikely that the drop in absolute CD4 count is HIV related. As a point of reference, in a patient with a normal white blood cell count, a CD4 count of 500 corresponds to a CD4 percentage of about 29%, and a CD4 count of 200 corresponds to a CD4 percentage of about 14%.

   - The CD4 count has traditionally been monitored every 3 to 6 months in patients with HIV. However, for patients who have been on ART for 2 years or more whose CD4 count has remained stable and viral load undetectable, the protocol can be relaxed.

Those with a count more than 300 cells/µL can be monitored annually. Monitoring can be performed even less often or even suspended (as long as there is no change in clinical status or other lab parameters) in those with a count more than 500 cells/µL.

2. **HIV genotype testing for drug resistance**

   Viral strains that are resistant to one or more antiretroviral drugs are relatively common, so this testing is recommended for any patient with newly diagnosed HIV to help guide treatment.

3. **Testing for common comorbid STIs and other complications**

   Associated STIs are common, and the presence of a comorbid STI may increase the risk of transmitting HIV. Patients are also at an increased risk of other noninfectious complications, notably cardiovascular disease. Typical testing at diagnosis therefore is broad and includes:

   - Comprehensive metabolic panel (CMP), hemoglobin A1c, and lipid panel

   - Urinalysis

   - Urine, pharyngeal, and rectal screening for gonococcal and chlamydia infection

   - Hepatitis A total antibody

   - Hepatitis B core antibody (IgM and IgG), surface antibody, and surface antigen

   - Hepatitis C antibody with reflex NAAT

   - Rapid plasma reagin (RPR) with reflex treponemal antibody (or vice versa; see page 236)

   - Varicella IgG antibody

   - TB testing, IGRA preferred

   - You should also consider a urine human chorionic gonadotropin (hCG) pregnancy test if the patient has a uterus and has childbearing potential.

SEXUALLY TRANSMITTED INFECTIONS

 Gonorrhea and Chlamydia

We group these two infections together because most of the time you will test for them together. Who are candidates for testing?

   - Patients with symptoms of an STI (eg, urethral discharge)

   - Sexual partners of patients with an STI, including those without symptoms (the majority of chlamydial infections are asymptomatic)

   - Individuals at high risk, such as those with a new sexual partner or multiple partners

- Screening recommendations keep evolving, but as of this writing annual screening is recommended for all sexually active women under the age of 25. Screening should also be considered for women over 25 who are at risk. Regular screening during pregnancy is standard of care.

- Current guidelines do *not* recommend routine screening for men, but it is reasonable to consider regular screening for men who have sex with men (MSM) or who otherwise are at high risk of infection.

The test of choice for both diagnosis and screening is a *PCR*.

- In men, the best specimen is a *first-catch urine*, that is, the initial 20 to 30 mL of urine, not a midstream sample. A urethral swab is an appropriate alternative. The patient should not have urinated for at least 1 hour prior to providing the sample.

- In women, the highest yield sample is a *vaginal or endocervical swab*; a first-catch urine sample will miss approximately 10% of infections that a swab will pick up. A single swab is sufficient. The swab should be rotated in place for 10 to 30 seconds. Patients who prefer can obtain the specimen themselves and then submit it for testing.

- In both men and women, *pharyngeal and rectal swabs* should also be considered if these are sites of possible exposure.

Test of cure 1 to 2 weeks after the completion of therapy is recommended for patients with oropharyngeal infection (cure rates are relatively low), but not for those with uncomplicated urogenital or anorectal infection. All patients, however, should be retested in 3 months because of the high rate of recurrent infection.

For patients with suspected disseminated gonococcal infection, *cultures* should be obtained from the blood, joint fluid (if arthritis is present), CSF (if you suspect meningitis), and any purulent skin lesions. However, the yield from all of these cultures is low, so it is important to obtain a *PCR* from any and all possible sites of exposure even in the absence of symptoms.

It is worth noting that for patients with suspected *pelvic inflammatory disease (PID)*, which is believed to be polymicrobial in origin, testing should be limited to looking for gonococcal and chlamydial infection.

 # Syphilis

Syphilis is diagnosed by serologic (antibody) testing, of which there are two types: *nontreponemal tests* and *treponemal tests.*

Nontreponemal Tests

There are two: the rapid plasma reagin (RPR) test and the venereal disease research laboratory (VDRL) test.

These tests are *nonspecific*, meaning they do not measure antibodies directed specifically against *Treponema pallidum*. Instead, they measure antibodies that the body produces as part of the general immune/inflammatory response to syphilis infection. Of the two tests, the RPR is the preferred blood test; the VDRL is most useful when assessing the CSF for neurosyphilis (see the box "Neurosyphilis"). The results of the RPR and VDRL are reported as a titer (1:2, 1:4, and so on).*

It can take several weeks after the first appearance of a chancre for the RPR and VDRL titers to rise. If you suspect the diagnosis and your initial testing is negative, repeat it in a few weeks. False negatives can also occur in as many as 30% of patients with tertiary syphilis.

False positives are also common. The higher the titer, the more likely the diagnosis is a true positive. False positives usually have a titer of 1:8 or lower.

Up to 2% of the healthy population have a positive RPR. Additional causes of false positives include:

- Pregnancy

- IV drug use

- HIV

- Acute illnesses (especially endocarditis)

- Chronic liver disease

- Chronic autoimmune disorders, notably systemic lupus erythematosus

The RPR (and VDRL) wanes over time following successful treatment and can therefore be used to monitor the patient's therapeutic response. A 4-fold decrease in the titer (eg, from 1:32 to 1:8) denotes an adequate response to treatment. In some patients, this can take up to a year, and others may remain RPR-positive for life despite successful treatment; in these instances, the RPR will then almost always hover below 1:8.

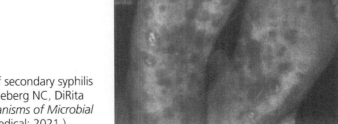

Figure 14.24 Cutaneous lesions of secondary syphilis on the soles of the feet. (From Engleberg NC, DiRita V, Imperiale M. *Schaechter's Mechanisms of Microbial Disease.* 6th ed. Wolters Kluwer Medical; 2021.)

---

*Because the process is done by serial dilution, the result is reported as a titer. The more dilutions in which the antibodies can be detected, the higher the titer (see Chapter 22 for more about titers).

Treponemal Tests

There are many, including the *fluorescent treponemal antibody absorption (FTA-ABS)* test, *microhemagglutination assay for Treponema pallidum antibodies (MHA-TP)* test, and *Treponema pallidum* enzyme immunoassay (TP-EIA).

These tests are *specific* for syphilis. False positives—while not unheard of—are rare.

Unlike the nontreponemal tests, these tests remain positive for many years after successful therapy, and therefore cannot be used to monitor a patient's response to treatment. For the same reason, these tests cannot be used to diagnose a new syphilis infection in someone with a prior history of the disease.

Two-Step Testing

The traditional way of testing for syphilis, still widely used, is a two-step process. First order a nonspecific nontreponemal test (eg, RPR). If it comes back positive, then it must be confirmed with a specific treponemal test (eg, FTA-ABS). If the specific test comes back negative, the patient can be presumed not to have syphilis. In most of these patients with discordant results, the RPR titer will be low.

Reversing the order of testing—so-called reverse treatment algorithms—have become increasingly popular. One advantage of this approach is the detection of early disease: the specific treponemal tests can generally detect infection earlier than the nontreponemal tests. However, because the specific treponemal test results remain elevated for years, positive tests must be followed by a nontreponemal test to distinguish an active or recent infection from a past infection.

One additional note: The CDC recommends that all patients diagnosed with syphilis should also be tested for HIV.

How Do You Diagnose Syphilis in Someone With a History of a Prior Infection?

Order an RPR or VDRL, then compare the results to the lowest previous titer. If you don't have previous RPR results on file, contact the appropriate health department which—as part of their function to track positive cases—should have these results on hand. If the new RPR is at least 4-fold higher, you can assume the patient has a new syphilis infection. Any patient whose RPR became negative after treatment for syphilis has a new diagnosis if any future RPRs are positive in the appropriate clinical context.

If you cannot get any previous RPR results, you can either monitor the RPR and see if it rises, indicating active infection (risky, because treating these patients early is the best way to avoid complications and prevent spread), or if your suspicion is sufficiently high, just treat them empirically.

Neurosyphilis

When neurosyphilis is suspected, a CSF VDRL is the test of choice. VDRL is specific but insensitive for neurosyphilis. The RPR should not be relied upon—it has an even higher rate of false negatives in the CSF. When testing the CSF, the treponemal tests do not have a sufficiently high specificity for neurosyphilis to be useful. PCR testing of the CSF is also available, but its sensitivity is too low to make it clinically useful.

Herpes Simplex

A diagnosis of genital herpes can usually be made clinically. Lab testing is not necessary except in those few cases where the diagnosis is uncertain.

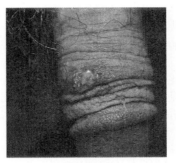

Figure 14.25 Genital herpes lesions. (From Goodheart, HP. *Goodheart: Goodheart's Photoguide of Common Skin Disorders*, 2nd ed. Wolters Kluwer Health; 2003.)

Testing the Lesion(s)

The best test for diagnosing active herpes infection is a PCR on a sample taken from the base of an ulcer. The lab will also test the specimen to see if the infection is caused by herpes virus type 1 or type 2. No other diagnostic testing is required unless you are concerned about resistance to therapy, in which case a culture is necessary.

Serologic Testing

Serologic (antibody) screening for asymptomatic adolescents, adults, or pregnant individuals tends to be unhelpful. Herpes infections are very common, so although the sensitivity of serologic testing for herpes type 2 is high (~99%), its comparatively low specificity (~83%) means that there are too many false positives. Nevertheless, the CDC recommends that herpes virus serologic screening can be considered for persons at risk. After initial infection, titers remain high for life.

As we discussed earlier in the book (see page 6), one question you always need to ask when ordering a test is what you and your patient will do with the information you obtain. A positive serologic test tells you little—too many false positives—and can cause undue anxiety and even disrupt ongoing relationships. However, there is one common situation where serologic testing can be helpful: patients who have learned that their partners have herpes type 2 may wish to know if they test negative (remember that the serologic test, while fraught with false positives, has few false negatives—you can rely on a negative result) and if so need to take precautions. The risk, again, is that the test will come back positive and you won't know if it is a true or false result.

The incidence of genital herpes caused by herpes type 1 is increasing and may have surpassed that caused by herpes type 2. Serologic testing for herpes type 1, however, cannot distinguish oral (prevalence of >50% in the United States) from genital disease.

 ## *Mycoplasma genitalium*

Although now recognized as a common cause of urethritis, there are no recommendations for general screening. There is an NAAT approved for use in patients with urogenital symptoms and their partners. Sensitivity is variable depending on the assay; specificity is very high.

> **Screening Recommendations for Transgender and Gender-Diverse Patients for Sexually Transmitted Infections**
>
> When screening is being considered, it is recommended that it should be based on the patient's sexual practices and anatomy. Self-collected specimens are perfectly acceptable for those who prefer that approach.

VAGINAL DISCHARGE

The common infectious causes of vaginal discharge can usually be diagnosed with a few simple tests. The three major diagnoses to consider are bacterial vaginosis (a disorder associated with an altered vaginal biome and *Gardnerella vaginalis* colonization, although many other organisms can also be detected), vulvovaginal candidiasis (yeast), and trichomoniasis.

 ## *How to Test at the Office*

- Start by examining the general appearance of the discharge. A normal vaginal discharge appears white and viscous and should not be homogeneous.

- Swab the discharge. The best place to obtain a sample is behind the cervix, in the posterior fornix. Mix the sample with 1 mL of saline, and agitate. Then place a drop of this mixture on a slide, place a cover slip over the sample, and examine it under a standard light microscope under both medium and high power. You are looking for yeast, clue cells (vaginal epithelial cells coated with coccobacilli, a sign of bacterial vaginosis; see Figure 14.26), and trichomonads. Warming the slide will enhance the motility of any trichomonads that may be present (see Figure 14.27) and increase your chance of detecting them.

- Next, place a second sample of the discharge on a slide with a drop of *KOH*, and top with a cover slip. If you detect a fishy odor when you add the KOH, that is considered a *positive whiff test*, the result of the aromatization of aromatic amines and evidence of bacterial vaginosis. The KOH dissolves much of the cellular material that may be in the sample, allowing for clearer visualization of any fungal elements. Also gently warm the slide, lysing any remaining cells. The warming should take only a few seconds; stop when you see tiny bubbles appear under the cover slip. *Candida* will appear as budding yeast, pseudohyphae, or hyphae.

- Test *the pH* by directly placing a small sample of the vaginal discharge on pH paper. Normal pH should be below 4.5. With infection, the pH may be increased, a result of decreased hydrogen peroxide production by *Lactobacillus acidophilus*, the major bacterium in normal vaginal flora that will have been displaced by any infecting organisms.

- A standard *Gram stain* of the discharge can be used to look again for yeast and clue cells (coccobacilli adherent to epithelial cells).

Table 14.5 summarizes the results associated with each of the different diagnoses.

Table 14.5 Diagnosing the Cause of Vaginal Discharge

Diagnosis	Appearance	KOH Whiff Test	pH	Microscopy
Normal	Viscous, white, and not homogeneous	Not fishy	3.8-4.5	No or only a few white blood cells (<10/HPF), some epithelial cells
Bacterial vaginosis	Thin, white or gray, and homogeneous	Fishy	5.0-6.0	Clue cells (>20% of epithelial cells), some but not many white blood cells (this is not an inflammatory disorder)
Vulvovaginal candidiasis	Thick, white, and often curdy	Not fishy	4.0-5.0	Budding yeast, hyphae, normal epithelial cells, some white blood cells
Trichomoniasis	White, yellow, occasionally green, and often frothy	Sometimes fishy, sometimes not	5.0-7.0	Motile trichomonads, many white blood cells

HPF, high-power field.

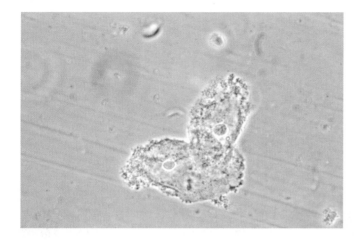

Figure 14.26 Clue cells in the vaginal discharge of a patient with bacterial vaginosis. (Courtesy of M. Rein/Centers for Disease Control and Prevention.)

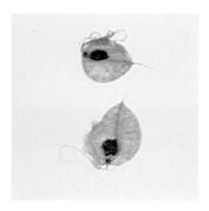

Figure 14.27 Trichomonads. The most notable feature of these protozoa are the flagella. (From Division of STD Prevention, National Center for HIV, Viral Hepatitis, STD, and TB Prevention, Centers for Disease Control and Prevention.)

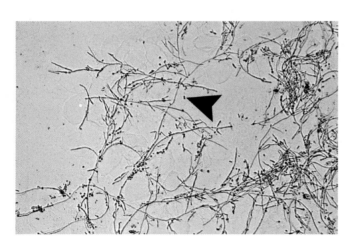

Figure 14.28 Yeast infection. Both budding yeast (black arrowhead) and pseudohyphae (everywhere) can be seen. (From Kroumpouzos G. *Text Atlas of Obstetric Dermatology*. 3rd ed. Wolters Kluwer Health/Lippincott Williams & Wilkins; 2014.)

Office Diagnosis Versus Molecular Testing

Combining all the criteria in Table 14.5, sensitivity is greater than 90% and specificity just below 80%. For confirmation, or when the diagnosis is uncertain or microscopy is not available, commercial labs offer *multiplex NAAT panels* for *Candida, Trichomonas,* and the most common organisms that are associated with bacterial vaginosis. Why not just order an NAAT and be done with it? Because office diagnosis is far less expensive and allows you to make a diagnosis that you can share with your patient on the spot.

TICK-BORNE INFECTIONS

 ## *Lyme Disease*

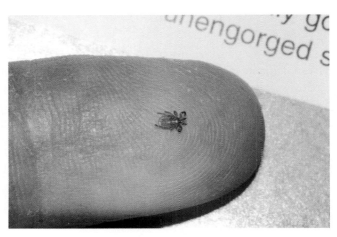

Figure 14.29 The deer tick, small but dangerous, transmits Lyme disease. (From Goodheart HP, Gonzalez ME, Gropper CA, Burgin S. *Goodheart's Same-Site Differential Diagnosis: Dermatology for the Primary Health Care Provider.* 2nd ed. Wolters Kluwer; 2023.)

Laboratory testing for Lyme disease consists of looking for antibodies against the spirochete, *Borrelia burgdorferi.**

___
*Occasionally in the United States, and especially outside the United States, other *Borrelia* species can cause the disease.

Two-Tiered Testing

Laboratory diagnosis requires a two-step process:

- Start with an *ELISA* (the technique is explained on page 198). The lab report will indicate whether or not antibody is present. If antibody is detected, the lab will then run separate IgM and IgG assays. ELISA testing is sensitive but not very specific; cross-reactivity to antibodies against other organisms can occur, so false positives are not uncommon.

- If the ELISA is negative, you are done. But if the ELISA is positive, a second test must be run for confirmation. This is usually a *Western blot test* (see page 199), which looks for antibodies against *specific* antigenic components of the spirochete. The Western blot is run for both IgM and IgG antibodies to various Lyme antigens. The test is considered positive if at least 2 of 3 specific IgM antibodies or at least 5 of 10 specific IgG antibodies are positive. IgG will persist for years; IgM usually fades within 30 days, although it can sometimes persist longer.

  - Note: The second confirmatory test, while usually a Western blot, can instead be a different ELISA directed against a different antigenic substrate.

Think of this two-step process as similar to the approach we discussed in Section 1 with our example of the airport check-in process. Start with a sensitive test, then confirm with a specific test.

Who Should Be Tested, and How

Early Localized Disease: Patients with Lyme disease present acutely with the classic rash of erythema migrans (EM) at the site of the bite (~80% of patients), along with flu-like manifestations such as fever, myalgias, and lymphadenopathy. *There is no need to order any lab testing at this point if you are confident in the clinical diagnosis.* If you are unsure, then by all means test, but antibodies may not be detectable at the time the rash first appears.

Early Disseminated Disease: If it is not treated in the early localized stage, the infection can spread systemically, resulting in diffuse EM and flu-like symptoms. It can also involve the heart (causing heart block or myocarditis) and the nervous system. *At this point, order the two-tier serologic profile.* If, more than 8 weeks into the course of the disease, only the IgM criteria on Western blot are positive, you are likely dealing with a false-positive result; you should expect to see IgG positivity by that point in the patient's course.

Late Disseminated Disease: If the patient is still untreated, the disease can progress to cause severe chronic arthritis and neurologic disease. Again, *two-tier testing should be performed.*

Some Additional Things You Should Know
- There is no reason to ever test a tick for Lyme disease; the findings will not (and should not) affect your management.

- Current guidelines recommend against screening asymptomatic persons who live in endemic areas for Lyme disease.

Patient Report

⬤ **YourLab**

Specimen ID: **059-992-3205-0**

Acct #: **90000999**   Phone: Rte: **00**

Control ID:

SAMPLE REPORT, 163600

|||₁₁||'₁₁₁₁|.|₁₁₁₁|₁₁|₁₁|₁||||||||₁₁.|||.₁|||₁||.|||₁₁|||₁₁

Patient Details	**Specimen Details**	**Physician Details**
DOB: **01/10/1984**	Date collected: **02/28/2023 0000 Local**	Ordering:
Age(y/m/d): **042/01/18**	Date received: **02/28/2023**	Referring:
Gender: **F**	Date entered: **02/28/2023**	ID:
Patient ID:	Date reported: **02/28/2023 0000 ET**	NPI:

General Comments & Additional Information
Clinical Info: ABNORMAL REPORT

Ordered items
Lyme, Line Blot, Serum

TESTS	RESULT	FLAG	UNITS	REFERENCE INTERVAL	LAB
Lyme, Line Blot, Serum					
Lyme Ab IgG by Line Blot:					
IgG P93 Ab.	Positive	Abnormal			01
IgG P66 Ab.	Negative				01
IgG P58 Ab.	Positive	Abnormal			01
IgG P45 Ab.	Positive	Abnormal			01
IgG P41 Ab.	Negative				01
IgG P39 Ab.	Positive	Abnormal			01
IgG P30 Ab.	Positive	Abnormal			01
IgG P28 Ab.	Negative				01
IgG P23 Ab.	Negative				01
IgG P18 Ab.	Positive	Abnormal			01
Lyme IgG Line Blot Interp.					
	Positive	Abnormal			01
		Abnormal			
		Positive: 5 of the following Borrelia-specific bands: 18, 23, 28, 30, 39, 41, 45, 58, 66, and 93.			
		Negative: No bands or banding patterns which do not meet positive criteria.			
Lyme Ab IgM by Line Blot:					01
IgM P41 Ab.	Negative				01
IgM P39 Ab.	Positive	Abnormal			01
IgM P23 Ab.	Positive	Abnormal			01
Lyme IgM Line Blot Interp.					
	Positive	Abnormal			01

Note: An equivocal or positive ETA result followed by a negative Line Blot result is considered NEGATIVE. An equivocal or positive ETA result followed by a positive Line Blot is considered POSITIVE by the CDC.
Positive: 2 of the following bands: 23, 39, or 41
Negative: No bands or banding patterns which do not meet positive criteria.

Figure 14.30 A typical Western blot report, illustrating what a positive test result looks like. Only certain antibodies are correlated with Lyme disease, and if five or more of these immunoglobulin (Ig)G antibodies and/or two or more of these IgM antibodies are positive, then the diagnosis of Lyme is likely.

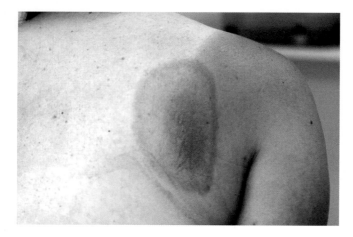

Figure 14.31 Erythema migrans in a patient with Lyme disease. Note the classic bullseye appearance of the rash. (From Goodheart HP, Gonzalez ME, Gropper CA, Burgin S. *Goodheart's Same-Site Differential Diagnosis: Dermatology for the Primary Health Care Provider.* 2nd ed. Wolters Kluwer; 2023.)

- It is also not recommended to screen persons for Lyme disease who present with only non-specific symptoms (eg, fatigue, headache) unless there is a reasonable history of possible tick exposure and a high level of clinical suspicion.

- In patients with a prior history of confirmed Lyme disease, subsequent serologic testing will be very difficult to interpret, because the IgG can remain elevated for many years. You likely won't know what to do with a positive result. You will have to rely on your clinical acumen—or the expertise of an infectious disease specialist—to determine whether the patient has a new case of Lyme disease and treat accordingly.

- Most patients with Lyme disease who develop nonspecific symptoms (eg, fatigue, mild cognitive impairment, and a modest fever) do not have actual neurologic infection. Instead, they are simply experiencing the usual symptoms that can accompany any systemic inflammatory condition, and a CSF analysis will be normal. However, in patients with symptoms more suggestive of actual meningitis or encephalomyelitis, the CSF should be sampled if only to rule out other causes. If the patient has CNS Lyme disease, the CSF will usually test positive for Lyme antibodies. Other common CSF findings in CNS Lyme disease include a pleocytosis and a mild elevation in the CSF protein along with a normal glucose.

 ## *Babesiosis*

Babesiosis is most commonly caused by the protozoan, *Babesia microti*. Suspect babesiosis in patients who have had a tick bite and who present with a clinical picture suggestive of Lyme disease but do not respond to Lyme-appropriate antibiotic therapy. Unlike Lyme disease, a rash is usually not present, and laboratory evidence of hemolysis (see Chapter 20) is a common finding.

Babesiosis can also be transmitted by blood transfusion, because the parasite likes to hang out inside red blood cells.

Start your evaluation with a *blood smear for parasites*. In patients with a high parasitic load, you may be able to see an intra-erythrocytic ring called the *Maltese cross*. However, you are unlikely to see this when the parasitic load is low, as is common early in the disease.

You therefore need to order serum *PCR testing*, which has a high sensitivity and specificity. *Antibody testing* may be negative early in the course, and when positive cannot distinguish acute from prior infection. Other laboratory findings, besides a hemolytic anemia, may include thrombocytopenia, increased liver transaminases, and proteinuria.

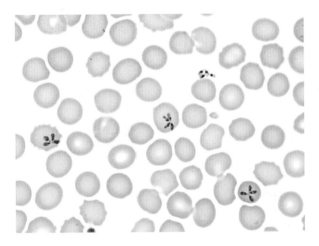

Figure 14.32 "Maltese cross" intra-erythrocytic inclusions in a patient with babesiosis. (From Pereira I, George TI, Arber DA. *Atlas of Peripheral Blood: The Primary Diagnostic Tool*. Wolters Kluwer Health/Lippincott Williams & Wilkins; 2012.)

 ## *Anaplasmosis and Ehrlichiosis*

Anaplasmosis and ehrlichiosis are caused by different pathogens but are virtually indistinguishable with respect to clinical presentation, laboratory diagnosis, and response to treatment. Test for them together, and beware that diagnosis can be difficult. On a *blood smear*, you may be able to see basophilic inclusion bodies called morulae in the cytoplasm of the white blood cells, but these are present in only a minority of patients with either disease. *PCR testing* should be considered. Sensitivity is less than 50%, although it may be higher early in the disease. You can check for *antibodies* as well, but they may be undetectable early in the course. You will want to obtain acute and convalescent antibody titers (the latter 2-4 weeks later); a 4-fold increase confirms the diagnosis, but by then you will probably have already instituted empiric therapy. As with babesiosis, other nonspecific lab abnormalities may include leukopenia, thrombocytopenia, and elevated liver transaminases.

Figure 14.33 Intracytoplasmic morulae in a patient with anaplasmosis. (From Stoller JK, Nielsen C, Buccola J, Brateanu A. *The Cleveland Clinic Foundation Intensive Review of Internal Medicine*. 6th ed. Wolters Kluwer Health; 2014.)

Rocky Mountain Spotted Fever

Caused by infection with *Rickettsia rickettsii*, Rocky Mountain spotted fever is now categorized as just one among several diseases referred to as the *spotted fever rickettsioses*. Among these, it remains the most common.

Acute and convalescent antibody titers can confirm the diagnosis (again, you are looking for a 4-fold rise in antibody titers over 2-4 weeks), but empiric treatment should not be delayed. *PCR testing* is rarely helpful, as the number of circulating rickettsial organisms is too low for detection unless there is severe, advanced disease. Other lab abnormalities that can occur with severe disease include thrombocytopenia, elevated liver transaminases, an elevated bilirubin, and hyponatremia due to the syndrome of inappropriate antidiuretic hormone (SIADH, see Chapter 19).

Direct immunofluorescence of a skin lesion has approximately 80% sensitivity early in the course of the illness and offers the additional advantage of rapid turnaround time. A positive result establishes the diagnosis. Once treatment has started, the sensitivity decreases dramatically.

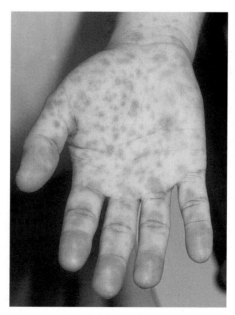

Figure 14.34 The rash of Rocky Mountain spotted fever. (Reprinted with permission from Hardin J. Cutaneous conditions. Knoop KJ, Stack LB, Storrow AB, Thurman R, *The Atlas of Emergency Medicine*, 4th ed. McGraw Hill; 2016. Copyright McGraw-Hill Education.)

Tick-Borne Disease Panels

Some labs offer comprehensive tick-borne disease panels. These may include molecular (PCR) panels and serologic (antibody) panels. They take the guesswork out of determining which tests to order, but you then run the risk of false positives and mounting cost. It is better to let your clinical judgment guide what tests to order. Take into account the patient's presentation, identification of the type of tick if possible, and your knowledge of what diseases are endemic where the patient lives and works. There will be times, though, when you may be totally baffled, and even the best infectious disease specialist may resort to this more generalized approach.

A FEW WORDS ABOUT PARASITES

Parasites account for a massive disease burden throughout the world. Developing nations are disproportionately affected. Patients who are immunocompromised are, not surprisingly, particularly susceptible to severe disease; your threshold for testing should be lower among these patients. When deciding on whether to test for a given parasitic infection, consider not only the clinical presentation but also the relevant geography and exposure history. Much more so than in cases of suspected "typical" bacterial infections, the decision to send testing for parasitic infections depends heavily on specific elements of the history such as recent activities (eg, swimming in a freshwater lake) and food ingestion (eg, ingestion of street food or undercooked meat).

Eosinophilia is a common—but not universal—laboratory feature of parasitic infections.

Important parasitic infections discussed elsewhere in this book include malaria (see page 257), babesiosis (see page 244), and trichomoniasis (see page 239). There are, of course, many others, but rather than tediously review every parasite one by one, we think it will be most helpful to discuss a few tests and principles that apply broadly to parasitic infections.

 The Power of Microscopy

Parasites tend to have complex life cycles and—fortunately for us—distinctive microscopic appearances. Think ova, cysts, larvae, trophozoites, worms, etc. This means that *microscopy* is almost universally helpful in the case of a suspected parasitic infection, with the one caveat that sensitivity can be limited (ie, false negatives are common). When a parasitic bloodstream infection (such as malaria or loa loa) is suspected, microscopy of the blood by *thick and thin smears* tends to be most helpful. When a GI infection is suspected, stool microscopy (often called a *stool ova and parasite examination*) should be sent.

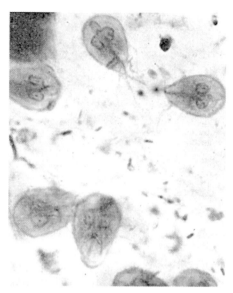

Figure 14.35 The distinctive "face-like" trophozoite form of *Giardia lamblia* seen on microscopy. (From Yamada T, Alpers DH. *Textbook of Gastroenterology.* Lippincott Williams & Wilkins; 2003.)

 ## Antigens, Antibodies, and Nucleic Acid Amplification Testing

Antigen and antibody testing are not available for all parasitic organisms, but when they are, they may improve sensitivity over microscopy alone. Notable parasitic organisms whose workup should include antigen and/or antibody testing include *Entamoeba histolytica, Cryptosporidium parvum, Giardia lamblia, Leishmania* species, *Strongyloides stercoralis, Schistosoma* species, and *Toxoplasma gondii.*

Antibody testing (ie, serology) of the blood is particularly important in cases of suspected toxoplasmosis, in which serology not only may provide knowledge of the timing of infection but may also help determine whether toxoplasma reactivation prophylaxis should be given in patients with HIV. Prophylaxis is typically indicated for those with a positive toxoplasma IgG and a CD4 count less than 100 cells/μL.

Keep in mind that patients who are severely immunocompromised may not mount antibody responses to many parasites—false-negative antibody testing is more likely to occur among such patients.

NAAT, typically performed by *PCR*, is not available for many parasitic organisms, but when it is, it tends to be very sensitive and specific. Consider sending PCR along with microscopy (ie, as adjunctive testing) when possible, especially if antigen and/or antibody testing is not available.

Cultures

Despite remaining the technical "gold standard" for the diagnosis of a few parasitic infections (eg, *Entamoeba histolytica*), parasite cultures are rarely performed and are often not available for clinical use. The process of cultivating a parasite in vitro tends to be slow, labor intensive, and complex (consider the many stages many parasites go through in their life cycles). Diagnosis is usually made by other means.

Enterobius vermicularis and the Cellophane Tape Test

No lab book would be complete without a brief discussion of the unique and elegant cellophane tape test. *Enterobius vermicularis* is a small roundworm ("pinworm") that causes intense perianal itching, a result of the deposition of embryonated eggs by female worms that have migrated from the anus. Because neither eggs nor larvae/worms are reliably released into the stool, stool microscopy tends not to be helpful in making the diagnosis. Examination of the blood tends to be equally unhelpful; eosinophilia and elevated IgE are typically not seen.

Enter the cellophane tape test: the diagnosis can be made with excellent sensitivity and specificity by applying clear tape to the perianal area first thing in the morning (egg deposition occurs overnight) and then inspecting the tape under the microscope for eggs and/or pinworms. Multiple tests should be performed; five successive tests yield a total sensitivity of nearly 100%.

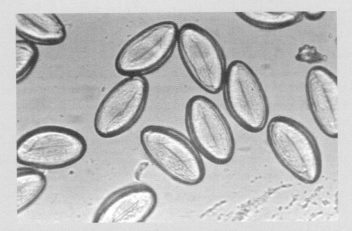

Figure 14.36 *Enterobius vermicularis* eggs stuck to a piece of tape under a microscope. This is a positive cellophane tape test. (From Procop GW, Church DL, Hall GS, et al. *Koneman's Color Atlas and Textbook of Diagnostic Microbiology.* 7th ed. Wolters Kluwer Health; 2017.)

CHILDHOOD INFECTIONS

 Varicella (Chickenpox)

The diagnosis of chickenpox can be made on a clinical basis alone without additional lab tests when the patient presents with the characteristic vesicular skin rash.

When the diagnosis is uncertain (or when the patient is immunocompromised, in which case laboratory confirmation of diagnosis is recommended), *PCR* is a very sensitive and specific first-line test for the identification of varicella-zoster virus (VZV). PCR is most commonly and conveniently run on fluid from an open vesicle, but can also be sent on other body fluids such as CSF or blood in cases of suspected disseminated disease (eg, in an immunocompromised patient).

Direct fluorescent antibody (DFA) testing (ie, immunofluorescence) may be run on skin lesion scrapings or vesicle fluid. Specificity is excellent, but sensitivity, although very good, lags behind that of PCR, making PCR the preferred first-line test in most scenarios. DFA results do come back quickly, usually within a few hours.

The main use of *varicella antibody testing (serology)* is in assessing immunity (eg, in the setting of a preemployment or student health physical). Most patients who test negative for varicella IgG antibodies are considered nonimmune and should be vaccinated.

Varicella viral culture is generally not favored as a diagnostic modality due to its insensitivity and long turnaround time.

 Measles

Measles should be suspected in any unvaccinated person presenting with rash (classically maculopapular and spreading downward from the face), fever, and cough. *Measles IgM*, the diagnostic test recommended by the World Health Organization, has high sensitivity and specificity for acute measles infection. False negatives may occur if the sample is obtained prior to the third day after the onset of the skin rash (it is around this time that IgM becomes detectable). False positives, although very rare, may occur in patients who instead have parvovirus B19, the cause of fifth disease (this occurs due to cross-reactivity of the assay with parvovirus B19 IgM).

Measles IgG starts to rise about 2 weeks after the appearance of the rash. An increase in measles IgG of at least 4-fold between acute and convalescent phases (about 10-14 days apart) confirms a diagnosis of acute measles infection when there is any uncertainty. In an asymptomatic patient, the presence of measles IgG correlates with immunity (either past exposure or vaccination).

PCR and, less often, *viral cultures* (oral, nasopharyngeal, urine, and/or serum specimens; conjunctival swabs may be obtained in those with conjunctivitis) are used to confirm the diagnosis and are also used for epidemiologic surveillance.

Mumps

Consider mumps in a patient with parotitis and/or orchitis along with nonspecific constitutional and GI symptoms, especially if they are unvaccinated. Neurologic manifestations such as meningitis or encephalitis may occur in those with severe disease.

A buccal swab specimen should be sent for *PCR*, which is very sensitive and specific. You can increase the yield by massaging the salivary gland region prior to obtaining the swab. False negatives may occur in those who have been symptomatic for less than 5 days. If the results are negative and clinical suspicion for mumps remains, testing should be repeated in 5 to 10 days. Those who are vaccinated, should they nevertheless get the disease, are at increased risk for false-negative results compared to unvaccinated individuals (no matter when the specimen is collected), so your threshold for repeat testing in vaccinated patients should be particularly low.

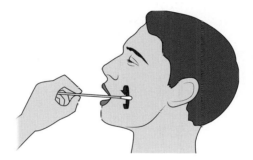

Figure 14.37 How to obtain a buccal swab.

Mumps antibody testing (serology) for IgM is another option and, when positive, confirms acute mumps infection. *ELISA testing* can return results quickly, but sensitivities are low (25%-50% depending on the manufacturer).

A CSF specimen should also be obtained if CNS involvement is suspected.

 ## *Rubella*

Because of the clinical and epidemiologic overlap among patients with measles and rubella (the latter is also called German measles)—for example, consider an MMR-unvaccinated patient with constitutional symptoms and a maculopapular rash—the laboratory may be the only reliable way to differentiate between the two.

Testing for rubella should start with *antibody testing (serology)* by ELISA. *Rubella IgM* becomes detectable about 4 days after the onset of rash and persists for several weeks. Specificity is excellent. Rare false positives can be seen in patients with parvovirus IgM, heterophile antibodies (seen most often with EBV infection), and rheumatoid factor (RF is commonly found not only in those with rheumatoid arthritis but in many healthy patients as well as in those with various acute and chronic illnesses). In cases of diagnostic uncertainty, antibody testing can be repeated 2 weeks later: an increase in *rubella IgG* of at least 4-fold over this time confirms the diagnosis.

If testing is obtained fewer than 3 to 4 days after the onset of rash—when false-negative antibody testing is common—*PCR* should be obtained and can be sent on oral, nasopharyngeal, and/or urine specimens. PCR has excellent sensitivity and specificity.

Rubella viral cultures have largely been replaced by the methods above, at least in part due to cultures' insensitivity and long turnaround time.

Measles, Mumps, and Rubella Immunity Profiles

Labs offer single panels that test for IgG levels against measles, mumps, and rubella. These are most often used to provide information regarding immunity when it is required, for example, for school or employment purposes.

≋YourLab   **Patient Report**

Specimen ID: 272-988-3205-0   Acct #: **90000999**   Phone: Rte: **00**
Control ID:

SAMPLE REPORT, 058495

Patient Details	**Specimen Details**	**Physician Details**
DOB: **01/10/1984**	Date collected: **09/29/2023 000 Local**	Ordering:
Age(y/m/d): **039/08/19**	Date received: **09/30/2023**	Referring:
Gender: **F** SSN:	Date entered: **09/30/2023**	ID:
Patient ID:	Date reported: **10/01/2023 0000 ET**	NPI:

General Comments & Additional Information
Clinical Info: NORMAL REPORT

Ordered items
Measles/Mumps/Rubella Immunity

TESTS	RESULT	FLAG	UNITS	REFERENCE INTERVAL	LAB
Measles/Mumps/Rubella Immunity					
Rubella Antibodies, IgG	2.43		Index	Immune >0.99	01
			Non-immune	<0.90	
			Equivocal	0.90 – 0.99	
			Immune	>0.99	
Measles Antibodies, IgG	95.0		AU/mL	Immune >16.4	01
			Negative	<13.5	
			Equivocal	13.5 – 16.4	
			Positive	>16.4	

Presence of antibodies to Rubella is presumptive evidence of immunity except when acute infection is suspected.

TESTS	RESULT	FLAG	UNITS	REFERENCE INTERVAL	LAB
Mumps Abs, IgG	180.0		AU/mL	Immune >10.9	01
			Negative	<9.0	
			Equivocal	9.0 – 10.9	
			Positive	>10.9	

A positive result generally indicates past exposure to mumps virus or previous vaccination.

Figure 14.38 Sample report of an immunity panel showing adequate immunoglobulin G levels to all three childhood diseases.

Parvovirus B19

Parvovirus B19 is the cause of fifth disease,* aka erythema infectiosum. In children, the diagnosis can almost always be made clinically by recognizing the classic "slapped cheek" rash and flu-like symptoms, and lab confirmation is rarely needed. In adults, the diagnosis can be more difficult because the rash may not be present and the disease often presents as a polyarthritis that can mimic rheumatoid arthritis.

When testing is indicated to confirm the diagnosis, serology is the best option. Detection of *parvovirus IgM* has good sensitivity (70%-100%) and specificity (76%-100%). The presence of *parvovirus IgG* indicates previous infection and immunity. *PCR testing* is useful in immunocompromised patients who may not be able to mount a detectable antibody response.

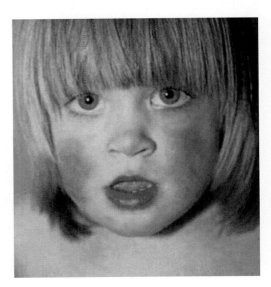

Figure 14.39 The "slapped cheek" rash characteristic of fifth disease in children. (From Kline-Tilford AM, Haut C. *Lippincott Certification Review: Pediatric Acute Care Nurse Practitioner.* Wolters Kluwer; 2015.)

ANTI-STREPTOCOCCAL ANTIBODIES: ACUTE RHEUMATIC FEVER AND POST-STREPTOCOCCAL GLOMERULONEPHRITIS

Major immune-mediated sequelae of group A streptococcus (GAS) infection include:

- **Acute rheumatic fever (ARF)**: migratory polyarthritis, carditis, chorea, skin nodules, and/or erythema marginatum, usually occurring about 2 weeks after an episode of untreated GAS pharyngitis. Thanks to the widespread use of antibiotics, ARF is no longer common, especially in developed countries.

---

*Why "fifth" disease? Because it was fifth in the classic listing of what were at one time considered the six major childhood exanthems. Only parvovirus B19 infection has retained its numerical assignment in popular terminology.

- **Post-streptococcal glomerulonephritis (PSGN):** nephritic syndrome caused by immune complex deposition, most commonly seen between 1 and 6 weeks after GAS pharyngitis or skin infection.

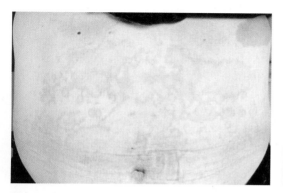
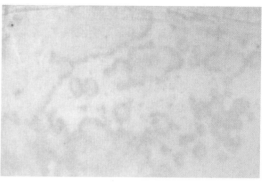

Figure 14.40 Erythema marginatum, the characteristic rash seen in acute rheumatic fever. Courtesy P. Witman, Mayo Clinic. (From Koopman WJ, Moreland LW. *Arthritis and Allied Conditions. A Textbook of Rheumatology.* 15th ed. Lippincott Williams & Wilkins; 2005.)

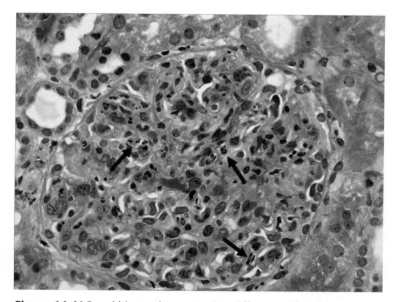

Figure 14.41 Renal biopsy demonstrating diffuse proliferative glomerulonephritis in a patient with post-streptococcal glomerulonephritis. The arrows point to inflammatory cells. (From Rennke HG, Denker BM. *Renal Pathophysiology.* 5th ed. Lippincott Williams & Wilkins; 2020.)

Although both diagnoses can often be made clinically (and/or with a renal biopsy in the case of PSGN), laboratory testing is used in both cases to confirm recent GAS infection.

Pharyngeal rapid strep tests and throat cultures should be sent in those with current or recent pharyngitis; however, these tests are likely to be negative during the "latent" period between acute infection and the development of ARF or PSGN.

The best tests to confirm recent GAS infection in those with suspected ARF or PSGN are *antistreptolysin O (ASO)* and *anti-DNase B (ADB)* antibodies. The sensitivity of these combined tests for antecedent GAS infection is high (>90%)—that is, if the patient has ARF or PSGN, at least one of these tests is very likely to be positive. Because the upper limit of normal for both tests varies significantly based on the patient's age, geographical location, and even the time of year, it is useful to repeat antibody levels after 2 to 4 weeks. Levels of ASO and ADB peak about 4 and 7 weeks after GAS infection, respectively; so levels that are significantly increasing after 2 to 4 weeks indicate recent infection.

The Streptozyme Screen

Some laboratories allow you to order a streptozyme screen, a panel of five anti-streptococcal antibodies:

1. ASO

2. ADB

3. Anti-hyaluronidase (AHase)

4. Anti-streptokinase (AKSase)

5. Anti–nicotinamide adenine dinucleotide (NAD)

Is it helpful to test for these three additional enzymes (aside from ASO and ADB)? The streptozyme screen is only slightly more sensitive for recent GAS infection than ASO and ADB alone. The added sensitivity is greatest after a recent GAS skin infection (eg, impetigo), when ASO antibodies tend to be negative.

Bottom line: ASO and ADB antibodies are usually sufficient to test for recent GAS infection in patients with suspected ARF or PSGN. Consider sending a streptozyme screen rather than ASO and ADB antibodies alone in patients with recent skin infections and/or without recent pharyngitis.

MALARIA AND OTHER TROPICAL DISEASES

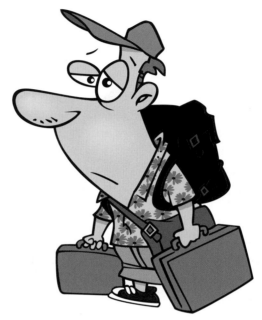

Figure 14.42 (Courtesy Ron Leishman/Shutterstock.)

Illness in the Returning Traveler

When we speak of illness in the returning traveler, we are usually talking about travelers returning from tropical destinations; it seems that most pathogens prefer tropical and subtropical regions to the glaciers and fjords of Scandinavia and the Antarctic. This observation, trivial at first glance, highlights the importance of obtaining a good history from anyone returning from abroad, whether for work or pleasure. You need to know more than just what their symptoms are, but also where they traveled, how long they were there, how soon after arrival or departure they became ill, what were their possible exposures, what precautions they took for protection, and—of course—what vaccines or medications they took to prevent infection. Once these questions have been answered and you've performed a good physical exam, it is often time to turn to the lab for answers.

The two most common presentations of illness in the returning traveler are fever and diarrhea, and we will divide our approach into these two categories. But remember that *travelers can get ordinary illnesses, too*—they just happen to have been away when they became ill. So don't just focus on the more exotic diseases; UTIs, respiratory infections, and viral hepatitis—to name just a few—can happen to anyone anywhere.*

*Diseases that can occur anywhere and everywhere are sometimes called *cosmopolitan diseases*.

Malaria

This is one diagnosis you never want to miss. There are several species of *Plasmodium* that can cause malaria; *Plasmodium falciparum* and *Plasmodium knowlesi* in particular can cause severe and even fatal illness. Malaria should be a consideration in any traveler with fever returning from an endemic area. Common laboratory abnormalities that can be seen in association with malaria (none are specific) include leukopenia, thrombocytopenia, hyperbilirubinemia, and elevated C-reactive protein.

Thin and Thick Blood Smears

Microscopic examination of *thin and thick smears of the peripheral blood* remains the definitive test for malaria. Some laboratories refer to thin and thick smears together as a *blood smear for parasites*.

Although suspected malaria is the most common reason for ordering thin and thick smears, this technique is also used to detect other intracellular parasites such as *Babesia* (like malaria, it can be found in red blood cells) and *Anaplasma* (in white blood cells). Thin and thick smears can detect even very low levels of parasites in the blood and can identify the particular species of malarial parasite. The thin smear is better for species identification, whereas the thick smear is more sensitive. Determining the degree of parasitemia and the infecting species is important for prognosis and guiding therapy.

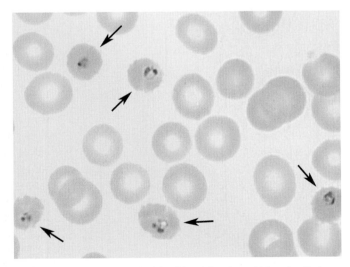

Figure 14.43 Malaria parasites can be seen inside this patient's red blood cells (arrows). The appearance of the parasite depends on the particular species and the stage of infection. (From Braun CA, Anderson CM. *Applied Pathophysiology: A Conceptual Approach to the Mechanisms of Disease*, 3rd ed. Wolters Kluwer; 2014.)

How to Make Thin and Thick Blood Smears

You will send blood specimens to the lab for these tests, but you can also perform them in your office. If the parasite is present in some of the patient's red blood cells, you are likely to find it. However, unless you have extensive experience doing these procedures, you won't be familiar enough with the different morphologies of the various malarial species to identify the precise parasite with confidence or make an accurate determination of the degree of parasitemia. But try if you can—making a diagnosis of malaria on the spot will allow you to initiate therapy while awaiting the final report from the lab.

To make a thin blood smear, place one drop of blood on a slide near the frosted end. Then quickly push the blood toward the unfrosted end with another slide angled at approximately 45°. The sample should thin out as you push the blood across the slide, creating a delicate, feathered edge. In this way you will create a monolayer of red blood cells ready for microscopy. Let the sample dry and fix it with absolute methanol.

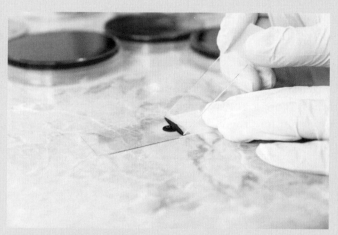

Figure 14.44 How to make a thin smear. It takes some practice but once you have it down it's easy. (Courtesy Zaharia Bogdan Rares/Shutterstock.)

To make a thick blood smear, we recommend what is called the scratch method. Spread the blood across the slide with another slide while applying downward pressure. This will create tiny scratches in the sample slide that lets the red blood cells adhere without disrupting them. Whereas a drop of blood can take hours to dry, this method allows drying to be complete within 30 minutes.

Both thin and thick smears are usually stained with Giemsa stain (Wright stain is a perfectly fine alternative).

You can't rule out malaria until at least three blood smears taken over 48 hours have come back negative. And even then, if you still suspect malaria, you should repeat testing every 12 to 24 hours.

Rapid Antigen Detection Tests

Rapid antigen detection tests (RDTs) are now part of the standard workup of suspected malaria at many institutions. They are run by placing a drop of blood on a test strip impregnated with antimalarial antibodies. Results are typically available within 2 to 15 minutes. The main role of these tests is to offer an alternative when lab personnel experienced in microscopy are not available. The World Health Organization continues to evaluate the performance of these test kits. There are a variety of different tests looking at different antigens, and their sensitivity and specificity vary greatly, so you need to know which test is being used and how accurate it is. The FDA has approved only one of these tests as of this writing, the histidine-rich protein 2 (HRP-2) assay, which is specific for *P. falciparum*. Unfortunately, the prevalence of HRP-2 negative *F. falciparum* is increasing worldwide, exceeding 20% in some areas, reducing the sensitivity of this test.

Polymerase Chain Reaction

PCR testing can be run on blood, saliva, or urine. It has a high sensitivity (>90%) and specificity (~100%) and can detect very low levels of parasites. It can also identify the specific malarial species that is causing the infection. However, PCR testing is not widely available, and results do not come back quickly enough to be of sufficient help in patients who are acutely ill. PCR testing is currently limited primarily to research settings.

Serology

Testing for antimalarial antibodies, either by immunofluorescence or ELISA, is not useful in the acute setting. It can identify prior infection.

Fever in the Returning Traveler

If there is an obvious source of infection—for example, the urinary tract or respiratory tract—then focus your attention there. Among the most common causes when a source is not apparent are *malaria, dengue fever,* and *typhoid (enteric fever)*. *Chikungunya* is also becoming increasingly common. The list will vary from year to year; for example, you will recall the surge of Zika infections a few years ago that fortunately has largely faded away with no major outbreaks since 2019.

All returning travelers with fever and no obvious cause who have traveled to a region where malaria is endemic should have the following lab tests:

- *CBC with differential and platelet count*
- *CMP*
- *Urinalysis*
- *Thin and thick blood smears for malaria*
- *Routine cultures of blood, urine, and/or stool depending on the presentation and how ill the patient is*

Dengue

Dengue is caused by various species of *Flavivirus* and, like malaria, is transmitted by mosquitoes. Dengue fever is self-limited, but dengue hemorrhagic fever, which occurs with a *second* infection with a flavivirus of a serotype *different from that of the first infection*, can be severe and life threatening.

As with malaria, leukopenia, thrombocytopenia, and elevated liver tests are common. An increased AST is almost always present. The hemoglobin may be elevated with hemorrhagic fever due to hemoconcentration. An abrupt rise in the hemoglobin and drop in the platelet count herald the onset of critical disease with plasma leakage and shock.

The diagnosis is made clinically, but laboratory testing can provide confirmation. *Rapid antigen tests* and *PCR* are available, and both have high specificity. However, sensitivity of both antigen and PCR testing declines starting a few days after symptom onset.

Serologic testing can also be helpful. IgM titers are elevated in 50% of patients by days 3 to 5. However, false positives are common due to cross-reactivity with other infections, including other flaviviruses such as Zika. IgG begins to rise after about a week and may persist for the lifetime of the patient.

 ## *Typhoid*

Enteric fever, caused by Salmonella enterica (serotypes typhi and paratyphi), can mimic malaria and dengue. Again, leukopenia, thrombocytopenia, anemia, and elevated liver tests are common. Diagnosis is made by *isolating the bacterium from cultures of the stool, urine, blood,* or—if all else proves negative and suspicion remains—the *bone marrow* (highest sensitivity at ~85%). After 1 week of illness, the chance of finding the organism anywhere declines dramatically. Antigen and antibody tests are available but are generally considered to be of limited utility.

 ## *Chikungunya*

Like typhoid, chikungunya is associated with leukopenia, thrombocytopenia, and elevated liver tests in most patients. The diagnosis can be confirmed by *serology* or *PCR testing*, both of which are very specific. The PCR is positive acutely, often as early as the first day of symptoms. However, if the patient is more than a week out from the onset of symptoms, serology is your best bet. IgM levels start to rise several days into the infection and remain elevated for weeks. Patients with chikungunya can develop prolonged (months to years) arthritis, so testing should be considered for persons with persistent arthritis and a travel history. In these cases, IgG antibodies can typically be detected, but do not differentiate chronic from resolved infection.

Zika

Zika first came to global attention in 2015-2016 when it swept through South and Central America (the virus was first isolated in Uganda in 1947). It usually causes only a mild febrile illness, but it is a potent teratogen. It is recommended that all asymptomatic pregnant women in regions where viral transmission is active should be tested.

Testing algorithms for Zika can get very complicated very quickly. In general, *PCR* is highly specific—a positive result confirms Zika virus infection—but sensitivity begins to wane about a week after exposure, when *serologic testing for Zika IgM* becomes more useful. A negative IgM rules out Zika with reasonable certainty, whereas a positive IgM typically entails further testing and involvement of an infectious disease specialist.

Current testing recommendations are as follows:

- For women less than 2 weeks postexposure, PCR screening of either the blood or urine is recommended. If the test is negative, then IgM levels should be measured 2 to 12 weeks from the time of exposure.

- For women 2 to 12 weeks postexposure, IgM levels are the test of choice. If positive or equivocal, then PCR testing should be done. Additional testing may also be indicated.

- Pregnant women with ongoing exposure should have serologic testing during each regular checkup.

 ## Yellow Fever

Yellow fever is often a mild or subclinical illness, but when severe has a high mortality rate. The diagnosis can be confirmed early in the disease by *PCR*. The presence of *IgM* antibodies is indicative of recent infection, although false positives may occur in the setting of infection with another flavivirus (eg, dengue) or in patients who have been vaccinated against yellow fever.

 ## Cholera

Cholera is caused by toxin-producing strains of *Vibrio cholerae*. Whereas most of the worrisome diarrheal illnesses are associated with bloody stools, cholera presents with profound watery diarrhea (often called rice-water stools) that can lead to the rapid development of severe, often life-threatening dehydration. Outbreaks frequently make the news, often a result of contaminated water supplies in regions affected by earthquakes, other natural disasters, or human-made catastrophes (ie, armed conflicts). The diagnosis can usually be made clinically. *Stool cultures* can confirm the diagnosis; however, alert the lab first, because they will need to provide special culture media. Numerous *rapid antigen tests* are also available, but they are less sensitive than stool culture.

Diarrhea in the Returning Traveler

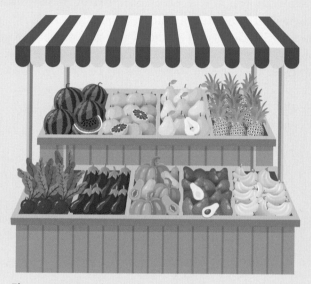

Figure 14.45 Within 24 hours, the large majority of travelers—despite best intentions—will do at least one thing that increases their risk of traveler's diarrhea. Eating unpeeled produce from a street vendor, however tempting, is best avoided (and first washing it with tap water doesn't help matters!) (Courtesy WinWin artlab/Shutterstock.)

Most travelers' diarrhea is either viral or caused by *Escherichia coli*, and the only question is whether or not to treat empirically for presumptive *E. coli* infection. On the other hand, travelers who return home with high fever, bloody stools, or evidence of dehydration require laboratory evaluation including:

- Stool tests:

  - Stool cultures

  - Fecal lactoferrin testing (see page 280) or stool exam for fecal leukocytes (the lactoferrin test is better)

  - Assay for Shiga toxin, looking for Shiga toxin–producing *E. coli* (STEC)

  - Molecular testing for enteric pathogens—multiplex testing (see page 280) is becoming more and more popular as a way to screen for multiple pathogens with a single specimen.

- Blood tests
  - CBC
  - CMP
  - Blood cultures; these can be helpful when salmonella is in your differential diagnosis.

If diarrhea has been present for 2 weeks or longer, you will also need to check additional stool tests for more persistent and chronic infections:

- Modified acid-fast staining for *Cyclospora* species
- Stool antigen tests for *Giardia*, *Cryptosporidium*, and *Entamoeba histolytica*
- Stool microscopy for ova and parasites

It is important to remember that not everyone who presents with fever and bloody diarrhea has an underlying infection. Although infection is by far the most likely cause of diarrhea in a returning traveler, there is no reason why other disorders—for example, Crohn disease or ulcerative colitis—can't develop while the patient is abroad. Think infection first, but keep your differential diagnosis wide open if your workup has not revealed a pathogen.

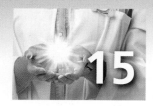

15 Cardiopulmonary Medicine

CARDIAC BIOMARKERS

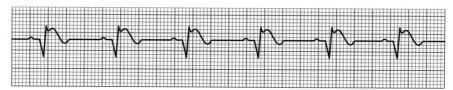

Figure 15.1 ST-segment elevation and T-wave inversion on the electrocardiogram (ECG) of a patient having an acute myocardial infarction caused by reduced coronary blood flow to the heart (cardiac ischemia). We won't be discussing ECGs here—that's a subject for another book.

The detection of myocardial injury and determination of its cause (eg, myocardial infarction [MI] or myocarditis) rely on the history and physical, electrocardiogram (ECG), and measurement of cardiac biomarkers. In some cases, imaging studies such as echocardiogram and cardiac magnetic resonance imaging (MRI) may also be required.

Cardiac biomarkers exist in high concentrations inside cardiac myocytes and spill out into the blood when these cells are damaged. Historically, a variety of different intracellular components have been measured to aid in the detection of myocardial injury. These include troponin I, troponin T, creatine kinase (the MB isoenzyme, CK-MB), lactate dehydrogenase (LDH), aspartate aminotransferase (AST), and myoglobin. Over time, it has become clear that the most clinically useful of these are the troponins.

 Troponins

By far the most common use of troponins is in the workup of a patient with a suspected acute coronary syndrome (ACS), an urgent situation caused by an acutely compromised blood supply to the heart. Patients with ACS can be divided into two broad categories:

- *Unstable angina*: Patients present with signs or symptoms of severe or worsening cardiac ischemia (eg, pressure-like chest pain at rest or occuring with increasing frequency), but troponin levels are normal (or only slightly elevated).

- *Myocardial infarction*: Patients present with signs or symptoms of cardiac ischemia and have elevated troponin levels. The urgency of coronary revascularization in these patients tends to be higher, especially if ST elevations are seen on an ECG.

Troponins therefore help us differentiate unstable angina from MI and, in a broader sense, help to determine the presence and extent of cardiac myocyte injury, thereby aiding in diagnosis and risk stratification.

Troponin results are often available within minutes and can be used to make key time-sensitive management decisions, such as if and when to perform coronary revascularization. Standard troponin levels start to rise 2 to 3 hours after myocardial injury, and even sooner when highly sensitive troponins are measured (see below). Levels remain high for several days.

Troponin I and Troponin T

The two commonly measured troponins are troponin I (often abbreviated cTnI, meaning cardiac troponin I; upper limit of normal 0.04 ng/mL) and troponin T (cTnT; upper limit of normal 0.1 ng/mL). These biomarkers are structurally similar and are both involved in regulating cardiac myocyte contraction. As diagnostic tests, they perform similarly in the workup of myocardial injury, with a few relatively uncommon exceptions:

- Whereas troponin I is found exclusively inside cardiac myocytes, troponin T may be found in small concentrations in skeletal muscle, particularly among patients with congenital or severe diseases of the skeletal muscle. In these patients, troponin T may be chronically (usually mildly) elevated. For similar reasons, troponin T may be elevated in patients with significant muscle breakdown (rhabdomyolysis).

- Troponin T can be cleaved by proteolytic enzymes that leak out of red blood cells in hemolyzed blood samples, leading to a false-negative result. This does not occur with troponin I.

- Troponin T may be more prone to chronic elevation than troponin I in patients with advanced chronic kidney disease (see the box "Troponins in Chronic Kidney Disease" on page 268), increasing the potential for false-positive results.

As a result of these factors, troponin I is slightly more sensitive and specific than troponin T for acute myocardial injury. In practice, troponin T is usually adequate. If your facility's lab defaults to troponin T, keep the above caveats in mind when interpreting the results.

High-Sensitivity Troponins

Most hospitals and labs have adopted *high-sensitivity* or *highly sensitive* troponin assays that can accurately detect very low levels of circulating troponins. These assays allow for the detection of a small degree of myocardial injury as early as 1 hour after the onset of an MI. They can also detect low, *chronic* troponin elevations in patients with:

- stable heart failure

- myocarditis and myocardial contusions

- noncardiac conditions including pulmonary embolism (PE) and chronic kidney disease

In many of these situations, results can be useful in determining prognosis and guiding therapy. For example, high-sensitivity troponin elevations in stable patients with heart failure are associated with increased mortality. Acute and chronic elevations can be distinguished by obtaining serial samples and seeing if there is a change.

The upper limit of normal for high-sensitivity troponins varies by specific assay but is usually about 15 ng/L (0.15 ng/mL) for troponin T and 25 ng/L (0.25 ng/dL) for troponin I. Many labs use a higher upper limit of normal for male patients than for female patients. False-negative results—that is, normal results in the presence of significant myocardial injury—are rare.

A positive result indicates myocardial injury, but it does not tell you whether that injury is clinically significant or, importantly, what the underlying cause of the injury is; these concerns of course are true for any troponin assay, highly sensitive or not.

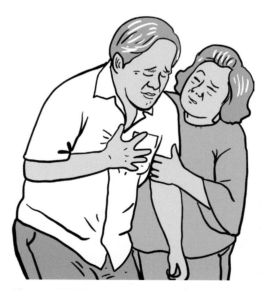

Figure 15.2 You must not miss a heart attack. High-sensitivity troponin assays were designed with that in mind. (Courtesy nottman cartoon/ Shutterstock.)

Interpreting Troponins

It is important to know that your classic type 1 MI caused by plaque rupture is not the only cause of an acutely elevated troponin:

Table 15.1 Common Causes of Acutely Elevated Troponins

Cause	Clues/Associations
Type 1 MI	Clinical signs of ACS Regional ECG changes Underlying CAD
Type 2 MI[a]	Severe systemic illness, coronary artery dissection, coronary artery spasm
Heart failure exacerbation	Volume overload
Myocarditis	Young patient without CAD Presentation highly variable
Stress (Takotsubo) cardiomyopathy	Clinical signs of ACS may or may not be present Troponin is only mildly elevated Normal coronary angiogram May have regional ECG changes May have preceding stressor
Supraventricular tachycardia	Marked tachycardia ECG showing SVT Patient may not have underlying CAD
Pulmonary embolism	Dyspnea Pleuritic chest pain DVT Hemoptysis Sinus tachycardia
Trauma (chest or head)[b]	Preceding chest or head trauma

ACS, acute coronary syndrome; CAD, coronary artery disease; DVT, deep venous thrombosis; ECG, electrocardiogram; MI, myocardial infarction; SVT, supraventricular tachycardia.

[a]Refers to myocardial ischemia and injury due to a mismatch between metabolic demand of the heart and coronary blood flow ("supply"). There are many reasons why such "supply-demand mismatch" can occur. One common example is in a systemically ill patient with underlying coronary artery disease whose baseline coronary blood flow is limited. Chest pain can occur but is not typical and is rarely prominent. The treatment is management of the underlying illness. There are other types of MI, too—but they are beyond the scope of this book.

[b]The mechanism of troponinemia in chest trauma is presumably cardiac contusion. The mechanism in head trauma is not as clear.

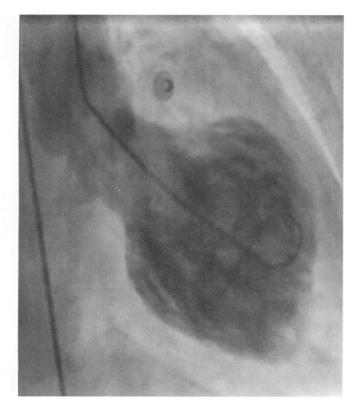

Figure 15.3 Left ventriculogram demonstrating the classic apical ballooning seen in Takotsubo ("octopus trap") cardiomyopathy, also called stress cardiomyopathy. The pathogenesis may involve catecholamine-induced microvascular spasm; coronary angiography will usually demonstrate no significant obstructive lesions. Although troponin levels may be elevated, they are rarely as high as in an acute myocardial infarction (MI). (From Klein JS, Brant WE, Helms CA, Vinson EN. *Brant and Helms' Fundamentals of Diagnostic Radiology*. 5th ed. Wolters Kluwer; 2019.)

Troponins in Chronic Kidney Disease

Chronic mild elevations in troponins (both troponin I and troponin T) are commonly seen in patients with chronic kidney disease. This phenomenon is incompletely understood; the etiology is likely multifactorial, involving both chronic microvascular injury and reduced renal clearance of troponins. The effects of hemodialysis on troponin levels are variable (troponins may slightly increase, decrease, or remain the same) and depend on the patient, dialysis method, and dialysis timing.

In the setting of suspected ACS, it is particularly important to obtain serial troponins over time among patients with chronic kidney disease (regardless of whether they are on dialysis); a single elevated troponin may simply reflect a patient's "baseline" level rather than acute myocardial injury. An elevated troponin that rises or falls by at least 20% over 2 to 6 hours in the right clinical setting (eg, chest pain, ECG changes) suggests evolution of an acute MI.

Dynamic Changes: Trending Troponins

Troponin levels rise and fall with a characteristic timing and pattern after an acute MI. By measuring troponin levels over time, you can determine if they are following this pattern and, if so, roughly how long it has been since the onset of the infarction. Timing matters, because our ability to intervene either medically or via a revascularization procedure to prevent or at least limit irreversible death of myocardial cells is greater the earlier we can start treatment.

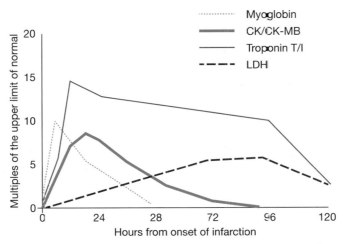

Figure 15.4 Troponins begin to rise shortly after the onset of an acute myocardial infarction (MI). Levels peak after 12 to 24 hours then return to normal after 1 to 2 weeks. The other cardiac biomarkers—discussed briefly on the next few pages— have slightly different patterns of rise and fall. CK-MB, creatine kinase-MB; LDH, lactate dehydrogenase. (From Irwin RS, Rippe JM. *Irwin and Rippe's Intensive Care Medicine*. 6th ed. Wolters Kluwer Health/Lippincott Williams & Wilkins; 2018)

Using Troponins to Guide Clinical Decision-Making

A negative troponin in a patient whose symptoms started several hours ago is reassuring that a type I MI is very unlikely. The same negative troponin in a patient whose symptoms started only 5 minutes ago doesn't tell you much—you should repeat the troponin in about 3 hours to make sure it is not rising.

What about when the initial troponin is positive?

If your suspicion for type I MI is high, your diagnostic work is usually done. Cardiology should be involved if they aren't already and management options (eg, coronary revascularization) quickly considered. In the meantime, it is prudent to continue trending the troponin; in cases of type I MI, the peak troponin correlates with the degree of myocardial injury and infarct size.

If your suspicion for type I MI is low to moderate (ie, not zero but not high enough to warrant immediate coronary angiography), check another troponin in about 3 hours.

- Serial troponins that significantly increase (commonly cited cutoffs for "significant" range from 5% to 20% over 1-6 hours; the lower the cutoff, the higher the sensitivity and the lower the specificity) shortly after the onset of symptoms should raise your suspicion for an acute MI.

- Because we expect troponins to continue to rise for at least several hours after the onset of an MI, a positive but decreasing troponin in a patient with very recent symptoms is a reassuring sign that there is not an ongoing infarction. When we begin to see this decrease or "downtrend," we consider the troponin level to have *peaked*. Unless symptoms recur in the meantime, it makes sense to stop trending troponins once they have peaked.

- Several risk stratification tools are available (eg, Thrombolysis in Myocardial Infarction [TIMI] or Global Registry of Acute Coronary Events [GRACE] score) that incorporate initial troponin results into a clinical calculator that spits out recommendations for next steps—their use is particularly helpful in the emergency room setting. There are also institution-specific algorithms for using serial troponins to rule in or rule out type I MI in patients with a positive or negative initial troponin, respectively.

 ## *Creatine Kinase-MB*

Once the gold standard for the laboratory diagnosis of myocardial injury and infarction, CK-MB has now taken a backseat to the troponins. CK-MB is one of three CK isozymes present in muscle cells. The upper limit of normal varies by lab but is usually between 3 and 10 ng/mL. Unlike its structurally related cousins, CK-MM and CK-BB (see Chapter 22), CK-MB is found in disproportionately high concentrations inside cardiac muscle cells. Like the troponins, CK-MB leaks out of cardiac myocytes when they are damaged and serves as an indicator of myocardial injury. However, CK-MB has several disadvantages compared to troponins in the workup of MI:

- Small amounts of CK-MB are found in skeletal muscle, leading to false positives in cases of skeletal muscle injury or even vigorous exercise.

- CK-MB levels tend to rise more slowly than troponins after the onset of acute MI. It may take anywhere from 4 to 12 hours for levels to rise, increasing the chances of a false-negative result when levels are measured shortly after symptom onset.

- CK-MB levels normalize about 2 days after an acute MI, leading to missed "late" diagnoses that would otherwise be caught with troponins.

Creatine Kinase-MB and Reinfarction

Given all of the advantages of troponins, many experts do not send CK-MB levels at all. Others, however, maintain that the rapid 2-day normalization of CK-MB makes it a useful marker for *reinfarction*, or recurrent MI. For example, 4 days after an acute MI, we expect CK-MB levels to have normalized while troponins remain elevated. A newly elevated CK-MB would then indicate reinfarction. CK-MB detractors point to the fact that troponins also increase in cases of reinfarction—they just do so from an elevated baseline. In our view, it is reasonable to send both troponins and CK-MB in the workup of reinfarction; the key is to understand their patterns of rise and fall (see Figure 15.4).

 ## Other Cardiac Biomarkers

Myoglobin, LDH, and AST are all found in cardiac myocytes. Because these biomarkers are also found in other tissues throughout the body, they are far less specific for myocardial injury than troponins and have little to no utility in the diagnosis of MI. Just know that levels are likely to be elevated in patients with a recent or ongoing myocardial injury.

NATRIURETIC PEPTIDES (B-TYPE NATRIURETIC PEPTIDE AND ATRIAL NATRIURETIC PEPTIDE)

The natriuretic peptides, B-type natriuretic peptide (BNP) and atrial natriuretic peptide (ANP), are released from the heart in response to volume overload. They increase urinary sodium excretion (*natriuresis*) and promote vasodilation, thereby increasing urine output (*diuresis*) and decreasing blood pressure.

Their primary use in the diagnostic lab is in the evaluation of patients with dyspnea. We expect these enzymes to be elevated in patients with decompensated heart failure (cardiac dyspnea) and normal in patients with other (usually pulmonary) causes of dyspnea.

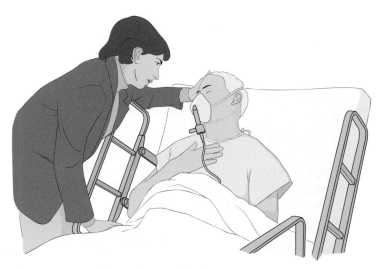

Figure 15.5 Cardiac and noncardiac dyspnea can look a lot alike. Which does this patient have? Impossible to tell just by looking at the picture. Natriuretic peptide measurement can help you tell them apart. (From LifeART image © 2023 Lippincott Williams & Wilkins. All rights reserved.)

What Do "B" and "A" Stand for in BNP and ANP?

The "B" in "BNP" originally stood for "brain," but ever since we learned that this peptide is primarily released from the ventricles of the heart, the "B" has come to stand only for "B-type." The "A" in ANP stands for atrial because ANP is released primarily by the atria of the heart. There is actually a C-type natriuretic peptide (CNP) as well, which can be found in the central nervous system and the peripheral tissues, but as far as we know, testing for CNP has no known clinical utility.

 B-Type Natriuretic Peptide

ProBNP is released primarily from the ventricles of the heart and is cleaved to N-terminal proBNP (NT-proBNP), which is biologically inert, and BNP, which is biologically active. Even though NT-proBNP is biologically inert, its levels correlate with volume overload just as well as those of BNP. As a result, either BNP or NT-proBNP can be used to help differentiate heart failure from other causes of dyspnea. The normal range for both varies significantly based on patient-specific factors such as age, sex (higher in women), and underlying comorbidities (see Table 15.2). In general, expect the following:

- The vast majority of *outpatients* with heart failure will have a BNP of at least 35 pg/mL and an NT-proBNP of at least 125 pg/mL.

- *Inpatients* with heart failure (who tend to be sicker with more comorbidities driving up natriuretic peptide levels) will have a BNP of at least 100 pg/mL and an NT-proBNP of at least 300 pg/mL.
- The above cutoff levels are more sensitive than specific. As the BNP and NT-proBNP increase above these cutoff values, the likelihood of heart failure tends to increase.

There are a few caveats:

- Patients who suffer from chronic volume overload (eg, advanced or poorly controlled heart failure) will often have a chronically elevated BNP and NT-proBNP; baseline values can be as high as the thousands. It is important in such patients to establish their baseline values so that, if and when they develop new dyspnea, you can compare the BNP and NT-proBNP to their "normal" values.
- Among patients in whom you do not have access to a baseline BNP or NT-proBNP, consider the potential confounding effects of the factors in Table 15.2.

Table 15.2 How Comorbidities Affect BNP and NT-proBNP Levels

	Renal Failure	Older Age	Obesity	Pulmonary Hypertension[a]	Neprilysin Inhibitor Use[b]	Atrial Fibrillation[c]
BNP	↑	↑	↓	↑	↑	↑
NT-proBNP	↑↑	↑↑	↓	↑	↔	↑

BNP, brain natriuretic peptide; NT-proBNP, N-terminal pro-BNP.
[a]Long-standing or severe pulmonary hypertension can cause right-sided heart failure; stretching of the right ventricle wall leads to the release of BNP and NT-proBNP.
[b]The neprilysin inhibitor sacubitril is a component of the medication sacubitril-valsartan used largely for its mortality benefit in patients with heart failure. Because neprilysin breaks down BNP, its inhibition leads to accumulation of BNP. NT-proBNP is unaffected and should be sent instead of BNP in these patients.
[c]Natriuretic peptide levels are often elevated in patients with atrial fibrillation even in the absence of related heart failure or volume overload.

BNP and NT-proBNP can still be useful in patients with one or more of the abovementioned conditions. You just need to take into account the direction in which you expect your results to be influenced and interpret accordingly. For example, a low BNP or NT-proBNP in a dyspneic patient with chronic kidney disease essentially rules out decompensated heart failure. An elevated BNP or NT-proBNP in an obese patient with dyspnea makes heart failure very likely. New and profound elevations in either BNP or NT-proBNP in any patient are likely to reflect heart failure, although—as always—use the clinical context as your guide.

B-Type Natriuretic Peptide and N-Terminal Pro–B-Type Natriuretic Peptide as Prognostic Markers

Higher BNP and NT-proBNP levels have been shown to correlate with a worse prognosis not only in patients with established heart failure but also in those with chronic obstructive pulmonary disease (COPD), PE, stable angina, and ACS (unstable angina and MI).

However, in patients with these conditions, we advise caution in using BNP alone to make specific management decisions (eg, changing your treatment approach in an otherwise stable patient with COPD due to an uptrending BNP).

A marked elevation in the BNP of a patient with an MI is a worrisome sign, indicating a higher mortality risk regardless of the degree to which the troponin levels are elevated or the presence of any other risk factors.

 ## *Atrial Natriuretic Peptide*

ANP is released primarily from the atria of the heart and functions similarly to BNP. Its levels have been shown to correlate well with volume overload, but it is not as well studied nor is it as widely employed in practice as BNP or NT-proBNP. As a result, cutoff values and guides to interpretation are not as well established. Mid-regional pro-ANP (MR-proANP)—a portion of the proANP molecule that can be selectively identified by immunoassay—has shown promise as a prognostic marker in patients with heart failure and as an additional diagnostic tool in patients with intermediate BNP or NT-proBNP values. For now, the use of ANP and MR-proANP remains largely restricted to the research setting.

D-DIMER

D-Dimer is the best studied of the *fibrin degradation products*, protein fragments released by the cleavage of fibrin, a key factor in the formation of a stable hemostatic plug (clot).

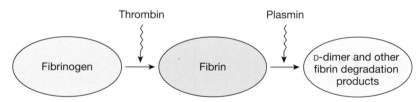

Figure 15.6 The formation and breakdown of fibrin.

D-Dimer is drawn in the same blue top tube containing sodium citrate that is used for other coagulation studies. Fasting is not required. Because of the acuity of many of the conditions that can elevate the D-dimer, the test is almost always ordered STAT.

Normal levels are less than 0.50 mg/L fibrinogen equivalent units, increasing slightly with age. For any patient over 50 years old, you can calculate the upper limit of normal (in mg/L) by dividing their age by 100. For example, the upper limit of normal for a 70-year-old patient would be $70/100 = 0.70$ mg/L fibrinogen equivalent units.

Elevated levels of D-dimer occur with ongoing coagulation and fibrinolysis (clot breakdown). As a result, D-dimer is helpful in the evaluation of:

- Deep venous thrombosis (DVT)

- Pulmonary embolism (PE)

- Disseminated intravascular coagulation (DIC)

- COVID-19, which predisposes patients to thrombosis*

- Primary hyperfibrinolysis (the term used to describe any of several congenital or acquired disorders associated with excessive fibrin degradation)

By far the most common use for this test is in the diagnosis of DVT and PE. An elevated D-dimer alone, however, does not confirm either of these diagnoses (it is not specific for DVT or PE); elevated levels must be followed by the proper imaging technique such as a duplex ultrasound in the case of suspected DVT or a computed tomographic (CT) angiogram of the chest in the case of suspected PE. The D-dimer is an acute phase reactant and thus can be misleadingly elevated in any cause of inflammation such as infection or malignancy, or after a serious injury or surgery. Elevations can also occur during pregnancy and with hepatic, renal, or cardiac failure.

The real power of the D-dimer test is in its ability to *rule out* a DVT or PE when the result comes back within the normal range; that is, it has a high sensitivity. It has also been used to follow-up patients with a DVT or PE once their course of anticoagulant therapy has been stopped: a persistently high level indicates an increased risk of recurrence.

Prediction Rules

There are numerous prediction rules that are widely used to guide the evaluation of patients with a suspected DVT or PE, and they all incorporate the D-dimer. The most commonly used are the Wells criteria for DVT and PE.

For all patients with suspected DVT, whatever their calculated risk, a D-dimer should be part of the initial evaluation. A negative result essentially rules out the diagnosis.

For patients with a suspected PE who have a calculated low or moderate risk, the D-dimer again is the test of first choice, with a negative result making the diagnosis unlikely. Some patients with no risk factors at all can have a second set of criteria applied—the so-called Pulmonary Embolism Rule-Out Criteria (PERC) rule—and if this is negative, the likelihood of a PE is extremely small and—barring compelling evidence otherwise—the workup can stop at that point.

For patients with a calculated high risk of PE, the diagnostic test of choice is not a D-dimer but rather a CT angiogram of the lungs.

---

*Elevated D-dimer levels in patients hospitalized with COVID-19 are associated with worse clinical outcomes.

ALPHA-1 ANTITRYPSIN DEFICIENCY

Alpha-1 antitrypsin (AAT) is an enzyme produced primarily in the liver that protects tissues throughout the body by inhibiting destructive proteolytic enzymes (eg, elastase). In AAT deficiency, unchecked activity of these proteolytic enzymes leads to tissue damage mostly in the lungs, liver, and skin, leading to complications such as emphysema, cirrhosis, and panniculitis, respectively.

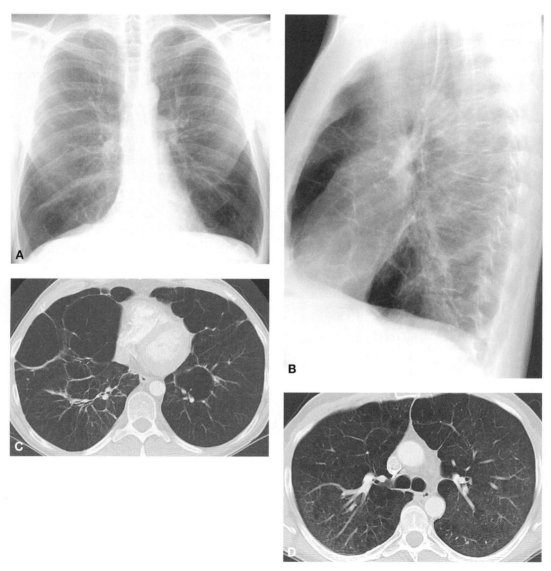

Figure 15.7 Emphysema associated with AAT deficiency tends to affect the lungs diffusely ("panlobular"): note the characteristic areas of basilar hyperlucency (chest x-ray images, A and B) and bullae (CT images, C and D). AAT, alpha-1 antitrypsin; CT, computed tomography. (From Collins J, Stern EJ. *Chest Radiology: The Essentials*. Wolters Kluwer Health; 2015.)

AAT deficiency is inherited in a codominant pattern, meaning that both parents' AAT alleles play into the ultimate phenotype (ie, both alleles are expressed). The result is that disease phenotype and severity are highly heterogeneous depending on the combination of alleles. The most common alleles that lead to clinically significant disease include "S" and "Z"; "M" is the normal allele. This clinical heterogeneity is at least in part why AAT deficiency continues to be underrecognized and underdiagnosed.

Consider checking *serum AAT concentration* in patients with emphysema, chronic hepatitis, or cirrhosis of unclear etiology, especially if they lack typical risk factors. For example, AAT testing may be indicated in a patient with emphysema who has little or no smoking history, or in a patient with cirrhosis who has no history of alcohol use, metabolic syndrome, or viral hepatitis. A strong family history of emphysema or chronic liver disease may also prompt testing, especially if any family members are known to have AAT deficiency or are carriers.

Many different assays are available; the most commonly used method is *nephelometry*, in which analysis of the turbidity (cloudiness) of an appropriately prepared sample allows for quantification of AAT concentration. Depending on the method and specific assay used, the lower limit of normal for AAT concentration varies. Levels below *57 mg/dL* reliably increase the risk for emphysema. Levels below *100 mg/dL* may cause clinically significant disease and generally warrant follow-up with genetic testing. *Genetic testing* is the gold standard test for the diagnosis and can identify both those with the disease and those who are carriers.

AAT is an acute phase reactant, meaning that levels increase with inflammation. As a result, the risk of a false negative (ie, a normal AAT concentration in a patient who is actually deficient) is increased in those who have an active infection, malignancy, or are otherwise acutely ill. Regardless of the clinical circumstances, false-negative results are extremely rare in those with severe AAT deficiency (eg, ZZ homozygous).

False-positive results (ie, a low AAT concentration in a patient who does not actually have AAT deficiency) are extremely rare.

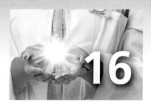

16 Gastroenterology

COMMON STOOL STUDIES

Laboratory examination of a stool specimen can be a critical component of the evaluation of many disorders affecting the gastrointestinal (GI) tract. Here is a look at those that are most widely used and that have proven to be the most helpful.

 Bacterial Cultures

Before we start talking about the how, why, and when of stool cultures, it is important to stress that stool is not sterile. You will always find normal colonizers that are not pathogenic, and this is a large part of why the accuracy of testing is limited. That being said, although they have never been patients' favorite test, stool cultures can be the key step in diagnosing many GI infections.

By far, the most common reason for ordering stool cultures is to discover the cause of diarrhea. However, by no means do all patients with diarrhea need to have stool cultures. For example, your average, run-of-the-mill diarrheal illness, however unpleasant, is almost always viral in origin and self-limited. Most guidelines recommend stool cultures in patients with diarrhea in the following cases:

- The stool is grossly bloody without obvious cause.

- There are signs or symptoms of significant inflammation (eg, high fever, marked abdominal pain, tenesmus, cramping, abdominal tenderness, very large volume stools).

- The patient is severely dehydrated.

- The patient is immunocompromised.

- You suspect a nosocomial infection.

- The diarrhea has lasted more than 3 to 7 days (how long you wait depends on how sick the patient is; if the illness isn't severe, many clinicians will wait even longer than 7 days).

Because collecting stool can be so unpleasant, the sample is often sent for several different tests at once, so the patient doesn't have to keep repeating the noxious procedure. However, you can't convincingly rule out a bacterial pathogen without two or three negative samples that have been obtained on separate days.

The usual lab requirement is 1 g or 1 mL of stool—the size of a thumbnail—submitted in a special Culture and Sensitivity (C&S) vial; do not overfill the vial. A rectal swab is also appropriate; make sure you pass the swab beyond the anal sphincter and rotate it thoroughly before withdrawing. Some organisms require special media for growth—for example, *Yersinia* species and *Vibrio parahaemolyticus*—so alert the lab ahead of time if you are looking for one of these pathogens. You may choose to have your patient fill a similar vial for O&P (see section on Ova and Parasites) at the same time if you have any suspicion of a parasitic infection.

If you are evaluating your patient for diarrhea, a liquid sample is far more likely to yield the pathogen than a solid specimen. What do we mean by liquid? It should be sufficiently soft and loose to take the shape of the container.

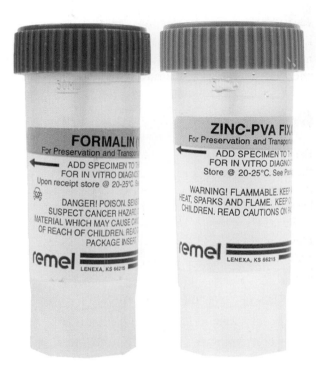

Figure 16.1 Typical stool sample collecting vials for Culture and Sensitivity (C&S) and Ova and Parasites (O&P).

 ## Ova and Parasites

As we just mentioned, you will usually order this test at the same time as a stool culture, and—because giardiasis is so prevalent—an enzyme immunoabsorbent assay (EIA) for *giardia antigen* as well. An ova and parasites (O&P) test is nothing more than a microscopic search for eggs and parasites. It is reasonable to order an O&P in a patient with diarrhea in the following cases:

- The patient has returned from a region where parasitic illnesses are endemic or where there has been a recent community-wide outbreak.

- The patient is HIV positive or is a male who has sex with men.

- The stool is grossly bloody.

- The diarrhea is persistent.

A stool test for O&P is, as you would expect, highly specific when an organism is identified, but the sensitivity varies greatly depending on the nature of the infecting parasite. To take just a few examples, the sensitivity of routine microscopic examination is almost useless for cryptosporidium, modest for entamoeba (~64% sensitivity when three specimens are evaluated), and reasonably high for giardia (as high as 90% with three specimens).

Stool Multiplex Assays

Multiplex polymerase chain reaction (PCR) panels (see general discussion on multiplex panels in Chapter 14) that test for numerous pathogens simultaneously can be run on a single stool specimen. Results are available within just a few hours. The diagnostic yield for bacterial pathogens exceeds that of stool cultures. However, these assays cannot distinguish between actual infection and colonization. Additionally, only cultures will allow you to assess antibiotic sensitivity and resistance.

Chronic or Persistent Diarrhea

The longer the diarrhea persists, the more likely it is that the usual viral and bacterial pathogens are not responsible, and the more you need to start thinking about inflammatory bowel disease (ulcerative colitis and Crohn disease), parasitic infections, malabsorption (including celiac disease), medication side effects, *Clostridium difficile* colitis, and microscopic colitis. Irritable bowel syndrome, which is often triggered by an infection that the body has cleared, must also be in the differential diagnosis.

Laboratory testing usually includes the following:

- Stool testing for O&P and giardia antigen
- Fecal calprotectin or lactoferrin (discussed next)
- Stool testing for *C. difficile* (see page 283)
- Complete blood count (CBC) with differential
- C-reactive protein
- Thyroid-stimulating hormone (TSH)
- Celiac disease screen (see page 285)

 ## *Fecal Lactoferrin and Fecal Calprotectin*

Lactoferrin and calprotectin are proteins that are present in leukocytes. Both are released when white blood cells are activated or damaged. Elevated levels in the stool are indicative of inflammation of the bowel. If their levels are not increased, the likelihood of an inflammatory process is extremely low. If they are elevated, then additional testing is indicated to pin down the cause. These tests have largely replaced microscopic examination of the stool for *fecal leukocytes*, once the standard test for inflammatory bowel diseases; the sensitivity and specificity of microscopic examination for white blood cells vary too widely from lab to lab and from patient to patient.

Fecal lactoferrin is most often used to distinguish bacterial causes of diarrhea from other infectious causes. Lactoferrin appears to be more specific for bacterial causes of acute diarrhea than calprotectin.

Fecal calprotectin is more often used to differentiate inflammatory bowel disease (in which it is elevated) from irritable bowel syndrome (in which it is not). Note that this test is not specific for Crohn disease or ulcerative colitis; it is merely a marker of inflammation.

 ## Stool Osmolality

Traditionally, diarrhea has been divided into two categories: osmotic diarrhea and secretory diarrhea. This distinction reflects the two major pathogenic mechanisms that underlie diarrhea—osmotic overload from too many solutes in the bowel, and enhanced secretion of water and chloride into the gut.

On rare occasions, distinguishing these two types of diarrhea can help determine the cause of unexplained diarrhea. Osmotic diarrhea is often caused by laxatives and malabsorption. Secretory diarrhea can be caused by infection, bacterial toxins, and hypersecretion of various substances such as bile salts, serotonin, vasoactive intestinal peptide (VIP), and—most famously—gastrin in patients with Zollinger-Ellison syndrome (see page 293).

Determining whether diarrhea is osmotic or secretory requires measuring stool osmolality, a procedure that is difficult for the patient and often the lab as well. The stool sample provided to the lab must be a frozen specimen of liquid stool submitted in a small plastic container. With osmotic diarrhea, the osmolality is high (>50 mOsm/kg greater than the plasma osmolality), whereas with secretory diarrhea it is close to the plasma osmolality. You may find this test useful someday, and it is often discussed on rounds—which are both reasons to briefly talk about it here—but distinguishing osmotic from secretory diarrhea is necessary on only rare occasions and is not a part of the routine evaluation of diarrhea.

 ## Fecal Fat and Elastase

A *fecal fat* can help you identify patients with malabsorption. Because patients who malabsorb fat also tend to malabsorb carbohydrates and protein, an elevated fecal fat serves as a good indicator for global malabsorption. Increased levels of fecal fat, referred to as *steatorrhea*, can occur with the following:

- Pancreatic insufficiency, a deficiency of pancreatic digestive enzymes that may be caused by pancreatic cancer, chronic pancreatitis, and cystic fibrosis

- A number of disorders affecting the small bowel: celiac disease, tropical sprue, small intestinal bacterial overgrowth (SIBO), inflammatory bowel disease, and Whipple disease

- Short-bowel syndrome due to surgical bypass or resection

- Cholestasis (with impaired circulation of bile acids) due to primary biliary cholangitis (PBC) or primary sclerosing cholangitis (PSC)

Diagnosis of steatorrhea requires a 24- to 72-hour stool collection while the patient is consuming 100 g of fat daily. If steatorrhea is diagnosed, a stool measurement of *elastase*, a pancreatic enzyme, can be used to test for pancreatic insufficiency. Elastase in the fecal specimen is detected by enzyme-linked immunosorbent assay (ELISA). Here, we are looking for abnormally *low* levels. **A measurement greater than 200 μg/g of fecal material is considered normal.** The sensitivity of this test for patients with moderate to severe chronic pancreatitis approaches 100% (very few false negatives) but is much lower in those with mild disease. False positives are rare—specificity exceeds 90% in patients with moderate to severe pancreatitis—but may occur when copious watery diarrhea dilutes the sample, lowering the concentration of detectable elastase. Because of the superior reliability and convenience of fecal elastase compared with fecal fat, some clinicians forgo the fecal fat measurement entirely when pancreatic insufficiency is suspected.

D-Xylose: Diagnosing the Cause of Malabsorption

Suppose you find that your patient with chronic diarrhea has steatorrhea. What is the cause? There are two basic mechanisms that can lead to malabsorption: problems with digestion (ie, inadequate breakdown of intraluminal contents; for example, pancreatic insufficiency) and problems with the intestinal wall itself (eg, Crohn disease or celiac disease). A *D-xylose test* can help differentiate between these two mechanisms of malabsorption.

D-Xylose is a simple carbohydrate that does not require any digestion before being absorbed across the wall of the small intestine and subsequently excreted in the urine. Therefore, a patient with a *digestive* problem will have no trouble absorbing D-xylose. However, a patient with an *intestinal wall* problem will. During a D-xylose test, 25 g of D-xylose is administered orally, then samples of serum and urine are collected at 1 and 5 hours. A serum D-xylose less than 25 mg/dL (at 1 hour) or urine D-xylose less than 4.5 g (over 5 hours) suggests intestinal mucosal pathology rather than maldigestion.

The concept of D-xylose testing makes sense, but there are several problems that make it unpopular. First, and perhaps most importantly, D-xylose testing is not very sensitive or specific for any particular disease; it only gives some idea of the *category* of disease. Several other tests—many of which are simpler and more reliable—allow us to more effectively rule in or rule out specific diseases (eg, tissue transglutaminase for celiac disease). In short, we have better tests. Second, D-xylose results are influenced by several confounding factors (renal dysfunction, gastroparesis, ascites, and several medications including aspirin and glipizide) that may lead to false positives—that is, a falsely low serum or urinary D-xylose. False negatives are not as common. Do not expect to make a final diagnosis without pairing a D-xylose test with appropriate disease-specific testing.

 ## *Fecal Occult Blood (and More)*

There are several tests that can be used to detect occult GI bleeding, that is, GI bleeding that is too small to be detected visually. They test for hemoglobin in the stool. *These tests have only been validated as a tool for colon cancer screening* and generally should not be used in the evaluation of other causes of GI bleeding, especially in the inpatient setting.

The samples can be obtained at home and then mailed directly to your office or the lab for testing. There are two basic types of test:

- The *fecal occult blood test (FOBT)* has been around for a long time. It is a chemical test in which a small sample of stool is applied to a paper slide that has been impregnated with guaiac, a naturally occurring brown resin. A few drops of hydrogen peroxide are then dripped onto the slide. In the presence of peroxidase-like activity, which is present in hemoglobin, the paper turns blue within seconds. The major drawback to this test is that there are many false positives (eg, it will detect hemoglobin in dietary meat, so the patient's diet must be restricted before testing) and false negatives (eg, vitamin C inhibits the enzymatic reaction).

- The *fecal immunochemical test (FIT)* is an immunoassay that employs monoclonal antibodies directed against the human globin chains of hemoglobin. Stool can be collected at home but the sample must be sent to a laboratory for testing. Unlike FOBT, FIT will only detect intact hemoglobin molecules and thus more accurately measures bleeding from below the stomach (stomach acid chews up hemoglobin molecules; however, when there is a massive upper GI bleed, sufficient hemoglobin may escape acid degradation in the stomach to reach the intestines intact).

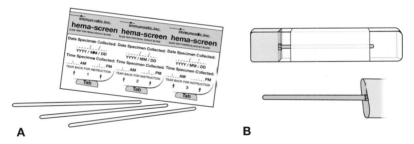

Figure 16.2 A. Fecal occult blood test (FOBT) collection kit. B. Fecal immunochemical test (FIT) collection kit.

Fecal Immunochemical Test Plus DNA Testing

There is another test that combines *multitarget stool DNA testing* with FIT. In addition to measuring hemoglobin in the stool, this test looks for DNA mutations associated with precancerous and cancerous lesions present in colonic cells that have been shed into the stool. It is more expensive than FIT alone, and although its sensitivity for colon cancer is higher, it may be less specific (more false positives). It is also not yet certain if the increased sensitivity of this test leads to better clinical outcomes.

 ## *Clostridium difficile*

The bacterium *C. difficile* elaborates two pathogenic toxins, A and B, that can be detected in the stool.* Although the organism itself is rarely invasive, these toxins can cause severe intestinal damage. Virtually any patient with severe or persistent diarrhea who has had exposure to an

---

*A minimum of 0.5mL of liquid stool should be sent to the lab in a screw-top container.

antibiotic in the preceding 3 months should be tested for *C. difficile*. The leading cause of hospital-acquired diarrhea, *C. difficile* infection can also result from even the most minimal exposure to an outpatient antibiotic. This association with antibiotic use occurs because antibiotics disrupt the normal intestinal biome, thereby allowing *C. difficile* to settle in and multiply.

There are various tests for *C. difficile*. Most of the time, *nucleic acid amplification testing (NAAT)* for *C. difficile* toxin genes is sufficient—it is both sensitive and specific—but only if the patient has had at least three unformed, otherwise unexplained stools in the preceding 24 hours. Otherwise, NAAT should be combined with an *enzyme immunoassay (EIA) for toxins A and B* and for *glutamate dehydrogenase* (GHD, an antigen elaborated by *C. difficile*). EIA for toxins A and B is specific but lacks sensitivity, whereas the EIA for GHD is sensitive but lacks specificity.

Recurrence of *C. difficile* after treatment is common, but the diagnosis can be difficult. Recurrent disease often presents just like irritable bowel syndrome, which occurs in as many as 25% of patients after *C. difficile* infection. Retesting for toxins A and B is usually not helpful, because many patients remain asymptomatic carriers and will test positive for up to a month after their disease has resolved. For this reason, testing for cure is not recommended unless symptoms persist without interruption for several weeks.

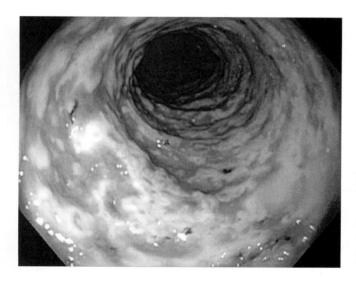

Figure 16.3 Endoscopy demonstrating the shiny white plaques of pseudomembranous colitis, a manifestation of severe *Clostridium difficile* infection. (From Riddell R, Jain D. *Lewin, Weinstein and Riddell's Gastrointestinal Pathology and Its Clinical Implications.* 2nd ed. Lippincott Williams & Wilkins; 2014.)

CELIAC DISEASE

 ## *Who Should Be Tested*

Screening the general population for celiac disease is not currently recommended, despite the high prevalence of the disease worldwide. Consider testing patients with:

- compatible GI symptoms, including most patients with suspected irritable bowel syndrome

- characteristic extra-GI manifestations: for example, unexplained iron deficiency anemia, autoimmune thyroiditis, unexplained elevated liver transaminases, or osteoporosis in the absence of obvious risk factors

- a high risk of having celiac disease (those with Down or Turner syndrome, type 1 diabetes, immunoglobulin A [IgA] deficiency, or a first- or second-degree relative with celiac disease), even in the absence of obvious signs or symptoms of the disease

 ## *The Tests*

Testing for celiac disease used to rely on seeing how a patient responded to a gluten-free diet. While this is still a reasonable approach, it is no longer considered necessary. Even the necessity of a duodenal biopsy is being questioned because of the high sensitivity and specificity of available lab tests.

The preferred tests today are *anti-endomysial IgA antibodies (EMA-IgA)* and *anti-tissue transglutaminase antibodies (anti-tTG IgA)*. These are both autoantibodies, the former directed against the connective tissue that covers smooth muscle cells, and the latter against the specific antigen in that connective tissue. Both have a very high sensitivity (around 90%) and specificity (approaching 100%).

- Testing should not be done on a patient who has been avoiding gluten. Several weeks of gluten avoidance allows the bowel to heal and can lead to false-negative results.

- In the United States, a positive small bowel biopsy is still required to confirm the result. However, elsewhere, including the United Kingdom, a positive antibody test—especially if the anti-tTG IgA is at least 10 times normal—in high-risk children is considered sufficient to establish the diagnosis. The trend of relying on a high anti-tTG IgA for diagnosis may be moving in this direction for all patients with suspected celiac disease.

Because patients with celiac disease are 10 to 15 times more likely than the general population to be IgA deficient, you should also measure a *total IgA level* when you screen for celiac disease. A low total IgA could cause a false-negative test with both EMA-IgA and anti-tTG IgA. If celiac antibody testing is negative and the total IgA is low in a patient in whom you suspect celiac disease, you have several options:

- Measure immunoglobulin G (IgG) levels of these autoantibodies

- Screen for two human leukocyte antigens (HLA): *DQ2* and/or *DQ8*. Almost all patients with celiac disease will have one of these HLAs. If they are both negative, celiac disease is very unlikely

- If despite everything your diagnosis is still uncertain, a duodenal biopsy can provide additional diagnostic information

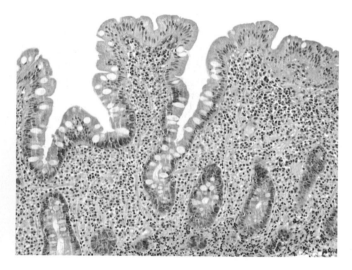

Figure 16.4 Duodenal biopsy of a patient with celiac disease. Note the villous blunting and the marked infiltration of inflammatory cells. (From Arnold CA, Lam-Himlin DM, Montgomery E. *Atlas of Gastrointestinal Pathology: A Pattern Based Approach to Non-Neoplastic Biopsies.* Wolters Kluwer Health; 2015.)

Antigliadin antibodies—gliadin is a component of gluten—were once the test of choice for celiac disease. Measurement of these antibodies is no longer recommended. This test's sensitivity and specificity are significantly lower than that of EMA-IgA and anti-tTG IgA.

HELICOBACTER PYLORI

Depending on what field of medicine you decide to pursue, tests for *Helicobacter pylori* may be among the more common ones that you order. More than one-third of persons in the United States and more than 50% worldwide are infected. *H. pylori* is the leading cause of peptic ulcer disease* (PUD) worldwide and is an important cause of GI bleeding and gastric malignancies.

 ## Who Should Be Tested

Despite its prevalence, screening the general population is *not* recommended. There are three general categories of patients in whom testing should be considered:

1. *Symptomatic patients*: those with active PUD, a past history of PUD who have never been tested, and patients under the age of 60 with unexplained dyspepsia (those over 60 or patients with alarm features such as GI bleeding or unexplained weight loss should proceed directly to endoscopy with biopsy); controversial—patients about to start long-term aspirin or NSAID therapy (because of the increased risk of bleeding), and those with idiopathic thrombocytopenic purpura (associated with *H. pylori* infection for unclear reasons) or unexplained iron deficiency anemia

2. *Patients at high risk of infection*: the most common example is household contacts of patients with active *H. pylori* infection

3. *Patients at risk of complications*: those with a family history of gastric cancer or peptic ulcer disease; patients with a history of a resection of early gastric cancer; those with a low-grade gastric mucosa associated lymphoid tissue (MALT) lymphoma

 ## How to Test

Testing can be done by a *stool antigen test* or a *breath test* in which the patient ingests urea—typically as a powdered solution, often fruit-flavored!—that has been labeled with radioactive C^{13}. *H. pylori* breaks down the urea, releasing labeled carbon dioxide in the breath. Both the breath test and stool antigen test have a very high sensitivity and specificity, each exceeding 90% for patients with active infection.

In one typical breath test protocol, patients are asked to breathe into a collection bag 15 minutes after ingesting the radiolabeled urea preparation. The contents of the bag are then analyzed by infrared spectroscopy. Patients must fast at least 1 hour before the test. They should also be off any proton pump inhibitor (PPI), antibiotic, or bismuth preparation for at least 2 weeks—all of these are used in the treatment of *H. pylori* and can therefore reduce the sensitivity of the test. The use of H_2 blockers does not impact the results. Active GI bleeding can yield a false-negative result.

---

*In case you are interested, #2 is the use of nonsteroidal anti-inflammatory agents (NSAIDs) and #3 is idiopathic peptic ulcer disease.

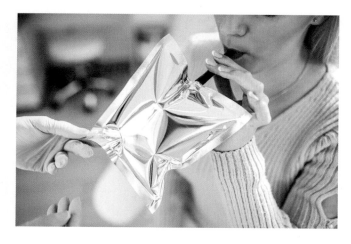

Figure 16.5 A patient performing a urea breath test. An alternative to the breath test is to test the stool for *Helicobacter pylori* antigen, with the same caveats as for the breath test. (Courtesy Dusan Petkovic/ Shutterstock.)

Measuring serum IgG levels against *H. pylori* is no longer recommended because this test cannot distinguish between ongoing and past infection.

In patients who are undergoing upper endoscopy (eg, for unexplained dyspepsia and weight loss), a gastric biopsy may reveal the organisms and thereby establish the diagnosis.

 ## *Testing for Cure*

Once the patient has been diagnosed and treated, retesting for cure is recommended because of the high rate of failure due to antibiotic resistance. Retesting should be done at least 4 weeks after the end of treatment with the patient off any PPIs.

Hydrogen Breath Tests

H. pylori infection is not the only disorder that can be diagnosed with a breath test. Others include the following:

- Although rarely needed, a *lactose breath test* can diagnose *lactase deficiency* (ie, lactose intolerance). This test looks for the production of hydrogen gas produced by colonic bacteria exposed to lactose that was undigested in the small intestine. The patient is usually asked to fast for 12 hours before ingesting a lactose solution and then blows into a series of collection bags over the course of several hours. Each bag is analyzed, and a curve is generated and compared to a normal standard.

- A similar test can detect overgrowth of colonic bacteria in the small bowel (SIBO). Here, the patient is often given a *lactulose* load, and—if the test is positive—two peaks of hydrogen gas are produced: one from digestion by bacteria in the colon (also seen in normal individuals) and one from digestion by bacteria in the small intestine (not seen in normal individuals).

PANCREATITIS: LIPASE AND AMYLASE

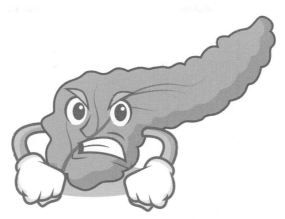

Figure 16.6 An inflamed pancreas. (Courtesy Kong Vector/Shutterstock.)

In acute pancreatitis, digestive enzymes leak out of the damaged pancreas and accumulate in the bloodstream. The most commonly measured and clinically useful of these enzymes are lipase and amylase.

 Lipase

Lipase breaks down fat in the intestines. The normal range is 13 to 60 U/L (with some variation by laboratory). Levels increase about 6 hours after the onset of acute pancreatitis, peak around 24 hours, and remain elevated for several days (sometimes up to 2 weeks). Order this test in any patient in whom you suspect acute pancreatitis.

In the right clinical context, an elevation in the serum lipase greater than 3 times the upper limit of normal is highly suggestive of acute pancreatitis (good specificity). False positives may occur in patients with peptic ulcer disease, acute or chronic renal failure (lipase is cleared by the kidneys), cholecystitis, bowel ischemia or obstruction, or recent surgical manipulation of the pancreas or surrounding structures. Very high elevations are unlikely to be due to reduced clearance from renal failure. Occasionally, certain medications may cause elevations in lipase even in the absence of drug-induced pancreatitis; examples include some opiates, cholinergics, and diuretics.

False negatives (a normal or near-normal lipase in a patient with acute pancreatitis) are occasionally seen in patients with underlying chronic pancreatitis with pancreatic insufficiency and decreased lipase production, but are rare. Because lipase hangs around in the serum for at least a few days after the onset of acute pancreatitis, levels are unlikely to be normal even when the presentation is delayed.

Amylase

Amylase is an enzyme that breaks down carbohydrates in the intestines. The normal range is 0 to 130 U/L (again with some variation by laboratory). As with lipase, an amylase level greater than 3 times the upper limit of normal is often seen in acute pancreatitis. However, lipase is the better test. Compared to lipase, amylase has less sensitivity for acute pancreatitis. There are a few reasons for this:

- Alcohol hinders the production of amylase, resulting in frequent false negatives in alcoholic pancreatitis.

- Very high triglyceride levels in the blood interfere with amylase assays, leading to false negatives in hypertriglyceridemia-associated pancreatitis.

- Amylase has a short half-life. Levels may return to normal within 1 to 3 days of the onset of pancreatic inflammation (which may precede the onset of symptoms). Because some patients do not seek care until they have had symptoms for a day or more, amylase levels may already have normalized (or nearly normalized).

- In patients with pancreatic insufficiency (eg, due to chronic pancreatitis), the relative decrease in the production of amylase is greater than that of lipase, resulting in high rates of "falsely normal" amylase in patients with acute pancreatitis superimposed on chronic pancreatitis.

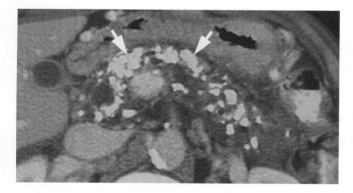

Figure 16.7 The pancreatic calcifications (arrows) in this patient with a history of chronic alcohol abuse indicate chronic pancreatitis. This condition tends to affect the production of amylase more so than lipase, although both enzymes may be "falsely" normal in acute-on-chronic pancreatitis. (From Brant WE, Helms CA. *Fundamentals of Diagnostic Radiology*, 4th ed. Lippincott Williams & Wilkins; 2012.)

Amylase is also less specific than lipase for acute pancreatitis. Common causes of false positives are similar to those for lipase: renal failure, cholecystitis, bowel ischemia or obstruction, recent surgical manipulation of the pancreas or surrounding structures, and (rarely) some medications such as nitrofurantoin, aspirin, and estrogens. But the specificity of amylase is further limited by the inability of assays to distinguish between different forms of amylase, which include *pancreatic amylase* (the one we care about), *salivary amylase*, and *macroamylase* (see the box "Macroamylasemia").

Salivary Gland Amylase

Just as the pancreas produces amylase in order to break down carbohydrates in the gut, the saliva contains its own amylase to break down carbohydrates while we are still chewing and swallowing. Salivary amylase can be elevated in multiple conditions including parotitis, salivary gland stones, malignancy (several solid tumors have been implicated—not just salivary gland tumors), eating disorders (including bulimia and anorexia nervosa), fallopian tube disease (including salpingitis, fallopian cysts, and ruptured ectopic pregnancy), and acidosis. The result is an elevated (total) amylase even in the absence of pancreatitis.

Macroamylasemia

Macroamylase forms when amylase binds to other molecules (usually immunoglobulins), resulting in bulky complexes that are poorly cleared by the kidneys and accumulate in the bloodstream. Amylase testing picks up this "macroamylasemia" as an elevated total amylase. Causes of macroamylasemia include HIV, malignancy (particularly multiple myeloma and lymphoma), and several autoimmune diseases (celiac, inflammatory bowel disease, and rheumatoid arthritis).

Overall, the ~ 75% sensitivity and ~ 90% specificity of amylase (when it is greater than 3 times the upper limit of normal) make it a reasonable test for acute pancreatitis. In practice, however, lipase is usually the only lab test you need to rule in or rule out pancreatitis. Adding an amylase may ultimately confuse the picture, especially given its poor sensitivity compared to lipase. If you do order amylase as part of the workup of acute pancreatitis, understand its limitations and interpret the results with caution.

Putting It All Together: Establishing a Diagnosis of Pancreatitis

Lipase and/or amylase can be combined with clinical and imaging findings to establish a diagnosis of acute pancreatitis. Patients must meet at least two of the following three criteria:

1. Lipase *or* amylase at least 3 times the upper limit of normal

2. Abdominal pain suggestive of acute pancreatitis (by history and physical; eg, epigastric pain radiating to the back)

3. Characteristic imaging findings (usually focal or diffuse enlargement of the pancreas seen on computed tomography [CT] or magnetic resonance imaging [MRI])

Note that, based on these criteria, a patient with classic signs and symptoms of acute pancreatitis and characteristic imaging findings can be diagnosed with acute pancreatitis even when both the lipase and amylase are normal.

Determining the Prognosis in Pancreatitis

There are several lab tests that are not particularly helpful in the diagnosis of pancreatitis but which inform prognosis once the diagnosis has been made. The higher these labs, the worse the prognosis:

- Hematocrit: elevations reflect hemoconcentration due to intravascular volume depletion ("third spacing").

- Blood urea nitrogen (BUN): correlates with mortality

- Creatinine: rising levels within the first 48 hours are associated with the development of pancreatic necrosis. The elevated creatinine probably reflects renal damage due to hypovolemia and hypotension.

- C-reactive protein (CRP): a level greater than 15 mg/dL after 48 hours suggests severe pancreatitis.

Some of these values can be plugged into validated prognostication scores, such as the APACHE II or BISAP. There is no firmly established consensus on if and when to trend these labs in patients with acute pancreatitis. In general, those with disease sufficiently severe to be hospitalized should have at least a daily basic metabolic panel (BMP) (including BUN and creatinine) and CBC (including hematocrit) checked; consider trending the CRP depending on the clinical scenario.

GASTRIN AND ZOLLINGER-ELLISON SYNDROME

Gastrin is a hormone produced mainly by the cells of the gastric antrum. Its major function is to stimulate acid secretion by the gastric parietal cells in response to feeding or a high gastric pH.

Elevated gastrin levels can be seen in a variety of conditions, but testing is primarily considered when the diagnosis of Zollinger-Ellison syndrome is on the table. This disorder is caused by a gastrin-producing tumor, usually located in the duodenum, less often in the pancreas. Zollinger-Ellison syndrome is rare, but it should be suspected in patients with peptic ulcer disease that is refractory to therapy (eg, PPIs), multiple peptic ulcers, ulcers distal to the duodenal bulb, or a family history of multiple endocrine neoplasia I.*

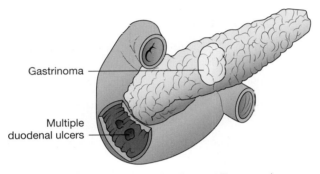

Gastrinoma

Multiple duodenal ulcers

Figure 16.8 Manifestations of Zollinger-Ellison syndrome.

The test of choice is a serum *fasting gastrin level.* Normal values should be less than 100 pg/mL. In the right clinical setting, the diagnosis of Zollinger-Ellison syndrome can be made when the gastrin level is 10 times higher than normal (at least 1000 or so, depending on the lab) and the gastric pH is less than 4.0.

A mildly to moderately elevated gastrin level can be seen in some patients with Zollinger-Ellison syndrome, but it is nonspecific; it is also seen in patients with pernicious anemia who have achlorhydria (an absence of acid in the stomach). When gastrin is mildly to moderately elevated and the diagnosis remains uncertain, a *secretin stimulation test* is the best next step. Secretin is a small peptide hormone that normally antagonizes the action of gastrin. However, it *paradoxically increases* gastrin release from gastrinoma cells. Secretin is given by a rapid intravenous (IV) infusion and gastrin levels are sampled every few minutes. A rise in the gastrin level of more than 120 pg/mL is 94% sensitive and approximately 100% specific for Zollinger-Ellison syndrome.

False negatives on the secretin stimulation test can occur in patients taking a PPI (eg, omeprazole). However, in patients with suspected severe Zollinger-Ellison syndrome, you should not stop the PPI; doing so risks provoking a sudden severe complication of peptic ulcer disease, such as perforation or bleeding. Before ordering this test, intense medical therapy should first be instituted to heal any active ulcerations.

*A rare genetic syndrome marked by a predisposition to GI endocrine tumors, such as gastrinoma, as well as pituitary adenomas and primary hyperparathyroidism.

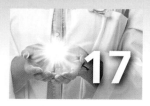

17 Hepatology

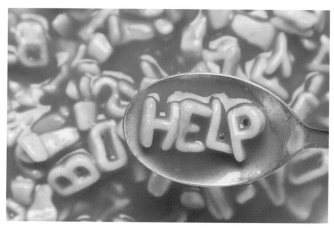

Figure 17.1 The alphabet soup of hepatitis viruses can be overwhelming. (Courtesy mattjeacock/iStock.)

Almost any virus can cause hepatic inflammation (hepatitis), many of which are discussed elsewhere in this book (if you have ever had infectious mononucleosis—and most of us have, or will at some point—then you probably had an inflamed liver). But certain viruses attack the liver as their prime target, and these are the ones we refer to as hepatitis viruses. They have been cleverly named hepatitis A, hepatitis B, hepatitis C, and so on. These viruses are common, and testing for them is a key step in the workup of patients with elevated hepatic aminotransferases (see Chapter 5, page 67). Appropriate interpretation of the results can dictate key management decisions.

Hepatitis A Virus

The most common presentation of hepatitis A virus (HAV) is an acute, self-limited hepatitis. Fever, abdominal pain, and jaundice are all common, but a significant minority of patients may be asymptomatic. Very rarely, progression to acute liver failure can occur. The diagnosis is made by antibody testing.

Immunoglobulin M Anti–Hepatitis A Virus Antibodies

These antibodies appear around the time of symptom onset—after an average incubation period of just under a month—and persist for up to 6 months. Rarely, anti-HAV immunoglobulin M (IgM) antibodies may persist for longer, or even permanently, in some patients who are no longer actively infected. However, it is safe to say that the presence of IgM antibodies is highly suggestive of acute HAV infection. A negative result makes a diagnosis of acute hepatitis A infection very unlikely.

Immunoglobulin G Anti–Hepatitis A Virus Antibodies

These typically become detectable as the patient begins to recover from acute HAV infection (the convalescent phase), usually a few days to weeks after IgM has become detectable. Immunoglobulin G (IgG) antibodies persist for many years, often for life, and indicate immunity either from prior infection or vaccination.

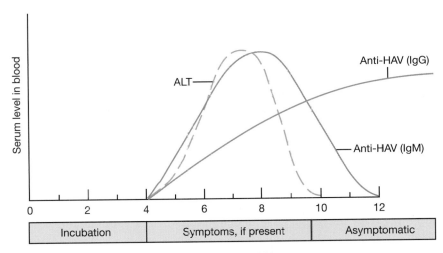

Figure 17.2 Anti-HAV IgG antibodies become detectable shortly after anti-HAV IgM antibodies. IgM antibodies usually decline to undetectable levels within weeks to months, whereas IgG antibodies persist for many years and indicate immunity. ALT, alanine aminotransferase; HAV, hepatitis A virus; IgG, immunoglobulin G; IgM, immunoglobulin M. (From Brown LJ, Coller RJ, Miller LT. *Pediatrics.* 2nd ed. Wolters Kluwer; 2019.)

Hepatitis B Virus

Hepatitis B virus (HBV) can cause both acute and chronic hepatitis. The virus has a long incubation period (up to several months), and even patients who have been infected for years can be asymptomatic. These facts, combined with the potentially devastating consequences of untreated disease—including progression to cirrhosis and hepatocellular carcinoma—mean that your overall threshold for testing should be low:

- The Centers for Disease Control and Prevention (CDC) recommends that all adults be screened once for HBV infection.

- Consider periodic testing in any patient (even if they have been vaccinated; not everyone responds to the vaccine) with ongoing risk factors for HBV (eg, multiple sexual partners, history of incarceration) or risk factors for severe disease (eg, immunosuppression).

- Otherwise unexplained signs or symptoms of acute or chronic hepatitis (eg, fever with jaundice) mandate HBV testing.

- Testing in the first trimester of pregnancy is also recommended.

Testing: Antigens, Antibodies, and DNA

When testing for HBV, sometimes we measure antigens, sometimes antibodies directed against those antigens, and sometimes both. There are three antigens of interest:

- *Hepatitis B Surface ("s") Antigen*: both the antigen itself (*HBsAg*) and antibodies directed against it (*HBsAb*) can be measured.

- *Hepatitis B Core ("c") Antigen*: only antibodies are measured, including IgM (*HBcAb IgM*) and total (*HBcAb total*). IgG antibodies exist but are never directly measured. Their presence is deduced by a positive HBcAb total with a negative HBcAb IgM.

- *Hepatitis B "e" Antigen*: the letter "e" doesn't actually stand for anything—it is not an envelope antigen as some mistakenly assume, but rather a protein secreted by the virus. Both the antigen (*HBeAg*) and antibodies directed against it (*HBeAb*) can be measured.

Why do we measure so many antigens and antibodies? It's not just because we can. Each test provides a unique piece of information that contributes to defining your patient's HBV status. Combining these tests allows you to determine whether your patient:

- Has an acute infection, chronic infection, resolved infection, immunity from vaccination, or no history of exposure or vaccination at all

- Is likely to be contagious or not

Each antigen and antibody has a characteristic pattern of rise and fall following infection with HBV. We can also directly measure HBV DNA via polymerase chain reaction (PCR).

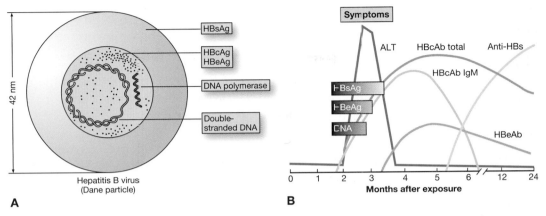

A

B

Figure 17.3 A. A schematic representation of hepatitis B virus (HBV) depicting its component antigens. B. The typical pattern of rise and fall of each HBV antigen and antibody in a patient who eventually clears the infection. HBsAg, HBeAg, HBV DNA, and HBcAb IgM all typically disappear with a resolution of the infection. The appearance of HBsAb indicates immunity. Importantly, HBcAb IgM may be the only positive HBV serologic test during the so-called "window period," when HBsAg has cleared but HBsAb has not yet appeared. ALT, alanine aminotransferase; HBcAb, hepatitis B core antibody; HBeAb, hepatitis B e antibody; HBcAg, hepatitis B core antigen; HBeAg, hepatitis B e antigen; HBsAg, hepatitis B surface antigen; IgM, immunoglobulin M.

In the following three tables, we will first go through what each test means (Table 17.1). We will then go over which tests to order depending on your clinical question (Table 17.2). Finally, we will look at how the results of these tests can be combined to determine a patient's HBV status (Table 17.3).

Table 17.1 What Each Hepatitis B Test Tells You

Antigen/Antibody	Clinical Interpretation	Caveats
HBsAg	Active infection (acute or chronic)	May be transiently positive after vaccination
HBsAb	Immunity (from vaccination or resolved infection)	Coexistence with HBsAg may indicate ineffective antibodies (carrier state). Can fade over many years
HBcAb total	Acute, chronic, or resolved infection	Not produced after vaccination Persists for lifetime
HBcAb IgM	Acute infection	Not produced after vaccination
HBcAb IgG	Remote infection (chronic or resolved)	Not produced after vaccination. No assay available; deduce presence by positive HBcAb total with negative IgM

(continued)

Table 17.1 What Each Hepatitis B Test Tells You (*continued*)

Antigen/Antibody	Clinical Interpretation	Caveats
HBeAg	Active infection with high infectivity Correlates with +PCR	Less useful than HBV PCR
HBeAb	Correlates with –PCR	Less useful than HBV PCR
HBV DNA (PCR)	Levels correlate with the degree of active viral replication/infectivity.	Low positive results (<300 copies/mL) may persist in both chronic and resolved infections.

HBcAb, hepatitis B core antibody; HBeAb, hepatitis B e antibody; HBsAb, hepatitis B surface antibody; HBeAg, hepatitis B e antigen; HBsAg, hepatitis B surface antigen; HBV, hepatitis B virus; IgG, immunoglobulin G; IgM, immunoglobulin M; PCR, polymerase chain reaction.

Table 17.2 Hepatitis B Tests to Order Depending on Your Clinical Question

Clinical Question(s)	Helpful Tests
Does this patient have HBV (acute or chronic)?	HBsAg HBsAb HBcAb total HBcAb IgM[a]
Has this patient ever had HBV?	HBsAg HBsAb[b] HBcAb total
Is this patient immune to HBV?	HBsAb
Is this patient with active HBV likely to spread it to others at this time (infectivity)?	HBV PCR HBeAg HBeAb
Is treatment indicated in this patient with HBV? Is the patient responding to treatment?	HBV PCR[c]

HBcAb, hepatitis B core antibody; HBeAb, hepatitis B e antibody; HBsAb, hepatitis B surface antibody; HBeAg, hepatitis B e antigen; HBsAg, hepatitis B surface antigen; HBV, hepatitis B virus; IgM, immunoglobulin M; PCR, polymerase chain reaction.
[a]HBcAb IgM may be the only positive HBV serologic test during the so-called "window period," when HBsAg has cleared but HBsAb has not yet appeared.
[b]HBsAb can become undetectable in some patients after many years.
[c]HBV PCR is most useful in patients in whom a diagnosis of HBV has already been established. In general, the higher the viral load, the lower the threshold to initiate treatment (treatment cutoffs vary and depend on HBeAg status as well as the presence or absence of transaminitis or cirrhosis). Once treatment has been started, a patient who is appropriately responding will tend to have a decreasing viral load. A viral load that fails to decrease or that is increasing raises concern for either a treatment-resistant virus or medication noncompliance. A persistently elevated viral load (> ~2,000 IU/mL) is associated with an increased risk of cirrhosis and hepatocellular carcinoma.

Table 17.3 Hepatitis B Test Results by Disease State

HBV Disease State	Expected Positive Tests
Acute infection	HBsAg (except in window period) HBcAb total HBcAb IgM HBeAg (usually) HBV PCR
Chronic infection	HBsAg HBcAb total +/– HBeAg HBV PCR
Resolved infection	HBsAb HBcAb total +/– HBeAb
Vaccinated	HBsAb

HBcAb, hepatitis B core antibody; HBeAb, hepatitis B e antibody; HBsAb, hepatitis B surface antibody; HBeAg, hepatitis B e antigen; HBsAg, hepatitis B surface antigen; HBV, hepatitis B virus; IgM, immuno-globulin M; PCR, polymerase chain reaction.

The patterns in Table 17.3 tend to hold true, but, as always, there are many exceptions. For example, patients transitioning between disease states (eg, gradually resolving acute or chronic infection) may have confusing or even seemingly nonsensical results. Use your clinical context and, if needed, repeat the labs again in a few days to weeks.

 ## *Hepatitis C Virus*

Most patients infected with hepatitis C virus (HCV) develop chronic hepatitis. High rates of asymptomatic infection and progression to cirrhosis (both higher than those for HBV) have led to the now standard practice of screening all adults between 18 and 79 years old for hepatitis C at least once.

Anti–Hepatitis C Virus Antibodies

There are several commercially available anti-HCV antibody tests. Although the specifics of different assays vary, these tests typically check for any of a group of antibodies to HCV, in particular against protein components of the virus such as core, NS3, NS4, and NS5.* The anti-HCV antibody test (regardless of specific assay—even home tests are available) has excellent sensitivity and specificity for HCV (each around 99%) and is the screening test of choice. A positive anti-HCV antibody test indicates either active (usually chronic) infection or prior (cleared) infection.

*NS stands for nonstructural.

The vast majority of patients with negative HCV antibody testing can be presumed to be HCV negative and do NOT need a follow-up HCV RNA test (discussed next). However, false negatives may occur in patients who were recently exposed (<2 months; this is about how long it takes for most people to generate antibodies) or who are immunocompromised and therefore have impaired antibody production.

Hepatitis C Virus RNA

Direct detection and quantification of HCV RNA is done using nucleic acid amplification techniques such as PCR. Results are typically given in IU/mL; most assays can detect HCV RNA levels as low as 10 IU/mL. Overall, HCV RNA testing has excellent sensitivity and specificity for active (acute or chronic) HCV infection. However, because HCV antibody testing is inexpensive and accurate, HCV RNA testing is not the preferred *initial* screen. Labs offer an HCV virus cascade that starts with an anti-HCV antibody and reflexes to RNA testing when the antibody titer is positive.

HCV RNA testing has several important clinical uses:

- *Differentiate active (acute or chronic) versus prior (cleared) HCV infection in any patient with a positive HCV antibody test.* In this scenario, the presence of detectable HCV RNA confirms active infection, whereas its absence indicates likely prior infection that has resolved. Rarely, patients who recently received blood transfusions may have positive anti-HCV antibodies with negative HCV RNA due to the passive transfer of anti-HCV IgG from the transfused blood. These antibodies typically wane and disappear within a few weeks.

- *Rule out HCV in patients with risk factors for a false negative HCV antibody test.* These risk factors include immunocompromise and suspected exposure within the preceding 1 to 2 months. The latter group includes any patients presenting with signs or symptoms of acute hepatitis, in whom you cannot rely on a negative HCV test alone to rule out HCV infection (they may not have developed antibodies yet). In any of these patients, the additional finding of negative HCV RNA testing makes active infection—either acute or chronic—very unlikely (sensitivity approaches 100%). A positive HCV RNA result makes HCV infection very likely.

- *Monitor patients who opt to forego immediate therapy and track for spontaneous clearance of the virus.*

- *Diagnose a second (or third, fourth, etc) HCV infection in a patient with a prior infection.* Antibody titers cannot be used to screen this population because they remain elevated after the initial infection. If you suspect reinfection in a patient with prior hepatitis C, the HCV RNA is the only test you can rely on.

 Hepatitis D Virus

Hepatitis D virus (HDV) requires HBsAg to form its envelope. As a result, only patients who are already infected with HBV can be infected with HDV.

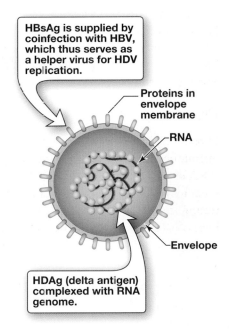

HBsAg is supplied by coinfection with HBV, which thus serves as a helper virus for HDV replication.

Proteins in envelope membrane

RNA

Envelope

HDAg (delta antigen) complexed with RNA genome.

Figure 17.4 Structure of the HDV virion. HBsAg forms the envelope. The only "native" antigen is aptly named the hepatitis D antigen (HDAg). HBsAg, hepatitis B surface antigen; HBV, hepatitis B virus; HDV, hepatitis D virus. (From Cornelissen CN, Fisher BD, Harvey RA. *Lippincott's Illustrated Reviews: Microbiology*. 3rd ed. Lippincott Williams & Wilkins; 2013.)

The presentation of HDV can range from fulminant liver failure to an asymptomatic carrier state. Most experts screen everyone with known HBV at least once for HDV, usually at the time of diagnosis. Otherwise, consider HDV testing in any patient with HBV who develops signs or symptoms of new or worsening liver disease. Do not send HDV testing on patients who are known to be HBV surface antigen negative.

Anti–Hepatitis D Virus Antibodies

The best initial test is the *total anti-HDV antibody*, which detects antibodies to HDAg. A negative result rules out chronic HDV infection in most patients. Because it takes about 4 weeks for anti-HDV antibodies to develop after infection, false negative results may be seen in those with early/acute HDV infection.

Depending on the laboratory, a positive total anti-HDV antibody result may include specific quantification of IgM anti-HDV and IgG anti-HDV. Because both IgM anti-HDV and IgG anti-HDV are associated with active HDV infection, the distinction between the two is less important than whether the total anti-HDV antibody result is positive.

Hepatitis D Virus RNA

A positive total anti-HDV antibody result should be followed by an *HDV RNA* test done by PCR. This test should also be sent whenever early/acute HDV infection is suspected. Most assays can detect levels of circulating HDV RNA as low as 10 copies/mL. Sensitivity and specificity for HDV infection (acute or chronic) are excellent.

Hepatitis E Virus

Hepatitis E virus (HEV) typically causes an acute, self-limited hepatitis. Testing is usually initiated in patients with otherwise unexplained acute or chronic hepatitis. Diagnosis is difficult because no standardized assay is available; sensitivity and specificity vary widely among the tests that do exist. Clinical context, then, is all the more important when interpreting your results.

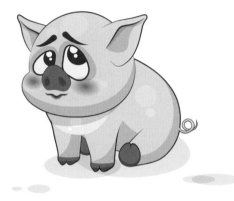

Figure 17.5 The most common mode of hepatitis E virus (HEV) transmission is fecal-oral, usually via consumption of contaminated water. Swine are a common viral reservoir. (Courtesy Stock_VectorSale/Shutterstock.)

HEV testing, like HCV and HDV testing, starts with an antibody test, followed by a confirmatory PCR.

Anti–Hepatitis E Virus Antibodies

Both IgM anti-HEV and IgG anti-HEV antibodies appear in the serum about 2 weeks after exposure in infected individuals (IgM shortly before IgG). IgM usually disappears after a few months. IgG may persist anywhere from a few months to many years.

The most common approach to testing is to start with an *IgM anti-HEV test*. A positive result suggests recent infection but, as mentioned earlier, sensitivity and specificity vary significantly depending on the assay. For this reason, either a positive IgM anti-HEV (in any patient) *or* a negative IgM anti-HEV in a patient with a moderate to high pretest probability of HEV should be followed by an HEV RNA assay.

Hepatitis E Virus RNA

Several tests are available that measure *HEV RNA in the stool*. Although performance characteristics are highly variable depending on the specific assay, the main advantage of these stool tests is the ability for early detection. HEV RNA can be found in the stool at or even just before the onset of symptoms in acute HEV. Expect results to remain positive for about 2 weeks.

HEV RNA can be detected in the serum beginning about 4 weeks after infection and typically persists a few weeks longer than stool HEV RNA. In rare cases of chronic HEV, serum HEV RNA may remain positive for years. Send a *serum HEV RNA* along with a stool

HEV RNA in any patient with positive antibody testing or with a moderate to high pretest probability of HEV. If either the stool or serum HEV RNA test is positive, active infection is highly likely.

The Acute Viral Hepatitis Panel

In practice, it rarely makes sense to test for only one of the above viral hepatitides at a time. Many of these diseases cause similar presentations and share multiple risk factors. In the case of a patient presenting with an acute hepatitis (eg, fever, right upper quadrant pain, elevated transaminases), testing for hepatitis A, B, and C is usually indicated. Remember that HEV testing is not widely available, can be unreliable, and thus is usually reserved for those with risk factors for severe disease or those whose diagnostic workup is otherwise unrevealing.

Most institutions have some version of an acute viral hepatitis panel, a "one-click" solution to quickly and efficiently test for acute hepatitis A, B, or C. The most commonly included tests are:

- Anti-HAV IgM

- HBsAg, HBcAb IgM

- Anti-HCV antibodies

YourLab — Patient Report

Specimen ID: 320-988-9014-0
Control ID:

Acct #: 90000999   Phone: Rte: 00

SAMPLE REPORT 2, 144000

Patient Details
DOB: 07/04/1978
Age(y/m/d): 045/04/12
Gender: M
Patient ID:

Specimen Details
Date collected: 11/16/2023 0000 Local
Date received: 11/16/2023
Date entered: 11/16/2023
Date reported: 11/16/2023 1500 ET

Physician Details
Ordering:
Referring:
ID:
NPI:

Ordered items
Acute Hepatitis

TESTS	RESULT	FLAG	UNITS	REFERENCE INTERVAL	LAB
Acute Hepatitis					
Hep A Ab, IgM	**Positive**	**Abnormal**		Negative	01
HBsAg Screen	Negative			Negative	01
Hep B Core Ab, IgM	Negative			Negative	02
HCV Ab	0.1		s/co ratio	0.0–0.9	02
Interpretation:					02

Negative
Not infected with HCV, unless recent infection is suspected or other evidence exists to indicate HCV infection.

Figure 17.6 Sample of an acute hepatitis panel. This patient tested positive for hepatitis A.

AUTOIMMUNE AND METABOLIC LIVER DISEASE

 Autoimmune Hepatitis

Patients with autoimmune hepatitis can present with acute liver failure, chronic liver disease, or without any symptoms at all. The variability in presentation, combined with the heterogeneity in associated laboratory findings, makes this diagnosis particularly challenging. Testing is often performed in a patient with abnormal liver function tests (hepatocellular pattern, cholestatic pattern, or mixed—see Chapter 5) when the workup for more common etiologies (eg, viral hepatitis, alcoholic liver disease) has been unrevealing.

As discussed in Chapter 22, antinuclear antibodies (ANA) are often positive in patients with autoimmune hepatitis and should be sent as part of the evaluation for this disease. The finding of a positive ANA, of course, is nonspecific. There are, however, a few tests that are more specific for autoimmune hepatitis.

Anti–Smooth Muscle Antibodies

These antibodies are directed against one or more antigens within muscle cells, such as actin and myosin. The test is usually done by immunofluorescence; a titer of at least 1:40 is considered positive. In general, the higher the titer, the higher the likelihood of autoimmune hepatitis. While anti–smooth muscle antibodies (ASMA*) are more specific for autoimmune hepatitis than a positive ANA, low ASMA titers can be seen in active (acute or chronic) viral hepatitis, primary biliary cholangitis (PBC), primary sclerosing cholangitis (PSC), infectious mononucleosis, and even in some malignancies (eg, ovarian cancer). The ASMA test is not sensitive—many patients with autoimmune hepatitis will test negative.

In recent years, some labs have replaced ASMA with *IgG anti-F-actin antibodies*, which are closely related to ASMA but may offer improved sensitivity and specificity. Consider a strongly positive ASMA or IgG anti-F-actin to be highly suggestive of autoimmune hepatitis in the appropriate clinical context. Neither should be used alone to rule out autoimmune hepatitis.

Anti–Liver-Kidney Microsomal-1 Antibodies

Anti–liver-kidney microsomal-1 (anti-LKM-1) antibodies are directed against one of the enzymes of the CYP450 system in the liver. Send this test along with an ANA and ASMA if you suspect autoimmune hepatitis. A titer of at least 1:10 is considered positive.

Like ASMA, this test is not sensitive. Specificity is not well established, but the presence of anti-LKM-1 antibodies in the appropriate clinical context is generally considered to be

---

*Do not confuse anti–smooth muscle antibodies (ASMA), which are associated with autoimmune hepatitis, with anti-Smith (anti-Sm) antibodies, which are highly specific for lupus. The shared "SM" in the abbreviation makes it all too easy to order the wrong test.

strongly suggestive of autoimmune hepatitis. Patients with autoimmune hepatitis who are anti-LKM-1 positive tend to be negative for ANA and ASMA and to have severe disease (sometimes fulminant hepatitis) that subsequently responds well to immunosuppression. This unique serologic and phenotypic profile is sometimes referred to as *type 2 autoimmune hepatitis* (patients with anti–liver cytosol antibody-1 [anti-ALC-1] antibodies are also included in this category; see the box below).

Other Laboratory Features of Autoimmune Hepatitis

Besides ASMA and anti-LKM-1 antibodies, what else might clue you in to a diagnosis of autoimmune hepatitis? Remember that neither ASMA nor anti-LKM-1 is sensitive, so a negative result on one or both tests does not rule out autoimmune hepatitis.

It is helpful to send *total immunoglobulin levels*, in particular *total IgG*, in a patient with suspected autoimmune hepatitis. Elevated IgG, although not always present, is strongly associated with autoimmune hepatitis and is thought to be a reflection of high levels of circulating autoantibodies (some of which we may not routinely check or may not even have discovered yet!). Other immunoglobulin classes (eg, IgA, IgM, IgE) are typically not elevated.

There are several other autoantibodies that are less commonly seen in patients with autoimmune hepatitis. These include antimitochondrial antibodies (*AMA*; more commonly associated with primary biliary cholangitis—discussed next), anti-*ALC-1*, anti-soluble liver antigen/liver pancreas antibodies (*anti-SLA/LP*), and atypical *perinuclear antineutrophil cytoplasmic antibodies* (p-ANCA; more commonly seen in ANCA-associated vasculitis, inflammatory bowel disease, and primary sclerosing cholangitis). Many experts send one or more of these tests when the initial workup with an ANA, total IgG, ASMA, and anti-LKM-1 is unremarkable and suspicion for autoimmune hepatitis remains.

 ## *Primary Biliary Cholangitis*

Consider PBC in a young middle-aged patient (>90% are female) with slowly progressive pruritus, fatigue, jaundice, and/or unexplained elevations in the alkaline phosphatase or direct bilirubin (cholestatic liver enzymes). Before testing for PBC, it is generally wise to rule out more common causes of liver disease such as infection or mechanical biliary obstruction (eg, choledocholithiasis or malignancy).

Antimitochondrial Antibodies

These antibodies are directed against one or more enzymes located inside the mitochondria and are typically measured either by immunofluorescence assay (IFA) or enzyme-linked immunosorbent assay (ELISA). An AMA titer of at least 1:40 is considered positive. AMA is an excellent test for PBC: the sensitivity and specificity are both estimated at around 95%.

Occasionally, a positive AMA may be seen in patients without PBC who have other autoimmune diseases, including autoimmune hepatitis, lupus, Sjögren syndrome, rheumatoid arthritis, and scleroderma. However, it is not clear to what extent these results are really false positives; some of these AMA-positive patients go on to develop PBC later in life, and others without signs or symptoms of PBC have been found to have histologic characteristics of the disease on liver biopsy. Patients with chronic graft versus host disease (GVHD) may also test positive for AMA for unclear reasons. Save yourself potential confusion by ordering AMA only in patients in whom you have clinical suspicion for PBC.

When an extensive workup has otherwise been inconclusive, it is reasonable to follow up a negative AMA with a liver biopsy in a patient whom you otherwise highly suspect may have PBC (ie, based on clinical presentation, other laboratories, and/or imaging). Remember that 95% sensitivity means that 5% (not 0%!) of patients with PBC have a negative AMA.

In a patient with established PBC, there is no utility in trending AMA titers over time—levels do not correlate with prognosis or clinical disease course.

Other Laboratory Findings Associated With PBC

No lab test approaches the sensitivity or specificity of AMA for PBC. However, a few other lab findings may point you toward the diagnosis:

- A positive ANA (particularly the multiple nuclear dots and rim patterns) is a common finding in PBC. This test, of course, is not specific.

- Hypercholesterolemia, often profound (and with an HDL predominance), is seen in more than half of patients with PBC. The HDL predominance may explain why this hypercholesterolemia does not seem to confer an increased risk of atherosclerosis in these patients.

- An elevated total IgM is often seen in PBC.

- Many autoantibodies besides AMA may be present in PBC, even in the absence of another autoimmune disease. Examples include antithyroid antibodies (eg, anti-TPO), anti-SSA/Ro, anticentromere, and anti-dsDNA. Their significance in the setting of PBC—both in terms of risk of associated autoimmune disorders and impact on prognosis—is unclear.

It may be helpful to send a lipid panel, ANA, and/or quantitative immunoglobulin levels (particularly IgM) as part of the workup of a patient with suspected PBC. However, remember that the diagnosis depends much more on the AMA.

 ## Wilson Disease

In Wilson disease, a defective copper transportation enzyme leads to inadequate copper excretion into the bile and impaired incorporation of copper into its carrier protein, ceruloplasmin. The result is that copper accumulates in places it shouldn't, particularly the liver and brain. This is a rare disease. Testing is typically indicated only when there is a known family history, when other more common etiologies of liver and/or neuropsychiatric disease have been ruled out, or when a patient has otherwise unexplained acute liver failure.

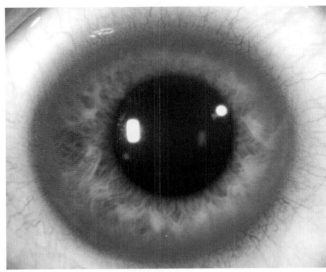

Figure 17.7 Kayser-Fleischer rings are copper deposits within the cornea that can be seen in some patients with Wilson disease. They may also occasionally be seen in patients with other chronic cholestatic diseases including primary biliary cholangitis. (From Gervasio KA, Fathy CA, Friedberg MA. *The Wills Eye Manual: Office and Emergency Room Diagnosis and Treatment of Eye Disease*. 8th ed. Wolters Kluwer; 2022.)

Ceruloplasmin

Serum ceruloplasmin is low* (<20 mg/dL) in about 90% of patients with Wilson disease, making this a fairly sensitive test. The lower the ceruloplasmin below 20 mg/dL, the higher the specificity for Wilson disease.

24-Hour Urinary Copper Excretion

Neither the sensitivity nor specificity of serum ceruloplasmin is perfect, so it is common practice to follow up a low or borderline ceruloplasmin with measurement of a 24-hour urinary copper excretion. A result of at least 100 μg is highly specific for Wilson disease; a result greater than 40 μg but less than 100 μg is less specific but still suggestive of Wilson disease in the appropriate clinical context. As with any timed specimen collection, precision is important in checking a 24-hour urinary copper excretion (see Chapter 8 for details on 24-hour urine testing).

> ### Genetic Testing for Wilson Disease
>
> Technologic advances have led to the increasingly common practice of using genetic testing to screen for and diagnose Wilson disease. The target mutation is in the *ATP7B* gene. Genetic testing is most commonly done in relatives of patients with known ATP7B mutations, those with inconclusive or a borderline ceruloplasmin and 24-hour urinary copper excretion, or those who cannot or will not undergo liver biopsy. For the vast majority of patients, serum ceruloplasmin and urinary 24-hour copper excretion remain the first-line tests.

---

*Ceruloplasmin that does not bind copper is not a happy protein; it has a shortened half-life and hence circulates in lower concentrations.

Hemochromatosis

This disease of iron overload is among the most common genetic disorders, particularly among persons of Northern European ancestry. Untreated, excessive iron deposition can damage the liver, pancreas, heart, endocrine glands, gonads, skin, and joints. Hemochromatosis is diagnosed most often in middle-aged males (it takes time for iron accumulation to cause signs and symptoms of disease) and postmenopausal females (prior to menopause, menstruation effectively removes excess iron from the body).

Testing is most often done in one of three scenarios:

- Following up an unexplained elevation in hepatic transaminases

- Evaluating a patient with organ dysfunction that remains unexplained despite initial testing and that could be related to hemochromatosis (eg, hypogonadism, hyperpigmentation, arthralgias)

- Screening patients with a family history of the disease, particularly first-degree relatives of someone with the disease

Screening of the general population is not recommended.

The initial workup includes a liver panel, complete blood count (CBC), transferrin saturation, and ferritin.

The earliest laboratory abnormalities to appear are elevations in the transferrin saturation and mean corpuscular volume (MCV). The ferritin and aminotransferases generally rise later in the course of the disease. The key finding for diagnosis is a *transferrin saturation more than 55% to 60%*. Those with a transferrin saturation of 45% to 55% should be retested in several months, although guidelines vary; some suggest ordering genetic testing in anyone with a transferrin saturation more than 45%. Using a threshold of 45%, the transferrin saturation has a sensitivity of more than 90% in men and more than 70% in women. A patient is highly unlikely to have hemochromatosis when both the transferrin level is less than 45% and the serum ferritin is normal.

If the diagnosis appears possible based on the above tests, order *genetic testing* looking for *mutations of the HFE gene** to confirm the diagnosis. Genetic testing should also be done on all first-degree relatives of patients with the disorder.

In patients with established hemochromatosis, a serum ferritin more than 1,000 mg/L should prompt a liver biopsy to assess the degree of liver damage and guide further management. Ferritin levels over 300 µg/L are the usual cutoff to consider initiating therapeutic periodic phlebotomy (the target is 50-100 µg/L).

---

*Most commonly the C282Y mutation, but there are others.

ACUTE LIVER FAILURE, HEPATIC ENCEPHALOPATHY, AND AMMONIA

Laboratory testing is vitally important in the diagnosis and workup of patients with hepatic encephalopathy and acute liver failure—so important that we feel it deserves its own chapter.

 ## Acute Liver Failure

In order to diagnose *acute liver failure (ALF)*, all four of these criteria must be met:

1. Severe acute liver injury (most commonly indicated by elevated transaminases; there is no strict cutoff that defines what is elevated and what is not)

2. Encephalopathy, without a readily identifiable extrahepatic cause

3. Impaired liver synthetic function indicated by an international normalized ratio (INR) ≥ 1.5

4. The patient's signs and symptoms must have developed within 26 weeks without previously known chronic liver disease (eg, cirrhosis).

Recognizing ALF is essential because of its high associated morbidity and mortality and the relatively short list of possible etiologies of which many are reversible.

Many patients with ALF have a readily identifiable cause based on their history and do not require a laboratory workup to establish the etiology; the most common example of this scenario is acetaminophen toxicity, which is the most common cause of ALF in the United States. However, even many of these patients should have additional laboratory studies sent. If a liver transplant is ultimately needed—and this may become apparent within days or even hours—results of a more extensive workup may be required in order to proceed.

Many providers test any patient with ALF for most or all of the following etiologies:

- *Toxins:* acetaminophen is by far the most common culprit, but many other medications and substances have been implicated. Alcohol is very unlikely to cause ALF on its own.

- *Infection:* the viral hepatitides (A, B, C, D, and E), herpes simplex virus (HSV), cytomegalovirus (CMV), Epstein-Barr virus (EBV), parvoviruses, adenovirus, and varicella-zoster virus (VZV)

- *Ischemia:* may occur in patients with shock (eg, septic or cardiogenic) or hepatic vein thrombosis/obstruction (Budd-Chiari syndrome)

- Autoimmune hepatitis

- Wilson disease

- HELLP (hemolysis with elevated liver enzymes and low platelets) in pregnant women

The lab is helpful in ruling in or ruling out several of these etiologies. We review many of the relevant tests elsewhere in this chapter. Take a look at Chapter 23 on Toxicology for more on acetaminophen testing. We review testing for several of the above viruses in Chapter 14 on Infectious Diseases.

 Hepatic Encephalopathy and Ammonia

Ammonia (NH_3) is a product of the digestion of nitrogen-containing foods (think proteins) and urea in the gut. Normally, ammonia is carried by the portal system to the liver where it is metabolized. But when the liver isn't working, ammonia accumulates in the bloodstream. The resulting hyperammonemia plays a significant role in the pathogenesis of hepatic encephalopathy: the gaseous form of ammonia crosses the blood-brain barrier and wreaks havoc on the central nervous system.

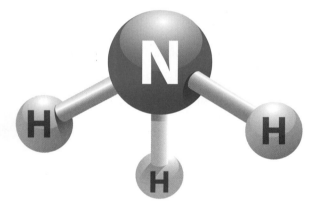

Figure 17.8 Depiction of an ammonia molecule. Real ammonia molecules are smaller and—to the best of our knowledge—rarely if ever labeled. (Courtesy EreborMountain/Shutterstock.)

The story above makes a compelling case for serum ammonia as a diagnostic test: detect an elevated ammonia, and—voila—you've diagnosed hepatic encephalopathy. Unfortunately, the clinical utility of measuring a serum ammonia level (either venous or arterial) is not so clear-cut. Here are a few reasons why:

- Hyperammonemia is nonspecific. Other causes of elevated ammonia include gastrointestinal (GI) bleeding, many medications (eg, some antiepileptics and diuretics), renal insufficiency, cigarette smoking, *Proteus mirabilis* infection (usually a UTI), and sometimes even vigorous exercise.

- Testing (including both venous and arterial tests) is susceptible to variability based on subtle changes in sample handling, timing of testing, and patient-specific factors (eg, dietary protein intake, tourniquet use, even fist clenching).

- Ammonia levels vary significantly from individual to individual, even among patients with cirrhosis with the same clinical grade of hepatic encephalopathy, in part because hyperammonemia is only one of multiple factors involved in the development of hepatic encephalopathy.

Experts do not all agree on if and when to measure a serum ammonia. If you are considering checking ammonia levels in a patient with suspected or known hepatic encephalopathy, you can use the following principles as a guide:

- The upper limit of normal for venous ammonia varies by laboratory but is generally around 50 to 55 μmol/L.

- Measurement of arterial ammonia does not seem to offer any significant advantages over the measurement of venous ammonia.

- Neither venous nor arterial ammonia can be used alone to rule in or rule out hepatic encephalopathy in any patient. One study found a sensitivity and specificity of venous ammonia (using a cutoff of 55 μmol/L) of 47% and 78%, respectively. In other words, many patients with hepatic encephalopathy have normal ammonia levels and many patients without hepatic encephalopathy have abnormal ammonia levels.

- Although both venous and arterial ammonia correlate moderately with the degree of hepatic encephalopathy in a given individual, this correlation is lost as ammonia levels rise to greater than twice the upper limit of normal.

- Resolution of hepatic encephalopathy symptoms may not be accompanied by normalization of ammonia.

The bottom line is that the measurement of serum ammonia as part of the diagnostic workup or monitoring of hepatic encephalopathy is controversial. The test has many limitations, and detecting an elevated ammonia is neither necessary nor sufficient to diagnose hepatic encephalopathy. Rather, the diagnosis is primarily based on clinical presentation and on ruling out other causes of encephalopathy.

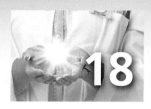

18 Nephrology and Urology

URINE ELECTROLYTES

Urine electrolytes are typically ordered in a panel that includes urine sodium, potassium, and chloride. This test can be a helpful tool in the evaluation of patients with acute kidney injury (AKI), unexplained electrolyte abnormalities, or acid-base disturbances. One of the more common uses is distinguishing *prerenal azotemia*—an increase in the blood urea nitrogen (BUN) and creatinine due to poor renal perfusion rather than intrinsic renal disease—from *intrinsic AKI*, most notably *acute tubular necrosis (ATN)*.

Often, it makes sense to pair the urine electrolyte panel with tests for urine osmolality, plasma osmolality, and plasma electrolytes (ie, the basic metabolic panel). We discuss plasma electrolytes and osmolality in Chapter 5.

Table 18.1 A Sample Report of Urine and Plasma Electrolytes

	Plasma	*Urine*
Osmolality	268 mOsm/kg	612 mOsm/kg
Sodium	128 mmol/L	106 mmol/L
Potassium	4 mmol/L	55 mmol/L
Chloride	98 mmol/L	89 mmol/L
Bicarbonate	22 mmol/L	

Urine and plasma electrolyte concentrations and osmolality are all closely related; it often makes sense to check all of these tests at the same time.

Urine Sodium Concentration and the Fractional Excretion of Sodium

The urine sodium concentration and fractional excretion of sodium (FENa) are the measurements most often used to help distinguish prerenal azotemia from intrinsic AKI.

Like the plasma sodium concentration, the urine sodium concentration depends on diet (primarily sodium and water intake) and the effects of hormones, including aldosterone and antidiuretic hormone (ADH). Most healthy individuals have a urinary sodium concentration of more than 20 mEq/L.

When the kidneys are inadequately perfused (prerenal azotemia), they "assume" that the body's intravascular volume is low. Aldosterone secretion is increased via the renin-angiotensin-aldosterone system, causing the reabsorption of sodium and water from the urine in an effort to restore the intravascular volume. The result is a decline in urinary sodium excretion that can be calculated from the concentrations of sodium and creatinine in the urine and plasma:

$$\text{Fractional excretion of sodium (FENa)} = [(U_{Na} \times P_{Cr})/(P_{Na} \times U_{Cr})] \times 100$$

where FENa is the percentage of sodium filtered by the kidneys that is excreted in the urine, U_{Na} and P_{Na} are urinary and plasma sodium concentrations, respectively; and U_{Cr} and P_{Cr} are urinary and plasma creatinine concentrations, respectively.

We measure the FENa and not the total urine sodium concentration because the latter depends on urine volume and the FENa does not.

An FENa less than 1% is classically associated with prerenal azotemia, whereas an FENa more than 3% is associated with intrinsic renal injury (most strongly with ATN). The higher FENa in intrinsic renal disease is in part related to impaired ability to reabsorb sodium due to tubular injury. Many patients with *post*-renal AKI (eg, obstructive uropathy) also have an elevated FENa. Because both hepatorenal syndrome and cardiorenal syndrome ultimately lead to poor renal perfusion without direct tubular injury (mechanistically, both are essentially forms of prerenal azotemia), both are associated with an FENa less than 1%.

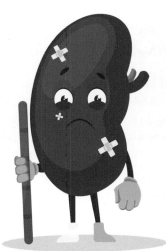

Figure 18.1 "A cute" kidney injury. Fractional excretion of sodium (FENa) can be a helpful part of the workup. (Courtesy Creative Hatti/Shutterstock.)

However, the FENa has significant limitations:

- An FENa less than 1% is not specific for prerenal azotemia. Other causes include glomerulonephritis, acute interstitial nephritis, rhabdomyolysis, early urinary tract obstruction, and contrast-induced nephropathy.

- The FENa is not reliable in patients with underlying chronic kidney disease, in whom sodium reabsorption is often impaired even in the case of prerenal azotemia. It is also unhelpful in patients on diuretics, in whom the urine sodium concentration is artificially elevated.

In any patient with AKI of unclear etiology, it is reasonable to check the urine and plasma electrolytes along with a urine and plasma creatinine in order to calculate an FENa, provided the patient is not on a diuretic and does not have advanced chronic kidney disease. Although the FENa can be helpful, the clinical history and response to treatment (eg, intravenous hydration) will likely weigh more heavily in deciding the etiology of AKI.

Fractional Excretion of Urea

As mentioned earlier, the FENa is unreliable in patients on diuretics, which artificially increase the urine sodium concentration. The effects of diuretics on urea, on the other hand, are much less pronounced. The fractional excretion of urea (FEUrea) can therefore be used instead of the FENa in patients with AKI who are on diuretics.

$$FEUrea = [(U_{Urea} \times P_{Cr})/(P_{Urea} \times U_{Cr})] \times 100$$

An FEUrea less than 35% suggests prerenal azotemia, whereas it is often more than 50% in patients with intrinsic AKI (eg, ATN). FENa remains the better test in patients who are not on diuretics.

 ## Urine Chloride Concentration

The most common use of the urine chloride is in the workup of patients with metabolic alkalosis. Urine chloride is typically less than 20 mEq/L if the metabolic alkalosis is due to hypovolemia (contraction alkalosis; see Chapter 9). Those with hypovolemia due to overdiuresis are an exception: the diuretic causes dumping of chloride into the urine in addition to intravascular volume depletion.

 ## Urine Potassium Concentration

The urine potassium concentration is highly variable depending on diet and the plasma potassium level. Consider 20 to 40 mEq/L to be the approximate normal range.

Patients with severe AKI may have impaired urinary potassium excretion resulting in a low urine potassium along with—more importantly—an *elevated* plasma potassium, a common indication for hemodialysis.

A high urine potassium is typically seen when aldosterone/mineralocorticoid levels are high: examples include hypovolemia, Cushing syndrome, and primary hyperaldosteronism.

In the absence of substances or medications affecting renal potassium handling, a patient whose kidneys are working normally should have a urine potassium concentration that roughly tracks with the plasma potassium. Thus, if the plasma potassium is high, the urine potassium should be high. A very low urine potassium in the setting of hyperkalemia or a very high urine potassium in the setting of hypokalemia should prompt concern for underlying renal pathology (eg, renal tubular acidosis).

KIDNEY STONES: METABOLIC EVALUATION

In a patient who presents with a kidney stone for the first time, it is important to do a thorough metabolic assessment to determine the underlying cause. This allows you to act proactively to prevent or at the very least limit the risk of future events. Interventions may include increasing urine volume, adjusting urine pH, altering diet, or in some cases prescribing medications.

The most common types of kidney stones are composed of *calcium oxalate* (the majority of all stones), *calcium phosphate* (most often apatite, less often brushite; the only difference between the two is in the ratio of calcium to phosphorus), *uric acid*, *cystine*, or *struvite* (magnesium ammonium phosphate).

The ideal test is to *capture the stone or fragments of the stone in a urine sample*, which can then be sent to the lab for analysis. However, this is often not possible—the stone may have passed or broken up into gravel by the time you begin your investigation. And even if you can identify the stone, you still want to determine if there are any underlying metabolic abnormalities that predisposed to stone formation.

A few blood tests and a urinalysis are helpful adjuncts in the evaluation. The comprehensive metabolic panel may reveal hypercalcemia or another electrolyte disturbance; you will also want to check the serum phosphate and uric acid. Urine microscopy may reveal crystals that reflect the nature of the stone (see Figure 18.2). However, often the real answer lies in a *24-hour urine collection.*

We described in Chapter 8 how to perform a 24-hour urine collection. Most labs offer a kidney stone panel, performed on a 24-hour urine specimen, that includes:

- Volume

- pH

- Creatinine

- Calcium, calcium oxalate, and brushite

- Sodium and chloride

- Phosphorus

- Uric acid

- Citrate

- Magnesium

- Ammonia

- Struvite

Do you really need all of these tests? Probably not, but it is reasonable to get them all at once so your patients don't have to go through the arduous process of spending a day collecting and storing their urine again and again.

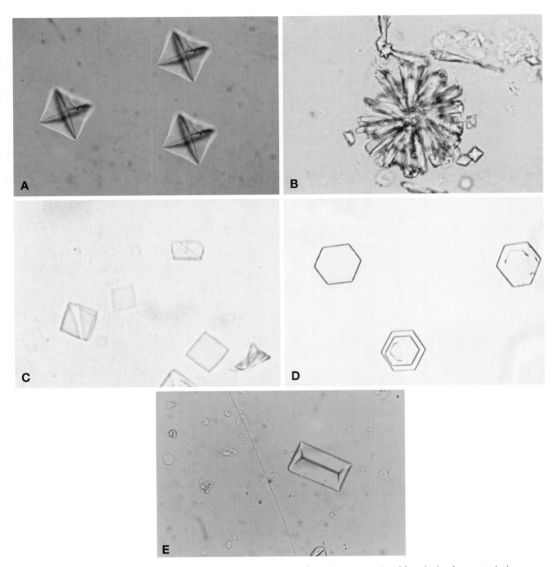

Figure 18.2 Different types of crystals in the urine can often be recognized by their characteristic shapes. A. Envelope-shaped calcium oxalate crystals. B. Needle-like calcium phosphate crystals. C. Rhomboid uric acid crystals. D. Hexagonal cystine ("SIX"tine) crystals. E. "Coffin-lid" shaped struvite crystals. (A, courtesy Schira/Shutterstock. B-D, from Mundt L, Shanahan K. *Graff's Textbook of Urinalysis*. Wolters Kluwer Health; 2016. E, courtesy Todorean-Gabriel/Shutterstock.)

The reasoning behind most of these tests, notably those tests that measure chemical constituents of different types of kidney stones, speaks for itself. Here is how the other tests can be helpful:

- Urine volume is important in the genesis of all types of kidney stones, as low urine flow increases the concentration of solutes and enhances the chances of crystallization.

- High concentrations of sodium and chloride in the urine enhance calcium excretion and increase the risk of calcium kidney stones.

- A low urine pH increases the risk of calcium phosphate stones. A high urine pH increases the risk of uric acid stones.

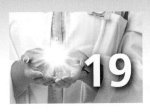

19 Endocrinology

HYPERGLYCEMIA, DIABETES, AND HYPOGLYCEMIA

You can't make the diagnosis of diabetes mellitus without the lab. You can suspect it, of course, by a patient's clinical presentation, but diabetes is defined by objective evidence of hyperglycemia. There are three standard ways to make the diagnosis.

 ### Fasting and Random Glucose

You met the serum glucose in Chapter 5 when we discussed the comprehensive metabolic panel (CMP). To reiterate, a fasting glucose less than 100 mg/dL is considered normal, whereas a fasting glucose ≥ 126 mg/dL is the threshold for diabetes. Anything in between is considered prediabetes, a term we do not like because it implies that this is an inevitable step on the road to frank diabetes (simply not the case); impaired glucose tolerance—while a bit of a mouthful—is a more accurate term.

A *random* blood glucose ≥ 200 mg/dL is also considered diagnostic of diabetes if it is accompanied by symptoms consistent with hyperglycemia, such as polydipsia, polyuria, or otherwise unexplained blurry vision.

When you are checking a fasting or random glucose for the purposes of the diagnosis of diabetes, a plasma glucose checked via venipuncture should always be used rather than a point-of-care finger stick.

 ### Oral Glucose Tolerance Test

Once the mainstay of diabetes diagnosis, this test has taken a backseat to the hemoglobin A1c (HbA1c; see page 320) for screening and diagnosis. The HbA1c is much simpler and far less of a hassle for the patient.

The Oral Glucose Tolerance Test and Pregnancy

The oral glucose tolerance test (OGTT) continues to be used in pregnant patients to screen for gestational diabetes. Patients with gestational diabetes are at increased risk of several complications of pregnancy, as well as developing diabetes later in life. Pregnancy is a state of relative insulin resistance, so patients who are otherwise normoglycemic may manifest hyperglycemia during pregnancy. Because the glycemic status of a pregnant patient can change quickly during the weeks of pregnancy, you need a test like the OGTT that can give you a view of the patient's glycemic status *at the moment*, rather than one—like the HbA1c—that averages things out over several weeks.

An OGTT is run at 24 to 28 weeks of pregnancy. It can be done in one of two ways:

- In a single step, in which the patient fasts for 8 to 14 hours and then consumes 75 g of glucose, or
- In two steps, in which the patient first consumes 50 g of glucose without needing to fast and a plasma glucose is checked 1 hour later. A glucose more than 140 mg/dL merits a follow-up 3-hour test in which 100 g of glucose is given after an overnight fast. This approach is generally preferred; although fewer patients meet the threshold for diagnosis, this does not appear to be associated with an increase in adverse events.

In the 75 g one-step test, gestational diabetes is diagnosed when one of these criteria is met:

- The fasting glucose is more than 92 mg/dL.
- At 1 hour, the fasting glucose is more than 180 mg/dL.
- At 2 hours, the fasting glucose is more than 153 mg/dL.

In the two-step test, gestational diabetes is diagnosed when two of these criteria are met:

- After the 50 mg dose, a 1-hour glucose is more than 135 to 140 mg/dL.
- After the 100 mg dose, the glucose is
  - more than 180 mg/dL at 1 hour,*
  - more than 155 mg/dL at 2 hours,* or
  - more than 140 mg/dL at 3 hours.*

 ## *Hemoglobin A1c*

This test is the most common way to establish the diagnosis of diabetes, even though it is a little less sensitive than a fasting glucose.

The hemoglobin inside red blood cells binds glucose irreversibly, and this glycosylated hemoglobin, referred to as hemoglobin A1c or HbA1c, can be measured by any of a variety of techniques, most commonly with an antibody directed against HbA1c. Red blood cells circulate for approximately 120 days, so the average red blood cell is approximately 60 days old. Hence, the HbA1c gives a good estimate of the mean plasma glucose over several weeks.

*These are the Carpenter-Coustan (CC) criteria. Slightly higher cutoffs of 190, 165, and 145 mg/dL are used by the National Diabetes Data Group. Women who meet only the CC criteria do appear to be at increased risk for some adverse outcomes compared to healthy controls, one reason why some providers prefer to use these cutoffs.

Patient Report

YourLab

Specimen ID: **285-988-9015-0**   Acct #: **90000999**   Phone: Rte: **00**
Control ID:

SAMPLE REPORT, 102004

Patient Details	Specimen Details	Physician Details
DOB: **02/14/1988**	Date collected: **10/12/2023 0000 Local**	Ordering:
Age(y/m/d): **035/07/28**	Date received: **10/12/2023**	Referring:
Gender: **F**	Date entered: **10/12/2023**	ID:
Patient ID:	Date reported: **10/12/2023 0000 ET**	NPI:

Ordered items
Gestational Glucose Tolerance

TESTS	RESULT	FLAG	UNITS	REFERENCE INTERVAL	LAB
Gestational Glucose Tolerance					
Glucose – Fasting	87		mg/dL	70-94	01
Glucose – 1 hour	159		mg/dL	70-179	01
Glucose – 2 hour	139		mg/dL	70-154	01
Glucose – 3 hour	124		mg/dL	70-139	01
Note:					01

For diagnosis of gestational diabetes, at least two values must meet or exceed normal limits, which is based on 100 g of oral glucose challenge.

Figure 19.1 This pregnant patient had a positive initial screen on the 1-hour 50 mg test, necessitating a follow-up 3-hour 100 mg test, which—as you can see—turned out to be normal/negative.

There are two major advantages of the HbA1c over a fasting glucose:

- Whereas a fasting glucose offers just a single snapshot in time, the HbA1c averages out a patient's glycemic status over a longer period. Although your patient may have a normal glucose today (at the moment you are drawing blood), they may have been running high much of the rest of the time; the HbA1c will detect that.

- The patient does not need to fast.

An HbA1c less than 5.6% is normal. An HbA1c ≥ 6.5% is defined as diabetes. Anything in between, similar to intermediate levels of the fasting glucose, reflects impaired glucose tolerance.

The HbA1c is not a perfect test. Patients with certain metabolic abnormalities—for example, iron, folate, or vitamin B12 deficiency—are slow to replace their worn-out red blood cells, so the red cell population is older, has had more time to bind glucose, and may yield a falsely elevated HbA1c. Chronic kidney disease, especially when advanced, can also raise the HbA1c. On the other hand, patients with high red blood cell turnover—for example, patients with hemolytic anemia or sickle cell anemia—have a younger population of cells in their circulation which have had less time to bind glucose and may have a falsely low HbA1c. Other causes of a falsely low HbA1c include red blood cell transfusions, erythropoietin administration, and advanced liver disease.

Hemoglobin A1c Versus the Oral Glucose Tolerance Test

How does the HbA1c compare to the OGTT? The OGTT, using the parameters cited earlier, is actually more sensitive than the HbA1c for detecting glucose intolerance. On the other hand, the presence of diabetic microvascular disease, specifically retinopathy, was found to correlate better with a positive HbA1c than with a positive OGTT, suggesting that the HbA1c may be a better gauge of *actual disease* than the more cumbersome OGTT.

In practical terms, the HbA1c is so much simpler to obtain than an OGTT that it remains the test of choice. But it is important to point out that some clinicians will also order an OGTT in an effort to help risk stratify patients and identify those who might benefit from aggressive modification of risk factors for developing diabetes and cardiovascular disease.

 ## Autoantibodies in Type 1 Diabetes

Type 1 diabetes is caused by autoantibody-mediated destruction of the pancreatic islet beta cells that normally produce insulin. It was once felt to occur only in children and young adults, but we now know this is not so. Patients with type 1 diabetes must be treated with insulin. Type 2 diabetes, on the other hand, is a disease of insulin resistance (insulin levels are often higher than normal). Once believed to be the sole province of adults, it also spans the entire age range. Although it may be treated with insulin, it is more often managed with lifestyle modification and non-insulin medications. Therefore, it is important to know which type of diabetes your patient has. Most of the time the answer is obvious, but not always, and this is where testing for autoantibodies becomes important.

Who and How to Test

Whenever the distinction between type 1 and type 2 diabetes is unclear, it is reasonable to check autoantibody titers. This issue comes up most often in adults who do not respond to non-insulin medications, adults with newly diagnosed severe hyperglycemia, and patients with a personal or family history of other autoimmune diseases. These patients can pose a significant management challenge until you consider the possibility that they are actually in the early stages of type 1 diabetes.

A positive test for autoantibodies in the setting of diabetes establishes a diagnosis of type 1 disease. When diagnosed in adulthood, this is often referred to as *latent autoimmune diabetes in adults (LADA)*. These patients can then be started on insulin right away, helping to preserve whatever β-cell function they have left and—more importantly—assuring that their next visit to a medical care provider will not be for diabetic ketoacidosis.

The two tests that are used most often are *islet cell antibodies (ICA)* and *antibodies against glutamic acid decarboxylase* (in particular the *GAD65* enzyme, produced primarily by the pancreatic islet cells). Both are highly specific for type 1 disease. Their combined sensitivity is also very good—most patients with type 1 diabetes will have at least one of these autoantibodies; anti-GAD65 antibodies appear to be the most sensitive, present in approximately 70% of patients with type 1 diabetes, and persist for many years.

More comprehensive panels are available for patients in whom the diagnosis is still in doubt, and while these increase sensitivity, they also increase cost. These panels include antibodies against *tyrosine phosphatase-like proteins* (including insulinoma-associated protein IA-2), *zinc transporter*, and *insulin*. You might expect that insulin antibodies would be particularly helpful—high in type 1 diabetes and absent in type 2 diabetes. However, these autoantibodies are present in only a minority of patients with type 1 diabetes. In addition, you can't check insulin autoantibodies once a patient has been on nonhuman insulin therapy for 2 weeks or more since this inevitably leads to the production of insulin autoantibodies.

Autoantibodies and Predicting/Preventing Type 1 Diabetes

With the advent of therapies that can delay the onset of type 1 diabetes in those at risk, testing for these autoantibodies may take on a whole new importance. The first drug approved for this indication is a monoclonal antibody that blocks T-cell activity. Treating patients with impaired glucose tolerance (but not yet meeting the criteria for frank diabetes) and who test positive for at least two of these autoantibodies has been shown to delay the onset of type 1 diabetes by an average of 2 years.

The question, of course, is who to screen. Only 0.4% of the general population eventually develops type 1 diabetes, so screening the general population is problematic at best. The initial study population all had a family history of diabetes, but only 15% of patients with type 1 diabetes have such a family history. Because the benefits to those who will eventually develop the disease are so great, this will be a topic of great interest in the years to come.

 ## Insulin, C-Peptide, and Hypoglycemia

We don't measure *insulin levels* very often in patients with diabetes; it doesn't add much to our management. However, along with C-peptide, it can be useful in patients with hypoglycemia.

C-peptide is a small protein that connects the α and β chains of proinsulin. Proinsulin is eventually cleaved into insulin and C-peptide, which are secreted in equal amounts. Unlike the serum insulin, which has a short half-life (5-10 minutes), C-peptide hangs around for more than half an hour, so the serum level is higher than that of insulin. Normal fasting levels are 0.9 to 1.8 ng/mL.

C-peptide and insulin levels are mostly used to assess the cause of *hypoglycemia*. In patients with factitious hypoglycemia due to covert insulin use, the insulin level will be high but the C-peptide will not. In patients with hypoglycemia due to an insulin-secreting tumor (insulinoma) or a medication that stimulates endogenous insulin secretion (eg, sulfonylureas), both the insulin and C-peptide levels will be elevated.

Table 19.1 Laboratory Evaluation of Hypoglycemia

Lab Test	Insulinoma	Sulfonylurea Use	Exogenous Insulin
Insulin	↑	↑	↑
C-peptide	↑	↑	↓
Proinsulin	↑	↑	↓ or ↔
Sulfonylurea levels (urine or plasma)	Negative	Positive	Negative

C-peptide can also be a useful addition to autoantibody testing in the evaluation of older patients with clinical features suggestive of type 1 diabetes, particularly if they have had hyperglycemia for more than 3 years. Levels will be elevated in patients with type 2 disease (who should still have functioning β cells) and decreased in those with type 1 (who do not).

MORE THYROID TESTS

For most things thyroid, the only test you will need—as we discussed in Chapter 7—is the thyroid-stimulating hormone (TSH), followed—as needed—by a Thyroid Cascade. There are, however, additional tests that can be helpful in specific situations. Two that you may have heard of—the *thyrotropin-releasing hormone (TRH) stimulation test* and *T3 resin uptake*—will not be discussed here because they have largely been supplanted by our ability to accurately measure the TSH, T3, and T4. But a couple of others deserve your attention.

Radioactive Iodine Uptake

The thyroid gland is the only organ in the body that uses iodine, a critical component in the manufacture of thyroid hormone. If you give a patient a dose of oral radioactive iodine, it will be taken up only by thyroid cells that are actively making thyroid hormone and nowhere else.

The *radioactive iodine uptake* (RAIU) is most often used in patients in whom you have already diagnosed hyperthyroidism. Your next step is to distinguish Graves disease or a toxic nodular goiter, in both of which thyroid hormone synthesis is increased, from subacute thyroiditis, in which it is not. Instead, in subacute thyroiditis, inflammation of the thyroid gland causes hyperthyroidism via the massive release of the gland's storehouse of preformed thyroid hormones.* Therefore, whereas in Graves disease or toxic nodular goiter the RAIU is high, in subacute thyroiditis it is low.

When the RAIU is elevated, the pattern of uptake can help you differentiate a toxic goiter(s), which will demonstrate focal uptake, from Graves disease, in which uptake will be increased diffusely.

The RAIU has several potential confounders, including a high iodine diet and recent exposure to iodinated intravenous (IV) contrast, both of which will yield a falsely low result.

It is also important to stress that the use of radioactive iodine is contraindicated in pregnancy.

Thyroid Nodules

The initial laboratory evaluation of a thyroid nodule, usually detected on physical examination or ultrasound, is designed to answer a single question—Is the nodule malignant or not? Hyperfunctioning, aka "hot," nodules that are churning out a lot of thyroid hormone are rarely malignant. Rather, almost all cancerous nodules are *not* hyperfunctioning (the term used to refer to these nodules is—you guessed it—"cold").

---

*Ultimately, once the inflamed thyroid has emptied out its supply of thyroid hormone, the patient becomes hypothyroid.

In a patient with a thyroid nodule, the first test you should run is a TSH. The result will guide your next steps:

- If the TSH is low, you may be dealing with a hot nodule that is producing high amounts of thyroid hormone, sufficient to suppress the pituitary gland's release of TSH. The next step then is to obtain an RAIU in combination with nuclear imaging (thyroid scintigraphy). If the RAIU is high and the image reveals a hot nodule, you can in most instances avoid a biopsy.

- If the TSH is normal or elevated, then you are probably dealing with a cold nodule. The next step is to obtain an ultrasound of the thyroid gland. Depending on the results of the ultrasound and the clinical context, a biopsy may also be indicated.

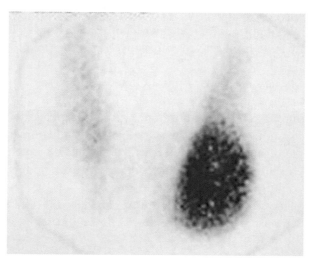

Figure 19.2 An example of a hot nodule on a thyroid scan. This nodule is producing so much thyroid hormone that it is suppressing thyroid-stimulating hormone (TSH) production and therefore the activity of the rest of the gland, which is barely detectable. (From Dimick JB, Upchurch GR, Sonnenday CJ. *Clinical Scenarios in Surgery*. Lippincott Williams & Wilkins; 2012.)

 Thyroglobulin

Thyroglobulin is an iodinated protein made by the thyroid gland. It is the main storage form of T3 and T4. It should not be measured as part of the routine assessment of thyroid function. The main reason to check a thyroglobulin level is to screen a patient with treated thyroid cancer for residual or recurrent disease. If therapy has been successful, the serum thyroglobulin should be undetectable. This test is only useful for well-differentiated follicular or papillary tumors because thyroglobulin is not synthesized by poorly differentiated malignancies.

A small but significant percentage of the general population has *antithyroglobulin autoantibodies* that can interfere with the standard assay for thyroglobulin, so these must be checked at the same time to rule out the possibility of a false negative result (many labs will do this reflexively). If the antibody titer is positive, the lab can assess thyroglobulin levels with other assays (more time-consuming and more expensive) that are less susceptible to antibody interference.

CORTISOL AND THE HYPOTHALAMIC-PITUITARY-ADRENAL AXIS

Cortisol is the most important of the glucocorticoids made in the adrenal gland. It contributes to the maintenance of blood pressure, gluconeogenesis, and downregulation of the immune system and the inflammatory response. The synthesis of cortisol is set in motion by the action of adrenocorticotropic hormone (ACTH), released from the anterior pituitary gland, on the adrenal cortex. There, it initiates the process by which cholesterol is metabolized into cortisol. Because ACTH has a diurnal pattern of secretion, cortisol levels are highest in the morning and lowest at night.

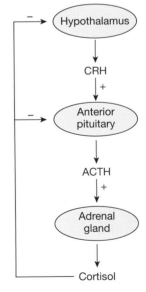

Figure 19.3 Regulation of cortisol secretion. The hypothalamus secretes corticotropin-releasing hormone (CRH) that stimulates the anterior pituitary to secrete adrenocorticotropic hormone (ACTH). This in turn stimulates the adrenal cortex to produce cortisol. As with everything endocrinologic, there is negative feedback as well, with cortisol limiting its own production by acting on both the anterior pituitary and hypothalamus.

We refer to higher-than-normal levels of cortisol as Cushing syndrome and lower-than-normal levels as adrenal insufficiency.

Cushing Syndrome

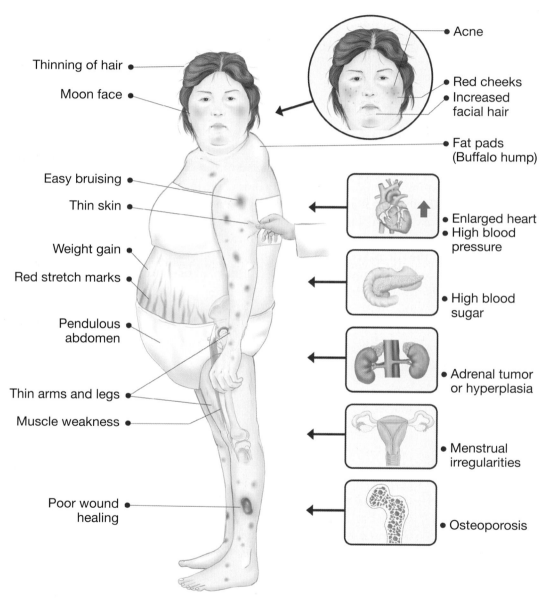

Acne

Thinning of hair

Moon face

Red cheeks

Increased facial hair

Fat pads (Buffalo hump)

Easy bruising

Thin skin

Enlarged heart

High blood pressure

Weight gain

Red stretch marks

High blood sugar

Pendulous abdomen

Adrenal tumor or hyperplasia

Thin arms and legs

Muscle weakness

Menstrual irregularities

Poor wound healing

Osteoporosis

Figure 19.4 Some of the sentinel findings of Cushing syndrome that should lead you to consider testing for excess glucocorticoids in the circulation. (Courtesy Chu KyungMin/Shutterstock.)

Causes

Cushing syndrome can arise from a process affecting any site in the hypothalamic-pituitary-adrenal (HPA) axis:

- The hypothalamus—This is extremely uncommon.
- The pituitary gland—This is the entity referred to as *Cushing disease* (yes, you need to distinguish this term from the more overarching term *Cushing syndrome*), and the cause is almost always a pituitary adenoma.
- The adrenal gland—Hypercortisolism can result either from an adenoma or carcinoma.

Additional causes include the following:

- Ectopic production of ACTH—Rarely, ACTH can be produced outside the HPA axis by an ectopic source, usually a small cell carcinoma of the lung, although other tumors can do this as well.
- Exogenous cortisol—The most common source would be a medication such as prednisone.

Testing

What steps should you take if you suspect that your patient may have Cushing syndrome?

1. Rule out the possibility that exogenous corticosteroid use is responsible for the patient's symptoms. This may be from medications taken appropriately for medical reasons, including oral, inhaled, and topical steroids, or taken covertly for performance enhancement. You need to take a careful medication/drug history.

2. Test for the presence of glucocorticoid excess; we'll describe how in a moment.

3. If the lab confirms glucocorticoid excess, establish the source of the problem. Is it at the level of the adrenals, pituitary gland, or hypothalamus? Could there be an ectopic source of excess cortisol?

Once you are ready to start testing, you have choices. No single test has sufficient sensitivity and specificity to be relied upon alone. You can start with any of the following three tests. All have a high sensitivity and specificity, but none are perfect. If the test you choose turns up positive, consider ordering a second, different test to confirm that what you are dealing with is indeed Cushing syndrome. If your initial testing is negative and you still have a high level of suspicion, order another test. The diagnosis of Cushing syndrome carries important therapeutic implications, so you must be as certain as you can and avoid both false negatives and false positives.

- *Midnight salivary cortisol*—Patients like this test because they can collect the sample at home. A special collecting device must be used—one in common use requires patients to keep a cotton pad in their mouth for at least 90 seconds until it is well saturated. The sample is then submitted to the lab. Because cortisol values fluctuate from hour to hour and day to day, two abnormal test results are required to consider this test positive. Normal values vary significantly among different laboratories. If the results are indeterminate (eg, a single weak positive), proceed with one of the other tests mentioned below.

- *24-hour urine free cortisol*—With this test, make sure you also order a 24-hour urine creatinine to ensure an adequate collection (see Chapter 8). As with the salivary test, two abnormal tests are needed to consider the test positive. The normal range for males is less than 60 μg/d; for females, it is less than 45 μg/d. In cases of mild to moderate elevations, Cushing syndrome is likely, but—again—consider ordering a different test to confirm.

- *1 mg dexamethasone overnight suppression test*—This test can be your first choice in any setting where Cushing syndrome is a possibility, but it is used most often—and is the test of choice—in the evaluation of an *adrenal incidentaloma*, that is, an adrenal mass detected on imaging done for some other reason. These patients may have no symptoms of Cushing syndrome at all or only mild manifestations for which the possibility of Cushing syndrome was previously not considered, such as hypertension, hyperglycemia, weight gain, or osteoporosis.* Dexamethasone, a synthetic corticosteroid, is given as a single dose late at night, between 11 PM and midnight. Cortisol levels are drawn between 8 and 9 AM. In patients who do not have Cushing syndrome, dexamethasone will suppress ACTH secretion, and thus the morning serum cortisol levels will be low (a level <1.8 μg/dL is considered normal). In patients with Cushing syndrome, the serum cortisol will not be suppressed. The values of cortisol that are considered diagnostic vary depending on whether you are more interested in maximizing sensitivity or specificity, but any result more than 1.8 μg/dL should be evaluated further.

Once you have established a diagnosis of Cushing syndrome, your next step is to figure out the cause. Start by measuring a *serum ACTH level*. This will allow you to divide the various causes into two general categories, those that are dependent on ACTH and those that are not:

- *ACTH dependent:* The ACTH is high (>15-20 pg/mL) and is driving the excess production of cortisol. The most common cause is an ACTH-secreting pituitary adenoma. However, you must also consider the possibility of ectopic ACTH secretion by a malignancy. In patients with confirmed Cushing syndrome and a high ACTH level, you need to distinguish between these two entities. Your next test should therefore be a *high-dose dexamethasone suppression test*. Eight milligrams of dexamethasone is given overnight (or 2 mg every 6 hours). Suppression of the serum cortisol level more than 50% suggests a pituitary origin. ACTH production by an ectopic (non-pituitary) tumor is typically not suppressed by dexamethasone—most ectopic tumors do not have glucocorticoid receptors that will respond to negative feedback from circulating glucocorticoids. Remember: *the low-dose dexamethasone test is used to establish the* diagnosis *of Cushing syndrome; the high-dose test is used to establish the* cause.

---

*Most adrenal incidentalomas are *nonfunctioning*—that is, they do not produce any excess hormone. *Functioning* incidentalomas are usually benign and most often produce cortisol. Despite cortisol being the most common hormone secreted by functioning adrenal masses, you still have to rule out the possibility that they are secreting other adrenal hormones such as catecholamines (pheochromocytomas, see page 346) or aldosterone (see page 336).

- *ACTH independent:* The ACTH is low (<5 pg/mL) and is not driving the excess production of cortisol. The cause lies in the adrenal gland and usually turns out to be a cortisol-secreting adrenal adenoma acting independently of ACTH. Other etiologies include adrenal carcinomas and adrenal hyperplasia. For patients with confirmed Cushing syndrome and a low ACTH, you will next proceed to adrenal imaging.

In some patients, the ACTH level will lie between the two diagnostic extremes of 5 and 20 pg/mL. It is best in these situations to repeat the ACTH level several weeks later and hope for some clarity. If you are still not sure what is going on at this point, reach out to your favorite endocrinologist for guidance.

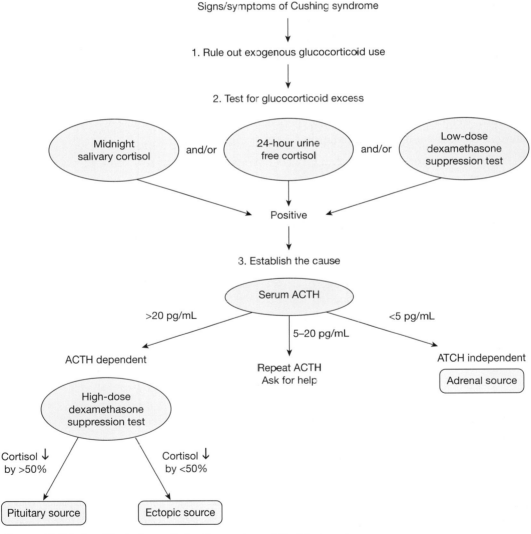

Figure 19.5 A simplified schematic for the workup of Cushing syndrome. ACTH, adrenocorticotropic hormone.

> **It's Hard**
>
> Testing for Cushing syndrome can be difficult. Sometimes, by following the testing algorithm we've outlined, the results will give you a definite answer, allowing you to determine that Cushing syndrome is present as well as where the problem likely resides. Unfortunately, this is not always the case, so never delay asking for help from a specialist who can guide you and your patient through what is often a labyrinthine process.

 ## *Adrenal Insufficiency*

As with Cushing syndrome, the cause of adrenal insufficiency may lie at the level of the adrenals ("primary" adrenal insufficiency), pituitary ("secondary" adrenal insufficiency), or hypothalamus ("tertiary" adrenal insufficiency).

Adrenal insufficiency can present as an acute emergency with sudden, life-threatening circulatory collapse (vasodilatory shock), or more subtly with mild hypotension, fatigue, weakness, weight loss, hyponatremia, hyperkalemia, hypoglycemia, and—when adrenal failure is the cause—hyperpigmentation.*

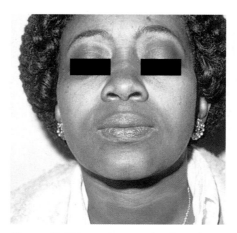

Figure 19.6 Hyperpigmentation in patients with primary adrenal insufficiency is often most apparent in sun-exposed areas such as the face, neck, and hands. (From *Goodheart HP. Goodheart's Photoguide of Common Skin Disorders.* 2nd ed. Lippincott Williams & Wilkins; 2003.)

---

*Why does hyperpigmentation only occur with primary adrenal disease? Because when the adrenal glands fail, the pituitary (which is working perfectly well) churns out excess ACTH in an attempt to stimulate the adrenal to up its game and produce more cortisol. In order to synthesize and release more ACTH, the pituitary must first make the prohormone proopiomelanocortin (POMC), which in turn is cleaved to ACTH and melanocyte-stimulating hormone (MSH). MSH drives melanin synthesis in the skin.

Causes

The most common cause of adrenal insufficiency today is withdrawal of synthetic glucocorticoids (eg, prednisone taken for an autoimmune disorder or severe asthma). This is actually a form of tertiary adrenal insufficiency because the problem lies at the very top of the HPA axis: the hypothalamus is so used to strong negative feedback from high levels of circulating exogenous steroids that it has fallen asleep on the job and is just not ready to start churning out corticotropin-releasing hormone (CRH) when the steroids are abruptly withdrawn. This is why, in patients who have been taking steroids for a prolonged period of time, especially if in high doses, they must be tapered rather than abruptly stopped.

The most common *intrinsic* medical cause of adrenal insufficiency is Addison disease, the term used to describe autoimmune destruction of the adrenal glands. Other causes of primary adrenal insufficiency include adrenal hemorrhage, infection (for much of human history, tuberculosis was the most common etiology of primary adrenal insufficiency), infiltrative diseases, and tumors. ACTH levels are high in all causes of primary adrenal insufficiency.

Any process affecting the pituitary (eg, infiltrative disease, tumor, aneurysm) can cause secondary adrenal insufficiency; in these cases, other pituitary hormones in addition to ACTH are usually also low.

> **Steroids and Stress**
>
> Patients under severe stress—whether from illness, trauma, or surgery—need their adrenal glands to pump out large amounts of cortisol to support their blood pressure. Without an appropriate adrenal response, circulatory collapse (adrenal crisis) can occur. With any of these stressors, adrenal crisis can occur in patients with adrenal (most often), pituitary, or hypothalamic dysfunction. It can also result, although rarely, from withdrawal of exogenous steroids in the absence of an acute stressor.

Testing

The essential steps involved in the diagnostic workup of adrenal insufficiency include the following:

1. *Establish the diagnosis.* There are several tests available and interpretation can be challenging.

2. *If adrenal insufficiency is confirmed, determine the cause.* Is the problem at the level of the hypothalamus (tertiary), pituitary (secondary), or adrenals (primary)?

The most widely used and convenient initial test is a *morning serum cortisol* checked between 6 and 9 AM. A value more than 18 µg/dL rules out adrenal insufficiency in almost all patients; a level less than 3 µg/dL is strongly suggestive of adrenal insufficiency and should be followed by a serum ACTH to determine the cause (see later). Intermediate levels—those between 3 and 18 µg/dL—typically demand further testing to determine whether adrenal insufficiency is present.

It is helpful to follow up an abnormal or intermediate-range morning cortisol with an *ACTH stimulation test*. Not only is this test considered the gold standard for the diagnosis of adrenal insufficiency, but it can also help you begin to localize the problem if adrenal insufficiency is present. The patient is given 250 µg of cosyntropin, a synthetic ACTH, either intramuscular (IM) or IV, and serum cortisol levels are measured 30 to 60 minutes later. In all patients with primary adrenal insufficiency, as well as in most patients with secondary adrenal insufficiency (in whom the adrenal glands often become atrophic over time from chronic understimulation), cortisol levels stay low (<18 µg/dL). A rise in cortisol to more than or equal to 18 µg/dL rules out primary adrenal insufficiency and makes secondary adrenal insufficiency less likely (although still possible).

Follow up an abnormal ACTH stimulation test with a *serum ACTH* to pinpoint the site of the problem. The ACTH will be high in primary adrenal insufficiency and low in either secondary or tertiary adrenal insufficiency. It makes sense to pair this testing with appropriate imaging to identify and/or further define the specific cause (eg, a pituitary mass).

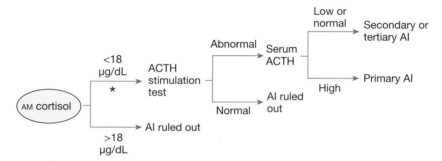

Figure 19.7 A simplified schematic for the workup of adrenal insufficiency. The reality is often much murkier: borderline and contradictory results are painfully common. Careful adherence to proper timing and collection is therefore all the more important. When results are unclear or don't make sense, have a low threshold to repeat one or more tests. ACTH, adrenocorticotropic hormone; AI, adrenal insufficiency. *Many clinicians consider an AM cortisol <3 µg/dL strong enough evidence of adrenal insufficiency that they skip the ACTH stimulation test and proceed with checking a serum ACTH.

You may have heard of *insulin-induced hypoglycemia* and *metyrapone*** testing. These tests are usually considered only when the results of the ACTH stimulation test are equivocal—for example, as may occur when only partial secondary adrenal insufficiency is suspected (often seen following pituitary surgery). The insulin-induced hypoglycemia test is potentially dangerous, should only be done in a setting monitored by experienced medical personnel, and is rarely performed. Patients with a normal response to these provocative tests do not have adrenal insufficiency.

**Metyrapone decreases cortisone secretion by blocking the final step in its synthesis.

You may be wondering why we don't simply measure a 24-hour urine or salivary cortisol like we do with Cushing syndrome. These tests have not been validated in the setting of adrenal insufficiency and are not currently recommended. They simply do not appear to be sufficiently sensitive to be used as a screening tool.

In patients in whom the adrenal gland has been identified as the source of the problem, you will want to sort out the different possible etiologies: Is it due to autoimmune destruction (Addison disease) or some other cause? It is helpful to measure *antibodies against 21-hydroxylase*, an enzyme present in the adrenal gland (see page 351 on Congenital Adrenal Hyperplasia). The vast majority of patients with autoimmune adrenal insufficiency will test positive for these antibodies. False positives can occur in patients with Graves disease and type 1 diabetes mellitus.

Patients with autoimmune adrenal insufficiency are at risk of other autoimmune disorders and should be screened for thyroid disease (get a TSH), parathyroid disease (check a calcium and phosphorus and, if abnormal, a serum parathyroid hormone [PTH]), and type 1 diabetes mellitus (see page 332).

Because aldosterone is also synthesized in the adrenal glands and can be affected by the same disease processes, all patients with primary adrenal insufficiency of any cause should also be evaluated for mineralocorticoid deficiency with a serum aldosterone and plasma renin activity (see page 336).

 ## *Now Take a Deep Breath*

If this chapter makes anything clear, it should be that cortisol testing can be challenging. However, if you understand the basic physiology of the HPA axis, you should be able to determine which tests are most useful, the sequence in which to order them, and the framework for how to interpret them. If you are lucky, a distinct diagnosis will emerge. If you are not—and all too often this is the case—you will find yourself dealing with indeterminate or even contradictory results. Repeat testing, and the expertise of a trusted endocrinologist, should eventually get you the answers you are seeking.

THE RENIN-ANGIOTENSIN-ALDOSTERONE SYSTEM

A picture—at least a picture with a caption—can certainly be worth a whole lot of words. Here in a nutshell is the renin-angiotensin-aldosterone system or RAAS:

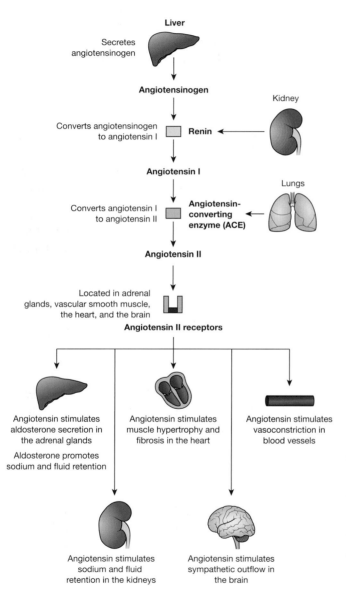

Figure 19.8 The endocrine renin-angiotensin-aldosterone system (RAAS). The kidneys secrete renin, primarily in response to low blood pressure, which converts angiotensinogen, which is made in the liver, to angiotensin I. The lungs produce angiotensin-converting enzyme (ACE) which then converts angiotensin I into angiotensin II. Angiotensin II acts on multiple organ systems; its major activity is to increase sodium and water retention via the stimulation of aldosterone secretion and to raise the blood pressure. However, you should know that there are local RAAS loops as well that, while not routinely measured by the lab, play a critical role in physiologic regulation.

The most common reason for evaluating the RAAS is in a patient with suspected *secondary hypertension*, defined as hypertension that ultimately proves to have an identifiable cause (see the box "Secondary Hypertension"). Hyperaldosteronism is the most common culprit. Hyperaldosteronism may also cause a low serum potassium and/or a high serum sodium, although most patients with this disorder have normal electrolytes. When you suspect hyperaldosteronism, start the workup by measuring a serum aldosterone level.

Because aldosterone secretion can be affected by posture, the patient should be upright for at least 30 minutes prior to the blood draw.

A normal standing aldosterone is 7 to 20 ng/dL (2 to 5 ng/dL when supine).

To diagnose the cause of hyperaldosteronism, check a *plasma aldosterone/plasma renin activity ratio*. Relying on this ratio, as many as 10% of patients with hypertension— that figure includes all comers with high blood pressure—will be found to have hyperaldosteronism.

- In patients with primary hyperaldosteronism—due to either bilateral adrenal hyperplasia or an adrenal adenoma—the aldosterone will be high and the plasma renin activity (PRA) suppressed, typically to less than 10 ng/mL/hr. (Why is there an hour in the units of PRA?—that's the period during which the lab measures the efficacy of the patient's plasma renin in the conversion of angiotensinogen to angiotensin I and II.) An aldosterone/PRA ratio more than 20 is considered positive (sensitivity is just below 90% and the specificity just over 70%).*

- In patients with secondary hyperaldosteronism, often the result of renal artery stenosis or fibromuscular dysplasia, the PRA is the driving force and it will be elevated along with the serum aldosterone.

The PRA can be increased in patients with a salt-restricted diet or who are taking medications that impact the RAAS (eg, such common antihypertensive medications as diuretics [especially aldosterone antagonists], angiotensin-converting enzyme [ACE] inhibitors, and angiotensin receptor blockers). For the most accurate results, patients should be off these medications for several weeks before testing.

Angiotensin II is rarely measured as it generally adds little to the evaluation.

If the diagnosis of primary hyperaldosteronism is uncertain, a 24-hour urine aldosterone should be obtained while the patient is consuming a high sodium diet. Normally the high sodium intake will suppress aldosterone secretion; in primary hyperaldosteronism, it will not.

Secondary Hypertension

Most patients with elevated blood pressure can be successfully managed with lifestyle changes and medications. In some, however, hypertension persists. When the blood pressure remains elevated despite ongoing treatment with three or more medications, one of which is a diuretic, patients are said to have resistant hypertension. They should be evaluated for secondary causes of high blood pressure. The most common of these are:

*Why is the PRA preferred over measuring the plasma renin concentration? The reason is simple: what we care about is what renin is doing, not how much of it is around. Because renin acts via angiotensinogen/angiotensin I and II and therefore impacts blood pressure only indirectly, there can be a divergence between its actions and its concentration.

- Primary hyperaldosteronism, as we just discussed
- Renal artery stenosis, either atherosclerotic or from fibromuscular dysplasia; many of these patients will have an elevated creatinine on their CMP.
- Sleep apnea

Other causes you may need to consider include medications (eg, oral contraceptives [OCPs]), pheochromocytoma (see page 346), and Cushing syndrome (see page 328).

Angiotensin-Converting Enzyme

ACE catalyzes the conversion of angiotensin I to angiotensin II in the lungs. The upper limit of normal varies by laboratory but is usually around 40 μg/L. The main reason to measure a serum ACE level is in the workup of suspected sarcoidosis, in which increased levels are thought to be due to ACE production by granulomas.

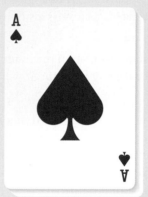
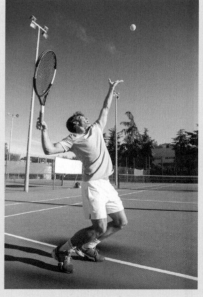

Figure 19.9 Neither of these aces will help you in the workup of sarcoidosis. Consider sending an angiotensin-converting enzyme (ACE) level instead. (Card image courtesy Stephen Marques/ Shutterstock; tennis image courtesy PabloBenii/ Shutterstock.)

The sensitivity of an elevated serum ACE for sarcoidosis is about 60% to 75%; specificity is about 90%. Thus, an ACE level should not be used by itself to rule in or rule out (especially the latter) sarcoidosis. Nevertheless, in the right clinical context, an elevated ACE does have good positive predictive value for sarcoidosis. Higher levels have been found to correlate with an increased incidence of extrapulmonary involvement (eg, sarcoidosis involving the liver or extrathoracic lymph nodes). Whether ACE should be monitored as a marker of disease activity in patients with established sarcoidosis remains controversial.

Other common laboratory findings in sarcoidosis include elevated levels of 1,25-dihydroxy vitamin D (calcitriol; also produced by granulomas), resulting in mild to moderate hypercalcemia and low or low-normal PTH levels. See Chapter 5 for more on calcium homeostasis.

TESTOSTERONE, ESTROGEN, AND THE HYPOTHALAMIC-PITUITARY-GONADAL AXIS

Figures 19.9 and 19.10 tell you pretty much all you need to know about the hypothalamic-pituitary-gonadal (HPG) axis in males and females and will serve as a useful guide to how, when, and why you need to interrogate it.

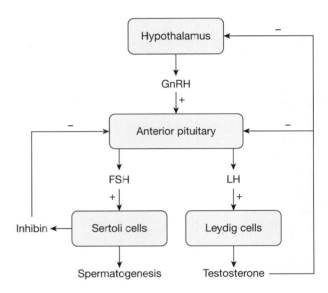

Figure.19.10 The hypothalamic-pituitary-gonadal (HPG) axis in males. FSH, follicle-stimulating hormone; GnRH, gonadotropin hormone-releasing hormone; LH, luteinizing hormone.

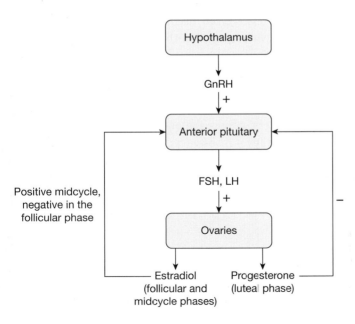

Figure 19.11 The hypothalamic-pituitary gonadal (HPG) axis in nonpregnant females. The feedback loops here are more complicated than in males, and we've simplified them a bit. Note that the feedback of estradiol on the anterior pituitary can be positive or negative, depending on the timing of the menstrual cycle. FSH, follicle-stimulating hormone; GnRH, gonadotropin hormone-releasing hormone; LH, luteinizing hormone.

Testosterone and the Hypothalamic-Pituitary-Gonadal Axis in Males

Although male patients may request a *serum testosterone* level for a variety of reasons—including concerns about low energy or diminished mental or physical functioning—the test is clearly indicated only when there is evidence of:

- Sexual dysfunction, such as diminished libido, erectile dysfunction, or hot flashes

- Physical signs of hypogonadism, such as gynecomastia, loss of body hair, infertility, or low bone mineral density

The reasoning here is simple: you are testing testosterone levels for one reason only: to see if replacement therapy may be helpful.* There is no convincing evidence that it helps men with nonsexual, nonspecific symptoms.

Testosterone levels reach a peak in the morning and decline to a nadir in the evening. The test should be drawn between 8 and 10 AM. It is important that the patient be fasting. The most accurate results—especially toward the lower limit of normal—are obtained when testing is done by liquid chromatography-mass spectrometry (LCMS) rather than immunoassay. Normal values for serum total testosterone are 300 to 1,200 ng/dL. Levels normally decline with aging.

If the result comes back normal, your workup is done. If it is low, repeat the test (some clinicians argue that you need three values below normal to diagnose a low testosterone).

If the total testosterone is still low, check a *free testosterone*. Testosterone is largely bound in the circulation to sex hormone–binding globulin (SHBG) and albumin, but it is only the free hormone that is biologically active. The free testosterone usually comprises less than 3% of the total testosterone and declines even faster with aging than the total testosterone. Levels below approximately 50 pg/mL are considered low.

Patients can have a low total testosterone with a normal free testosterone if their SHBG levels are low, in which case they do not have hypogonadism. The most common cause of a low SHBG is obesity, followed by hypothyroidism and anabolic steroids. Conversely, normal total testosterone with a low free testosterone can be seen in patients with elevated SHBG levels, which may be caused by pregnancy, OCPs, liver disease (eg, cirrhosis), HIV, and hyperthyroidism.

There are various methods for measuring the free testosterone, but the most accurate is a technique called equilibrium dialysis,** and this technique should be requested whenever possible.

---

*And safe; no reason to check the testosterone level if there is a contraindication to treatment, such as sleep apnea, polycythemia, or prostate cancer.

**In brief, the technique exploits the fact that unbound hormone can move across a dialysis membrane whereas bound hormone cannot. Once the sample reaches equilibrium, it is easy to measure the percent of free hormone compared to the total hormone in the sample.

Once you have confirmed a low testosterone, you need to find out why it is low. You will want to order the following lab tests:

- *Follicle-stimulating hormone (FSH)* and *luteinizing hormone (LH)*—Measuring these pituitary hormones allows you to determine if the cause is primary (testicular) or secondary (pituitary or, rarely, hypothalamic). A high FSH and LH are consistent with primary testicular disease, whereas low or normal levels suggest a pituitary disease, hypothalamic disease, or anabolic steroid use. In males, a normal FSH is 5 to 15 mU/mL, and a normal LH is 3 to 15 U/L.

- *Prolactin*—Hyperprolactinemia is relatively common, and prolactin can lower the FSH and LH and in this way lower the testosterone. See page 344 for more on prolactin.

- *TSH*—Hypothyroidism lowers the SHBG and thus the total testosterone. In some men, hypothyroidism may also directly affect the hypothalamus and pituitary and cause a decrease in the free testosterone as well.

- *Iron studies*—Hemochromatosis is a common cause of low testosterone in relatively young males.

- *AM cortisol*—A low AM cortisol can be a sign of pituitary dysfunction and therefore secondary hypogonadism. See page 333 for more on cortisol testing.

- *Urine toxicology screen*—Marijuana and opioids can lower the testosterone.

Once you have started patients on testosterone therapy, you will need to monitor their serum testosterone levels. The goal is generally a level within the low-to-normal range. You should also consider monitoring the complete blood count (testosterone raises the hemoglobin) and prostate-specific antigen (PSA) (see Chapter 20).

 ## Estrogen and the Hypothalamic-Pituitary-Gonadal Axis in Females

Estradiol is the major circulating estrogen prior to menopause. It is synthesized within the ovaries. Estradiol is most often measured as part of an infertility workup and in the evaluation of menstrual irregularities.* Normal values fluctuate with the menstrual cycle:

- Days 1 to 10: 14 to 27 pg/mL

- Days 11 to 20: 14 to 54 pg/mL

- Days 21 to 30: 19 to 41 pg/mL

---

*In males, where estradiol is produced in the testes, it is part of the evaluation of gynecomastia.

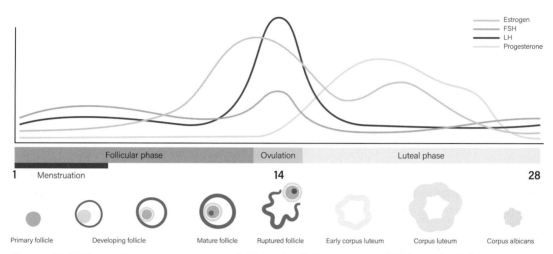

Figure 19.12 How estrogen, progesterone, follicle-stimulating hormone (FSH), and luteinizing hormone (LH) fluctuate with the menstrual cycle.

Normal *FSH* levels also vary with the menstrual cycle; typical normal values are 5 to 20 mU/mL in the follicular or luteal phase and 30 to 50 mU/mL at midcycle peak. Levels persistently over 35 mU/mL are consistent with menopause. *LH* levels also vary, with normal values of 5 to 22 mU/mL in the follicular or luteal phase, 30 to 250 mU/mL at midcycle peak, and persistently more than 30 mU/mL consistent with menopause.

Menopause

As estrogen levels decline with menopause, feedback inhibition on the pituitary gland declines and *FSH* and *LH* levels rise. However, measurement of these parameters is not required to make the diagnosis of menopause when a woman 45 years old or above presents with more than or equal to 12 months of otherwise unexplained amenorrhea.

An FSH measurement may be helpful in females approaching menopausal age who are still on OCPs and who therefore may not exhibit symptoms of menopause such as hot flashes. However, OCPs also prevent the usual menopausal rise in the FSH, so one approach is to have the patient stop their OCP (and use an alternative method of contraception) for 2 to 3 weeks and then check an FSH. A high level confirms menopause, but a normal level tells you little, as the anterior pituitary may remain suppressed for many weeks.

Amenorrhea

Primary Amenorrhea: Evaluation for primary amenorrhea is recommended for women who have not started menarche by the age of 15. The most common cause other than pregnancy is gonadal dysgenesis (eg, Turner syndrome), so a pelvic ultrasound and a human chorionic gonadotropin (hCG) are typically the first tests that are ordered.

A karyotype analysis for congenital disorders is needed if there is no uterus present.

If a uterus is present, laboratory evaluation should focus on other causes of primary amenorrhea, including hyperprolactinemia, hypothyroidism, polycystic ovary syndrome, gonadal hormone-releasing hormone deficiency, and hypopituitarism. Laboratory testing therefore includes an FSH, LH, prolactin, and TSH. Karyotype analysis is needed if the FSH and LH are elevated. Women with symptoms suggestive of congenital adrenal hyperplasia (see page 351) should be tested for 17-hydroxylase deficiency with a serum 17-hydroxyprogesterone (17-OHP) level.

Secondary Amenorrhea: Secondary amenorrhea is defined as the absence of menses for 3 months in women who have previously had normal menstruation. Women with secondary amenorrhea should always be tested first for pregnancy with an hCG. If pregnancy is ruled out, the next steps include the same lab tests as mentioned earlier—an FSH, LH, prolactin, and TSH. In women with normal lab results, a *progestin challenge* can be performed to evaluate if the patient has outflow obstruction (eg, due to intrauterine adhesions). Ten milligrams of medroxyprogesterone is given once a day for 10 days; if bleeding occurs after the withdrawal of progesterone, then outflow obstruction is not present.

Female Infertility and Ovarian Reserve

One of the key steps in the evaluation of female infertility is to measure ovarian reserve, that is, the number of healthy oocytes remaining in the ovaries. Knowing a patient's ovarian reserve is particularly important in predicting the likely success of in vitro fertilization. There is no single test that can do this accurately, and even when used together they do not give a definitive answer:

- *Antimullerian hormone (AMH)*: AMH is produced by the ovarian follicles and its level correlates with the number of oocytes. It therefore declines with age. Levels of greater than 1.0 ng/mL predict a good response to stimulation with in vitro fertilization techniques. However, AMH levels are not predictive of a successful pregnancy. This test is discussed more on page 357.

- *Day-3 FSH[a]*: The logic here is that women with a high ovarian reserve—that is, many viable oocytes—should be producing sufficient hormones to suppress the FSH. Those with a low reserve should have a high FSH. A normal result tells you little, but a high result suggests that pregnancy is unlikely using the woman's own oocytes.

- *Day-3 estradiol*: Very low levels are associated with a very low chance of pregnancy.

[a]Day 1 is the first day of menstrual flow.

PROLACTIN

The major function of prolactin, a polypeptide hormone secreted by the anterior pituitary gland, is to stimulate the production and secretion of milk. The most potent stimuli to its release are pregnancy and breastfeeding. Like many hormones, it regulates its own secretion:

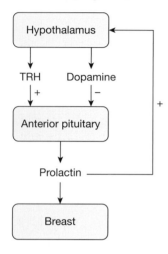

Figure 19.13 Prolactin secretion by the anterior pituitary is controlled by the hypothalamus. In patients who are neither pregnant nor lactating, the inhibitory effect of dopamine is more powerful than the stimulation induced by thyrotropin-releasing hormone (TRH). Prolactin increases hypothalamic production of dopamine, thereby limiting its own secretion.

Normal prolactin levels are less than 20 ng/mL in nonpregnant, non-breastfeeding females and less than 15 ng/mL in males.

Many of the effects of a prolactin level that is too high or, rarely, too low, are related to its impact on the HPG axis.

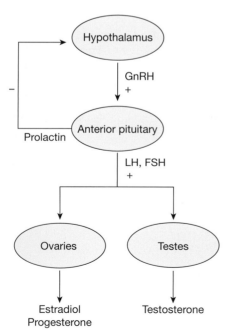

Figure 19.14 High levels of prolactin inhibit hypothalamic secretion of GnRH, which ultimately leads to decreased testicular secretion of testosterone or decreased ovarian secretion of estradiol and progesterone. FSH, follicle-stimulating hormone; GnRH, gonadotropin hormone-releasing hormone; LH, luteinizing hormone.

- In *premenopausal women*, elevated levels can cause infertility, menstrual cycle dysfunction, and galactorrhea.

- In *postmenopausal women*, symptoms of hyperprolactinemia are rare; endocrinologic effects on fertility and menstrual function are not an issue in this population.

- In *men*, prolactin decreases testosterone levels which in turn can cause diminished libido, erectile dysfunction, infertility, gynecomastia, and rarely galactorrhea.

Many patients with hyperprolactinemia, both women and men, have no symptoms at all. Causes of abnormally high levels of prolactin include:

- *Pituitary tumors*—Prolactinomas are the most common cause of hyperprolactinemia. They comprise about half of all pituitary adenomas; these can be microadenomas (<1 cm in diameter) or macroadenomas (>1 cm in diameter). The degree of prolactin elevation roughly correlates with the size of the adenoma. Very high levels of prolactin (>500 μg/L) are very specific for pituitary macroadenomas but are not sensitive (~35%).

- *Hypothyroidism*—Low thyroid hormone levels drive up TRH, stimulating prolactin secretion.

- *Decreased prolactin clearance* from the circulation, most often as a result of renal failure.

- *Macroprolactinemia*—In this condition, prolactin forms large clumps because of the binding of anti-prolactin antibodies. These clumps are clinically inactive and are important only because they can lead to falsely elevated prolactin readings by the lab. Consider macroprolactinemia in a patient with hyperprolactinemia in the absence of symptoms or abnormal imaging findings.

- *Various medications that oppose the action of dopamine*—The resulting prolactin elevation is usually small; the most common causes are antipsychotic drugs, selective serotonin reuptake inhibitors, and metoclopramide.

If you detect elevated levels of prolactin, always make sure you have first ruled out pregnancy as a cause. And, as should be apparent from the list mentioned earlier, you must also rule out medication side effects and check a TSH to assess thyroid function. Only then should you focus your attention on the pituitary gland.*

The only situation in which we speak of abnormally low prolactin ("hypoprolactinemia") is with breastfeeding, where it is associated with low breast milk production. Otherwise, even an undetectably low prolactin is typically not cause for concern.

Prolactin and Seizures

Measuring prolactin levels has been suggested as a possible way to distinguish generalized tonic-clonic seizures from psychogenic nonepileptic seizures. The hypothesis is that prolactin levels would be high in the former and low in the latter. However, there turns out to be a great deal of overlap in the prolactin values between these two entities, compromising the utility of measuring prolactin in this setting.

---

*One other caveat when it comes to hyperprolactinemia: extremely high levels of prolactin can paradoxically cause falsely normal or low readings via interference of the assay by the prolactin itself. If you suspect this so-called "Hook" phenomenon, repeat the test on a diluted sample.

CATECHOLAMINES AND METANEPHRINES

There may be no testing that is done with a lower rate of return than these tests, which are used to screen for a pheochromocytoma, a rare neuroendocrine tumor that secretes the "fight-or-flight" hormones known as the catecholamines (epinephrine, norepinephrine, and dopamine). Nevertheless, testing does make sense in several scenarios when more likely diagnoses are not apparent:

- Patients who present with palpitations, headache, diaphoresis, tremor, and pallor with or without hypertension, especially if occurring in self-limited episodes ("hyperadrenergic spells"). Very few of these patients will prove to have a pheochromocytoma.

- Patients with suspected secondary hypertension (see page 337)
  - A pheochromocytoma is—yet again—rarely the culprit

- Patients with a family history of a confirmed or suspected condition that predisposes to a pheochromocytoma (eg, multiple endocrine neoplasia type 2)

The screening test that is most often ordered is either a *plasma metanephrines* or a *24-hour urine metanephrines*. Metanephrines are breakdown products of norepinephrine, epinephrine, and—one step further back in the metabolic pathway—dopamine. A normal serum metanephrine level is less than or equal to 205 pg/mL. A normal 24-hour urine metanephrine level is 224 to 832 µg/24 hr.

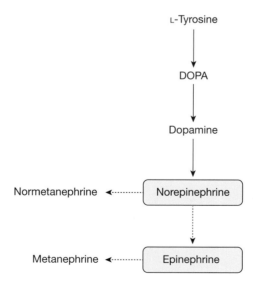

Figure 19.15 The catecholamine metabolic pathway. DOPA, dihydroxyphenylalanine.

Measurement of plasma metanephrines has a high sensitivity (over 96%) for a pheochromocytoma, but a lower specificity, especially in older patients (77% in those over the age of 60). The plasma metanephrines are elevated more than 4-fold in about 80% of patients with a pheochromocytoma. False positives can be seen in the setting of stress, exhaustion, acute illness, or—importantly—various medications and drugs.* A positive result is therefore often a false positive, but a negative test is useful in ruling out the diagnosis. Patients with hyperadrenergic spells that occur intermittently for a short period of time should undergo 24-hour urine testing that overlaps with one of their spells even if their plasma test is negative.

Because upright posture can lead to elevated catecholamine secretion—the effect is small but real—serum metanephrines should be drawn after the patient has been supine for at least 30 minutes. To avoid the catecholamine release stimulated by the blood draw itself (if you have ever been the recipient of a difficult blood draw, you know that it can elicit the catecholamine-mediated "fight-or-flight" response), the test can be done with a cannula placed before the 30 minute rest period and the blood then pulled from the cannula at the proper time.

Other tests, such as *plasma or 24-hour urine fractionated catecholamines and vanillylmandelic acid* (another catecholamine metabolite), are preferred by some experts and have reasonable sensitivities. However, most expert guidelines recommend testing for metanephrines as the first-line screen.

---

*Medications and drugs that can cause falsely elevated plasma and/or urine metanephrines include tricyclic antidepressants, monoamine oxidase (MAO) inhibitors, sympathomimetics (eg, phenylephrine, methylphenidate, cocaine), labetalol, sotalol, buspirone, sulfasalazine, levodopa, and even acetaminophen.

GROWTH HORMONE AND INSULIN-LIKE GROWTH FACTOR-1

Growth hormone (GH) is secreted by the anterior pituitary. Levels change dramatically with age, rising during childhood, plateauing during adolescence and young adulthood, and then slowly declining. Prior to adulthood, the normal range is approximately 1 to 15 ng/mL. In adult males, it is 0 to 4 ng/mL, and in adult females 0 to 18 ng/mL. Among its many actions, GH exerts powerful anabolic effects on virtually every organ in the body, stimulating cellular growth, differentiation, and proliferation.

The primary reasons to worry about GH levels in adults are:

- When you are considering the diagnosis of *acromegaly*. As a result of excess GH secretion, acromegaly is characterized by excessive growth of the body's tissues. The symptoms that typically bring the patient to clinical attention are skin thickening, coarse facial features, enlargement of the tongue, and diffuse joint pain.

- When you are considering the diagnosis of *hypopituitarism*, in which case GH secretion is low. Symptoms of GH deficiency may not be dramatic; the most notable consequence for many patients is low bone mineral density.

The primary reasons to worry about GH levels in children are:

- *Gigantism*, from excess GH secretion
- *Short stature*, from low GH secretion

The anterior pituitary secretes GH in pulsatile bursts approximately every 2 hours, a pattern that can be modulated by a large number of factors; for example, fasting and exercise stimulate its secretion, whereas obesity and hyperglycemia inhibit it. A random GH level can therefore be at best unreliable and at worst misleading about the patient's GH status.

Instead, it is preferable to measure levels of *insulin-like growth factor (IGF-1)* when GH-related problems are suspected. A small peptide secreted by the hypothalamus, IGF-1 is similar in structure to insulin. Its main action is to mediate the effects of GH. Like GH, its levels first rise and then fall with age; adult levels range from 245 to 737 ng/mL. However, unlike GH, its levels remain constant throughout the day.

Biotin, a commonly used over-the-counter supplement, can interfere with the IGF-1 assay. Hypothyroidism, use of oral estrogens, hepatic or renal failure, or poorly controlled type 1 diabetes can all lower IGF-1. On the other hand, hyperthyroidism, pregnancy, and certain diets (those very high in sugar, protein, and some dairy products) tend to raise IGF-1. These factors should all be considered in the interpretation of IGF-1 results.

 Acromegaly

In adults, the most common indication for measurement of IGF-1 is suspected acromegaly. In the appropriate clinical context, an elevated IGF-1 confirms the diagnosis of acromegaly. If IGF-1 comes back normal, it is highly unlikely the patient has acromegaly. Borderline results or suspected false negatives or false positives (see potential confounding factors mentioned earlier) should be followed by measurement of GH before and 2 hours after oral glucose administration. Failure to suppress GH—as demonstrated by a post-glucose GH concentration more than 1 ng/mL—establishes the diagnosis of acromegaly.

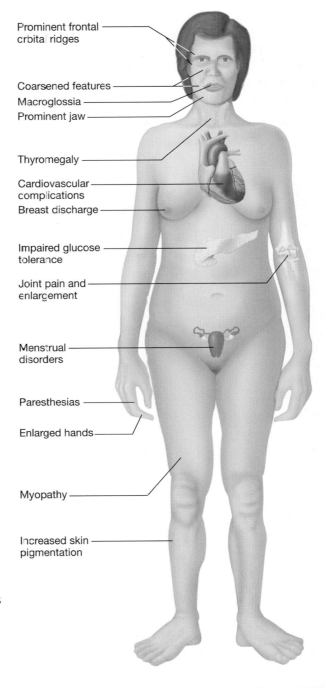

Prominent frontal orbital ridges

Coarsened features
Macroglossia
Prominent jaw

Thyromegaly

Cardiovascular complications

Breast discharge

Impaired glucose tolerance

Joint pain and enlargement

Menstrual disorders

Paresthesias

Enlarged hands

Myopathy

Increased skin pigmentation

Figure 19.16 Some of the major features of acromegaly. (Adapted from Braun CA, Anderson CM. *Applied Pathophysiology: A Conceptual Approach to the Mechanisms of Disease*. 4th ed. Wolters Kluwer; 2022.)

Growth Hormone Deficiency in Children

In children, the most common reason to check IGF-1 is suspected GH deficiency. It is recommended to check both IGF-1 and *IGFBP-3* (insulin-like growth factor binding protein-3), the major plasma carrier of IGF; expect both to be decreased in GH deficiency.

If the levels of IGF-1 and IGFBP-3 are sufficiently low and the clinical picture is consistent with GH deficiency, you are done. If there is any question, however, the diagnosis can be confirmed with a *GH stimulation test*, typically using glucagon, clonidine, or arginine; a blunted rise in GH levels to less than 7.5 μg/L is considered a positive test for GH deficiency. However, even this test is not perfect and, by inducing fluctuations in blood glucose or hypotension (arginine has the fewest side effects), can be quite unpleasant for the patient. The cutoff of what is considered a normal response—generally a GH concentration more than 7.5 μg/L—cannot be relied on for all patients, and a subnormal response is not necessarily indicative of GH deficiency.

Measurements of IGF-1 and IGFBP-3 are also used to monitor patients, usually children of short stature with GH deficiency, who are receiving recombinant GH therapy.

17-HYDROXYPROGESTERONE AND CONGENITAL ADRENAL HYPERPLASIA

Congenital adrenal hyperplasia (CAH) is a genetic disorder affecting the synthesis of the hormones produced by the adrenal cortex. A deficiency of the enzyme 21-hydroxylase underlies more than 90% of cases. We do not test for the enzyme itself but rather for its substrate, *17-hydroxyprogesterone (17-OHP)*, which builds up due to the enzyme deficiency. For accurate results, the blood sample must be collected early in the morning due to the significant drop in 17-OHP as the day goes on.

You can see from Figure 19.16 that a deficiency of 21-hydroxylase will compromise the synthesis of aldosterone and cortisol. Another consequence is that the precursors in these pathways are shunted toward the production of androgens.

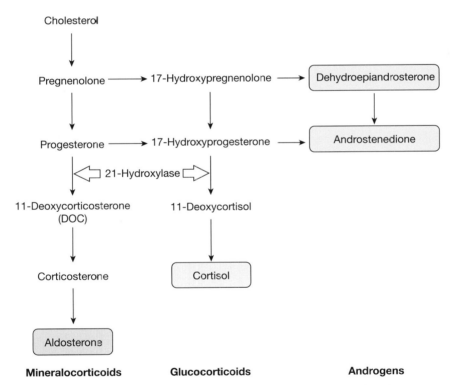

Figure 19.17 The metabolic pathways of the adrenal cortex. 21-Hydroxylase is involved in the pathways leading to cortisol and aldosterone synthesis. 17-Hydroxyprogesterone (17-OHP) builds up when the enzyme is deficient, forming the basis of how we diagnose congenital adrenal hyperplasia (CAH). Adrenal hyperplasia results from chronic stimulation of the glands by the pituitary as it tries to drive (fruitlessly) the production of cortisol.

- In the classic—severe—form, enzymatic activity is nearly undetectable. Diagnosis is almost always made shortly after birth through routine neonatal screening demonstrating 17-OHP levels that are extremely high (usually >3,500 ng/dL). Affected neonates most often present with evidence of mineralocorticoid deficiency (eg, hyponatremia, hypotension).

- In the more common nonclassic form, 20% to 50% of enzymatic activity is maintained and the disease is less severe. Presenting symptoms include early onset puberty and accelerated growth; female patients may exhibit virilization and menstrual abnormalities. Some patients may have no symptoms at all. In children, a 17-OHP cutoff of 200 ng/dL is very sensitive and specific for this form of CAH. Specificity approaches 100% at levels more than 1,500 ng/dL. When the diagnosis is in question, retesting for 17-OHP is the best next step. The diagnosis can be confirmed with a high-dose (250 μg) ACTH stimulation test; levels of 17-OHP will skyrocket in patients with CAH. If the diagnosis is still uncertain, genetic testing is recommended.

SEMEN ANALYSIS

Semen analysis is done both to evaluate male infertility and to confirm the completion of a successful vasectomy. An acceptable lab specimen should include approximately 0.5 mL of ejaculate collected in a sterile container. The patient should abstain from any sexual activity for at least 2 days prior to the collection. The sample must be kept at room temperature and analyzed within 1 hour of collection.

A basic semen analysis looks for a low *quantitative* sperm count as well as *qualitative defects* in the sperm that are present. Testing includes:

- Semen volume, viscosity, and pH

  - Why check the pH? A pH range of approximately 7.2 to 7.8 is necessary for a healthy environment for sperm to thrive within the seminal vesicles. Deviations from this range correlate well with poor motility and a low sperm count. An abnormal pH often indicates either inflammation or an anatomic lesion of the genital tract.

- Microscopic evaluation of

  - Sperm count and concentration
    - A low sperm count (oligospermia) is typically defined as fewer than 20 million sperm/mL.

  - Sperm motility (total motility and progressive motility*) and morphology
    - In a normal ejaculate, total motility should exceed 40% of sperm and progressive motility should exceed 32%.

    - Teratozoospermia (abnormal morphology) is diagnosed when fewer than 30% of sperm appear normal.

  - The presence of white blood cells, which may indicate infection or inflammation

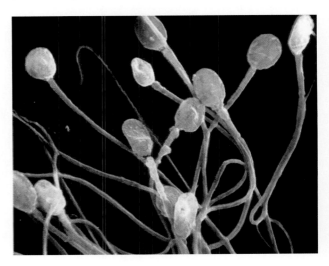

Figure 19.18 Normal sperm seen under the microscope. (Courtesy of Dr. Judi Nath.)

---

*Total motility measures all sperm movement. Progressive motility refers to the percent of sperm that move effectively in large circles or straight lines.

Some key points to note:

- A low volume of ejaculate with a normal sperm concentration is most often the result of an incomplete collection. A second major reason is retrograde ejaculation. If both the volume and concentration are low, there may be some blockage to the movement of sperm within the genital tract.

- A low sperm count in a normal volume of ejaculate should prompt an evaluation for hypogonadism (see the box "Male Infertility").

- Sperm autoantibodies may cause agglutination that can be seen under the microscope; however, these antibodies have not been convincingly implicated as a cause of infertility.

- In a patient who has undergone a vasectomy, the presence of more than 100,000 nonmotile sperm/mL or any motile sperm suggests the possibility that the procedure has failed.

Male Infertility

Defects of spermatogenesis are only one cause of male infertility. Others include:

- Endocrine disorders, primarily a deficiency of gonadotropins

- Other systemic disorders, such as renal failure, hepatic cirrhosis, hemochromatosis, sickle cell disease, and infections (most notably mumps orchitis)

- Testicular injury

- Various drugs (such as antiandrogens and chemotherapeutic agents)

- Anatomic disorders affecting the transport of sperm

- Varicoceles

As many as 20% of cases remain unexplained.

If there is no reason to suspect an underlying systemic illness, the laboratory evaluation typically starts with:

- Semen analysis, as discussed above

- Endocrinologic testing: serum testosterone, FSH, and LH (see page 339); consider a prolactin and TSH as well.

- Genetic testing: among the most common genetic disorders underlying male infertility are Klinefelter syndrome (XXY) and cystic fibrosis (mutations in the CFTR [cystic fibrosis transmembrane regulator] gene).

PREGNANCY TESTING

The role of the laboratory in determining whether someone is pregnant can be summed up in one word (well, technically three words): *human chorionic gonadotropin (hCG)*. hCG, a hormone that is made primarily by the placenta, begins to rise after implantation, usually 6 to 10 days after ovulation. hCG levels in the blood then begin to double approximately every 1 to 3 days until 4 to 6 weeks gestation, after which the rate of rise decreases until levels plateau around 8 to 11 weeks gestation. Levels then gradually decline.

Once it begins to be produced, hCG is almost immediately detectable by *serum testing*, which can detect levels as low as 1 to 2 mIU/mL. hCG can also be measured in the urine. Because of their convenience, *urine tests* are by far the most common method by which pregnancy is diagnosed. However, urine tests are not as sensitive as serum tests, first detecting levels in the 20 to 50 mIU/mL range. A urine pregnancy test typically does not become positive until at least 3 to 4 weeks gestation (~1-2 weeks after conception). All urine tests are able to detect a pregnancy by one week after the first missed menstrual period (~5 weeks gestation).

Table 19.2 Typical Levels of hCG During the First Month of Pregnancy

Weeks Since Conception	hCG (mIU/mL)
0.2-1	5-50
1-2	50-500
2-3	100-5,000
3-4	500-10,000

hCG, human chorionic gonadotropin.

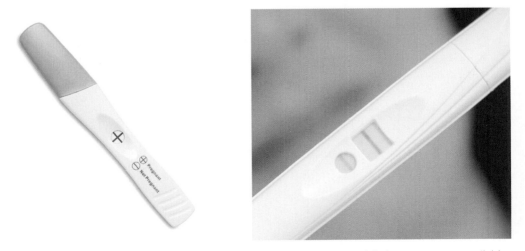

Figure 19.19 Two examples of positive home urine pregnancy tests. Digital tests are now available and, despite their high-tech appearance, work in exactly the same way. (Left image is from O'Meara AM. *Maternity, Newborn, and Women's Health Nursing: A Case-based Approach.* Wolters Kluwer; 2019. Right image from Pillitteri A. *Maternal and Child Health Nursing: Care of the Childbearing and Childrearing Family.* 4th ed. Lippincott Williams & Wilkins; 2002.)

Home urine pregnancy tests use an immunometric technique to detect hCG. A sample of urine is placed on test paper and exposed to anti-hCG antibodies that are tagged with an enzyme. Tagged antibody-hCG complexes bind to different anti-hCG antibodies that are fixed to the paper in what is referred to as the test zone. This creates an antibody-hCG-antibody sandwich, and the enzyme alters the color of the test line. Meanwhile, antibodies that have not bound hCG bind to a second population of antibodies that are fixed to the control line. Thus, if sufficient hCG is present, two lines will be detected; if not, and the test was done properly, only the control line will change color.

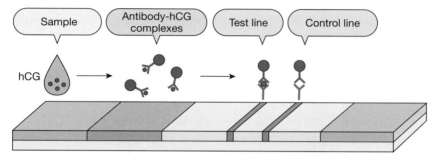

Figure 19.20 How a pregnancy test is run. hCG, human chorionic gonadotropin.

False negatives can occur early in pregnancy, in which case repeat testing should be performed 1 week later. False positives are rare, but they can occur because of operator error, secretion of hCG from a tumor instead of a pregnancy, and recent pregnancy loss (after implantation) when hCG levels have not yet declined to zero.

ANTI-MÜLLERIAN HORMONE

Anti-Müllerian hormone (AMH) is secreted by growing ovarian follicles and is a measure of how many oocytes a woman has in her ovaries, that is, her *ovarian reserve*. The number declines over time as follicles go through their terminal stages of maturation. Fertility clinics rely on harvesting as many oocytes as possible, and a very low AMH (below 1 ng/mL) is a good predictor of the number of eggs available for retrieval in women seeking in vitro fertilization. However, it is not a good predictor of a successful live birth.

Among women *without* a history of infertility, the likelihood of pregnancy is identical among women with normal and low (<0.7 ng/mL) AMH levels.

It only takes a single ovum to make a successful pregnancy, and it appears that the total number of oocytes is less important than the quality of the remaining oocytes, especially when there are no infertility issues.

A number of at-home fertility tests are now available, claiming that they can accurately assess a woman's chances of becoming pregnant. They measure several hormones including the AMH. Outcome data assessing their accuracy in predicting pregnancy are not available, and this poses a problem. When home testing seems to indicate that their chance of pregnancy is low, women may stop trying to conceive. On the other hand, a woman with a normal AMH may decide to wait to conceive and be falsely reassured that her fertility won't decline naturally over time.

MARKERS OF BONE TURNOVER

There are serum and urine tests that can assess the ongoing levels of bone formation and bone resorption. However, only the measures of bone resorption have been shown to have clinical utility and even that is quite limited.

The markers that are used most often look at breakdown products of collagen and include *urinary N-telopeptide crosslink (NTx)* and *serum C-telopeptide crosslink (CTx)*. Levels of these markers rise with increased bone resorption, such as occurs in postmenopausal women, and fall with successful therapy of osteoporosis.

Normal values vary from lab to lab but are roughly:

- Urinary NTx (units are nmol bone collagen equivalents per mmol creatinine)

  - Males: 21 to 83

  - Premenopausal women: 17 to 94

  - Postmenopausal women: 26 to 124

- Serum CTx (units are pg/mL)

  - Males: 60 to 700

  - Premenopausal women: 40 to 465

  - Postmenopausal women: 104 to 1,008

Although these tests are fairly predictive of the future rate of bone loss and fracture risk, neither test is recommended as a screen for who should be tested or treated for osteoporosis. We have clinical guidelines incorporating dual x-ray absorptiometry (DEXA) scanning that do a more than adequate job.

Bone marker testing can be useful in assessing adherence and response to antiresorptive therapy for osteoporosis (eg, a bisphosphonate). However, do not rely on these tests when patients are on medications such as recombinant parathyroid hormone that increases bone formation. If you use NTx or CTx for the purpose of monitoring response to antiresorptive therapy, make sure to get baseline levels prior to starting treatment. A fall of approximately 30% to 50% in NTx and/or CTx after initiating treatment is considered an indicator of a good therapeutic response. Some clinicians also use these tests to see when patients who have stopped antiresorptive therapy need to restart, but interpretation of the results in this context can be challenging.

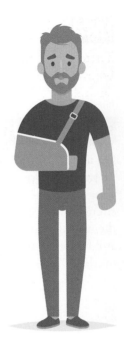

Figure 19.21 Markers of bone turnover are typically elevated for several weeks after a fracture as the bone remodels in an effort to heal itself. (Courtesy stickerama/Shutterstock.)

Both NTx and CTx should be run on morning samples after an overnight fast; bone metabolism has a distinct diurnal pattern: high in the morning and low in the evening. The urinary NTx should be run on the second void of the morning. Although standardization of these tests across laboratories is improving, it remains far from perfect; any repeat testing should be run by the same lab on the same equipment.

Paget Disease of the Bone

Bony overgrowth is a hallmark of Paget disease, and the serum alkaline phosphatase (see chapter 5) is usually the only serum marker of increased bone turnover that you need to assess disease activity. In some patients, however, the serum alkaline phosphatase may be normal, especially if only one area of bone is involved, and then it can be helpful to order a bone-specific alkaline phosphatase as well as an NTx and CTx, which may be elevated.

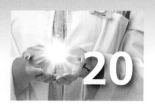

20 Hematology/Oncology

IRON STUDIES

On a biochemical level, iron metabolism can get immensely complicated. But for those of us on the clinical side, there are only a few things we need to know. Iron is absorbed from the gut and then binds to transferrin, a glycoprotein made in the liver, for its sojourn in the circulation. It is then either stored as ferritin or utilized for various cellular processes, such as the manufacture of hemoglobin in the bone marrow. These components—iron, transferrin, and ferritin—are what we look at first when we suspect either iron deficiency or iron overload.*

 Iron Deficiency

Ferritin

For patients with anemia in whom you suspect iron deficiency as the cause (see our discussion of the complete blood count [CBC] in Chapter 4), the only test you will need most of the time is a serum *ferritin*. Circulating ferritin levels correlate very well with total body iron stores. The ferritin is a more accurate measure of the body's total iron storage than the serum iron and will decline before the serum iron does, making it a more sensitive indicator of iron deficiency.

Normal values are in the range of 15 to 200 ng/dL. In patients with anemia, the threshold for what is considered a low ferritin, while not written in stone, is commonly cited as less than 45 ng/mL. Using this number, the serum ferritin has a sensitivity of approximately 85% and specificity of approximately 92% for diagnosing iron deficiency. As you can see from these less-than-perfect percentages, the ferritin is not always reliable. The primary reason is because ferritin is an acute-phase reactant. Ferritin levels rise with inflammation, as well as with infection, malignancy, liver disease, and chronic renal disease, so patients who have both iron deficiency and one of these underlying disorders may have misleadingly high levels of ferritin. For these patients you will need to order additional testing.

---

*There are many, many pieces of the iron puzzle that contribute to its regulation. One component you may have heard of, *hepcidin*, downregulates the absorption and recycling of iron and plays an important role in the anemia of chronic disease. However, there is no readily available clinical test for it.

Iron, Total Iron-Binding Capacity, and Transferrin Saturation

Normal levels of serum iron are 60 to 160 μg/dL. As you would expect, the serum iron is low in patients with iron deficiency. And yet, perhaps unexpectedly, a serum iron in isolation is not a reliable marker of iron deficiency in patients with anemia. There are several reasons for this: (1) the serum levels vary throughout the day (they tend to peak at the stroke of midnight); (2) they are very sensitive to dietary intake; and (3) they are frequently low in patients with anemia of chronic disease.

Transferrin levels can also be measured and are usually reported as *total iron-binding capacity (TIBC)*. Normal TIBC ranges between 250 and 460 μg/dL. The TIBC is high in iron deficiency (lots of binding sites are unoccupied and free) and often normal or low in anemia of chronic disease. You can then use the iron and TIBC to calculate the *transferrin saturation* as follows (the lab will typically do this for you):

$$\text{Iron concentration} \div \text{TIBC} = \text{Transferrin saturation}$$

For patients with possible iron deficiency anemia and an equivocal ferritin, the transferrin saturation can be a useful test to move your diagnostic needle; most labs use a cutoff of less than 20% to be indicative of iron deficiency. Levels of 20% to 50% are considered normal. The lower the percentage, the more likely the patient has iron deficiency.

 ## Iron Overload

Hemochromatosis, an autosomal recessive disease, is common, with as many as 10% of the White population carrying at least one mutation. It is especially common in people of northern European ancestry. You do not want to miss this diagnosis, since early intervention can prevent severe complications from iron deposition in organs throughout the body. Testing involves first demonstrating an elevated *transferrin saturation*—more than 60% in men and less than 50% in women—followed by confirmation with genetic testing. We discuss hemochromatosis further in Chapter 17.

VITAMIN B$_{12}$ (CYANOCOBALAMIN) AND FOLATE

Deficiencies of vitamin B$_{12}$ (cyanocobalamin) and folate are the most common causes of macrocytic anemia. These vitamin deficiencies cause a particular type of macrocytic anemia termed *megaloblastic anemia* in which the red blood cell (RBC) precursors in the bone marrow are larger than normal due to delayed nuclear maturation and cell division. The neutrophils are also large and their nuclei typically have an increased number of lobes.

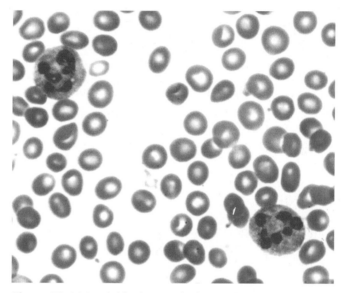

Figure 20.1 Megaloblastic anemia due to vitamin B$_{12}$ deficiency. Note the large red blood cells and the multilobed nuclei in the neutrophils. (From Strayer DS, Saffitz JE. *Rubin's Pathology: Mechanisms of Human Disease.* 8th ed. Wolters Kluwer; 2020.)

You will most commonly screen for these vitamin deficiencies when you discover that your patient has a macrocytic anemia. However, this is not the only reason to test for vitamin B$_{12}$. Vitamin B$_{12}$ deficiency is also an important cause of a *distal, symmetric peripheral neuropathy* and, less often, various *neuropsychiatric disorders* (including cognitive impairment and depression) and a very specific spinal cord syndrome called *subacute combined degeneration*. Testing for vitamin B$_{12}$ deficiency is indicated in patients with neurologic signs or symptoms compatible with these diagnoses. Folate deficiency does not cause neurologic complications.

You can screen for folate deficiency by ordering a *serum folate* (normal, 4.0-20 ng/mL) and for vitamin B$_{12}$ deficiency with a *serum vitamin B$_{12}$* (normal, 200-800 pg/dL).

However, in the case of vitamin B$_{12}$ deficiency, a serum *methylmalonic acid* (normal, 0-0.4 μmol/L) may be a more reliable test. Vitamin B$_{12}$ is a cofactor in the conversion of methylmalonic acid to succinyl-CoA, a mitochondrial enzyme involved in adenosine triphosphate (ATP) generation, and deficiency of vitamin B$_{12}$ therefore leads to *increased* levels of methylmalonic acid. Whereas vitamin B$_{12}$ levels can fluctuate substantially over a period of weeks, methylmalonic acid levels do not. *Bottom line:* in most instances, a serum vitamin B$_{12}$ will get the job done, but if you suspect B$_{12}$ deficiency in a patient with levels that are hovering in the low range of normal, order a methylmalonic acid to confirm the diagnosis.

There is some evidence that *RBC folate* is a better marker of the body's total folate stores than the serum folate, and thus is a better indicator of long-term folate deficiency. However, in the absence of strong evidence showing that testing for RBC folate leads to better clinical outcomes, there is little indication for running this test.

Both folate and vitamin B$_{12}$ deficiency are associated with elevated serum levels of *homocysteine* (normal, 5.0-15.0 μmol/L). Homocysteine is an amino acid, and vitamin B$_{12}$ and folate serve as cofactors in its conversion to methionine. This test is rarely needed in the evaluation of macrocytic anemia. However, in some cases, it may be elevated before the blood tests for vitamin B$_{12}$ and folate fall below normal, and thus can be an early indicator of deficiency. It may also help to confirm vitamin B$_{12}$ and folate deficiency when their levels are borderline low.

A Bit More About Homocysteine

Elevated levels of homocysteine are associated with an increased risk for cardiovascular disease. However, including this test in routine screening for cardiovascular risk factors—although it is done and often requested by patients—is generally not recommended. Although folate or vitamin B$_{12}$ supplementation will lower homocysteine levels, decreasing the serum concentration of homocysteine has not been shown to protect against the development of cardiovascular disease.

 ## *Parsing Out the Cause of Vitamin B$_{12}$ Deficiency*

With folate deficiency, once you have identified low serum levels, your job is essentially done; the cause is almost always dietary insufficiency (although, if you haven't already checked for vitamin B$_{12}$ deficiency, make sure you do because the two conditions can coexist). Not so with vitamin B$_{12}$ deficiency, which has multiple potential causes. Determining the reason for vitamin B$_{12}$ deficiency is important for appropriate clinical management.

Table 20.1 Causes of Vitamin B_{12} Deficiency

Common Causes
Pernicious anemia
Achlorhydria (decreased stomach acid, often seen in elderly patients with atrophic gastritis)
Malabsorption (many bowel diseases; celiac disease is increasingly being diagnosed in this setting)
Long-term use of metformin
Strict vegan diet (vitamin B_{12} is only present in animal products, including eggs)
Less Common Causes
Bacterial overgrowth in the bowel
Tropical sprue
Tapeworm infection

As you can see from Table 20.1, the evaluation of B_{12} deficiency may veer off into several directions (eg, screening for celiac disease or other bowel diseases, gastric biopsy for atrophic gastritis and achlorhydria), but efforts are usually first directed at ruling in or out the diagnosis of pernicious anemia.

Pernicious Anemia

Pernicious anemia refers to impaired vitamin B_{12} absorption due to deficient intrinsic factor activity. It is the most common cause of vitamin B_{12} deficiency. Intrinsic factor, a glycoprotein secreted by the gastric parietal cells, binds vitamin B_{12} and enhances its absorption in the terminal ileum. About 90% of patients with pernicious anemia have detectable *antibodies against parietal cells*, and about half (50%-60%) have *antibodies against intrinsic factor* (yes, some have both).

Anti-parietal cell antibodies are not specific for pernicious anemia and can be seen in patients with atrophic gastritis and other autoimmune conditions. Anti-intrinsic factor antibodies, although less sensitive, are highly specific for pernicious anemia. Both of these tests should be ordered once you have established the diagnosis of vitamin B_{12} deficiency.

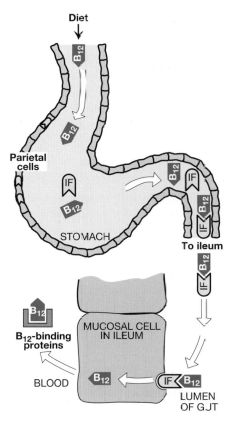

Figure 20.2 The pathway by which vitamin B$_{12}$ gets absorbed from the gut.

Too Much of a Good Thing

Do we ever need to worry about excess vitamin B$_{12}$ or folate? These are both B vitamins, meaning they are water soluble, and the body does a great job of getting rid of any excess in the urine. Some people do run higher than normal levels, but there is no evidence that these are harmful. Rarely, an elevated B$_{12}$ level may be seen in the setting of an occult malignancy (in and of itself, it remains harmless).

HEMOLYSIS

There are many causes of hemolysis—*mechanical* (eg, shearing of RBCs on a mechanical heart valve), *autoimmune* (eg, warm autoimmune hemolytic anemia [AIHI]), *hereditary* (eg, sickle cell disease, hereditary spherocytosis), *medication or toxin-related,* and others (eg, disseminated intravascular coagulation [DIC]). Hemolysis can occur within the blood vessels (intravascular) or outside the vessels (extravascular) in the spleen, liver, bone marrow, or lymph nodes via the reticuloendothelial system. Some degree of hemolysis is normal in healthy individuals—this is part of how we turn over our RBC supply (out with the old, in with the new). When we use the term hemolysis in clinical practice, however, we are typically referring to the *premature* or *excessive* destruction of RBCs resulting in anemia.

The *reticulocyte count, peripheral blood smear,* and *bilirubin* are mandatory parts of the workup of hemolysis.

- Expect a patient with a hemolytic anemia to have an elevated corrected reticulocyte count consistent with a hyperproliferative anemia (remember from Chapter 4 that, when peripheral destruction of RBCs is the problem, the bone marrow churns out reticulocytes in an effort to compensate).

- Examination of RBC morphology on the smear can help differentiate among various causes of hemolysis (see Table 4.1).

- Bilirubin is a breakdown product of RBCs (see Chapter 5). Its unconjugated form (indirect bilirubin) is usually elevated in patients with hemolysis.

Additional lab tests can also be helpful in establishing the diagnosis of hemolysis: the *lactate dehydrogenase (LDH), haptoglobin,* and—less often—*plasma-free hemoglobin.* A *Coombs* (aka *direct antiglobulin [DAT]*) test is also often a part of the initial evaluation.

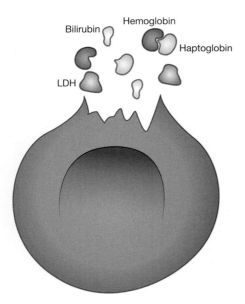

Figure 20.3 When red blood cells hemolyze, their contents spill into the circulation. The lactate dehydrogenase (LDH), plasma-free hemoglobin, and unconjugated bilirubin will all rise. Haptoglobin, on the other hand, which binds hemoglobin in the circulation, falls; the hemoglobin-haptoglobin complex is rapidly cleared by the liver.

Lactate Dehydrogenase

Lactate dehydrogenase (LDH) is an enzyme that plays a key role in anaerobic cellular respiration, the process by which we convert glucose to energy when oxygen is in short supply (eg, during vigorous exercise). The normal range of serum LDH varies by laboratory, but is typically around 60 to 100 U/L.

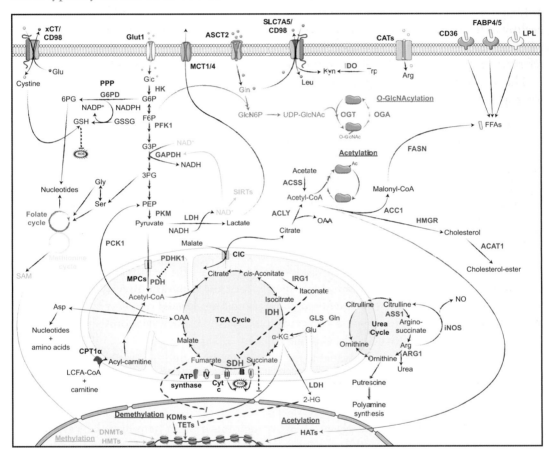

Figure 20.4 Remember all of the pathways involved in cellular respiration? Neither do we. For our purposes, it will suffice to understand that lactate dehydrogenase (LDH), like cellular respiration, is found in many cells throughout the body, including the red blood cells. When hemolysis occurs, LDH spills out of the red blood cells and serum levels rise. You will find LDH at the bottom and mid-left of this illustration. (From Flajnik M. *Paul's Fundamental Immunology*. Lippincott Williams & Wilkins; 2022.)

The LDH will most likely be high in any patient with hemolytic anemia. A normal LDH makes hemolytic anemia very unlikely, especially if other labs that would be abnormal in the setting of hemolysis are all normal (see later). However, because LDH is found in so many types of cells, an elevated LDH is not specific for hemolysis.

Haptoglobin

Haptoglobin is an enzyme synthesized by the liver that plays several important physiologic roles (it wears many "hapts?"*): it acts as an antioxidant, helps to fight infections (it is an acute-phase reactant), and—most importantly for our purposes here—binds free hemoglobin which would otherwise accumulate and damage the kidneys. The normal range for serum haptoglobin is 50 to 150 mg/dL.

In the setting of hemolysis, large amounts of free hemoglobin spill out of the RBCs and bind haptoglobin, causing serum haptoglobin levels to fall. A haptoglobin ≤ 25 mg/dL is more than 95% specific for hemolysis, although rare false positives—a low haptoglobin in the absence of hemolysis—may be seen in patients with severe liver disease. Unlike LDH, haptoglobin is not very sensitive for hemolysis. Because haptoglobin is an acute-phase reactant, false negatives—a normal or high haptoglobin in the setting of hemolysis—may be seen in states of inflammation.

Both the sensitivity and specificity are improved when haptoglobin is used in conjunction with the LDH to rule hemolysis in or out. It therefore makes sense to order these tests together.

 Plasma-Free Hemoglobin

Since the vast majority of hemoglobin resides within the RBCs in healthy individuals, the normal plasma-free hemoglobin range is typically very low, around 0 to 5 mg/dL. In the setting of hemolysis, the plasma-free hemoglobin should be elevated. However, it is usually *not* elevated in patients with chronic low-grade hemolysis, presumably because it is produced slowly enough not to overwhelm the binding capacity of haptoglobin.

Although several methods are available for measurement, including spectrophotometry and (less commonly) enzyme-linked immunosorbent assay (ELISA), plasma-free hemoglobin is not often measured in routine clinical practice because it is more expensive and involved than other hemolysis labs and often unnecessary.

It may make sense to order a plasma-free hemoglobin if other hemolysis labs are conflicting (eg, a low LDH with low haptoglobin) or potentially confounded by other factors (eg, a low haptoglobin in a patient with hepatic cirrhosis, which can impair haptoglobin synthesis). Plasma-free hemoglobin is also ordered in certain special clinical situations—for example, it is used to monitor hemolysis in patients on extracorporeal membrane oxygen (ECMO).** In general, the plasma-free hemoglobin is not a necessary part of the evaluation of most patients with suspected hemolysis.

---

*Sorry.
**Hemolysis is caused by mechanical shearing of red blood cells

Direct Antiglobulin Test and Autoimmune Hemolytic Anemia

The *direct antiglobulin test (DAT)*, also called the *direct Coombs test*, is often part of the initial workup of hemolytic anemia. It allows for detection of autoimmune hemolytic anemia (AIHI) and for differentiation between the two main forms of AIHI:

- *Warm agglutinin disease*: This is the most common cause of immune-mediated hemolysis. Antibodies, usually immunoglobulin (Ig)G, bind RBC surface antigens at warm temperatures (≥37 °C, or 98.6 °F—whichever scale you prefer, we are talking normal core body temperature). This process may be idiopathic or associated with underlying systemic disease, most commonly infection (eg, human immunodeficiency virus [HIV], hepatitis C, or Epstein-Barr virus), autoimmune disease (eg, lupus), or lymphoproliferative disorders (eg, chronic lymphocytic leukemia).

- *Cold agglutinin disease*: Antibodies, usually IgM, bind RBC surface antigens at cold temperatures (ie, in the relatively cooler distal extremities, often resulting in bluish discoloration of the hands and feet from decreased oxygen delivery, a condition called *acrocyanosis*). This process is often associated with infection, particularly with *Mycoplasma pneumoniae* or Epstein-Barr virus. Much less commonly it is seen in lupus, rheumatoid arthritis, and lymphoproliferative disorders.

Because AIHI is relatively common, usually treatable, and often associated with one or more specific underlying diseases (aforementioned), your threshold for sending this test should be low in any patient with highly suspected or confirmed hemolytic anemia. If another cause of hemolytic anemia is apparent or likely (eg, if many schistocytes are seen on a blood smear, indicative of a microangiopathy such as thrombotic thrombocytopenic purpura [TTP] or DIC—see page 371), a DAT is usually not indicated.

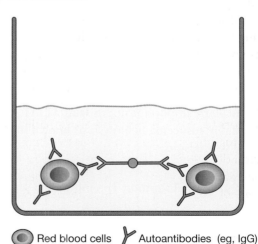

Figure 20.5 When Coombs reagent is added to the washed red blood cells of a patient with autoimmune hemolytic anemia, agglutination occurs. IgG, immunoglobulin G.

Here is how the DAT works:

1. Add antibodies: The patient's RBCs are washed and combined with anti-IgG and anti-C3d antibodies ("Coombs reagent").

2. Check for agglutination:

   • If the patient has warm AIHI, meaning their RBCs are coated with IgG, RBC *agglutination* will occur when anti-IgG is added. The anti-IgG binds the IgG on the RBCs, making "bridges" between the RBCs that can be detected upon microscopic examination.

   • If the patient has cold AIHI, then their RBCs will be coated with C3d, a complement component left behind by the complement activation cascade initiated by IgM cold agglutinins. The added anti-C3d antibodies will bind to the C3d coating the RBCs and agglutination will occur. Much more rarely, IgM cold agglutinins themselves may be detected directly with anti-IgM antibodies.

   • Agglutination with both anti-IgG and anti-C3d is usually due to warm AIHI but may also represent mixed warm and cold agglutinin disease, particularly if the cold agglutinin titers are very high (see later).

3. Measure titers: When agglutination occurs, serial dilutions are performed until agglutination can no longer be appreciated. Whereas even low warm agglutinin titers (eg, 1:32) suggest clinically significant disease, those with clinically significant cold agglutinin disease usually have cold agglutinin titers of at least 1:512. In the absence of compelling clinical evidence of AIHI, lower titers of isolated cold agglutinins may be an incidental finding.

Lack of agglutination with either anti-IgG or anti-C3d makes AIHI unlikely but not impossible. The sensitivity of most assays is around 90% to 95%, meaning that 5% to 10% of AIHI is "DAT-negative." More sensitive assays are available but usually unnecessary.

False positives are more common than false negatives and most often result from the recent administration of immunoglobulins, such as intravenous immunoglobulin (IVIG) or RhD immune globulin.

Importantly, the presence of warm or cold agglutinins does not always result in clinically significant disease, especially if the agglutinins are present in low titers. It is therefore particularly important not to send a DAT without a clear clinical indication (eg, confirmed or highly suspected hemolysis or known lupus); if you do so, you may not know what to do with your results.

Putting It Together: The Initial Lab Workup of Suspected Hemolytic Anemia

The labs that are usually ordered in a patient with suspected hemolytic anemia include:

• CBC

• Peripheral blood smear

- Reticulocyte count

- Liver function panel (to check total and indirect bilirubin)

- Lactate dehydrogenase

- Haptoglobin

- +/− DAT (aka direct Coombs)

Sometimes it makes sense to proceed directly to testing for specific causes of hemolytic anemia (eg, hemoglobinopathy such as sickle cell disease) when such a cause seems likely. See page 379 for more on hemoglobinopathies.

 ## Microangiopathic Hemolytic Anemia

Microangiopathic hemolytic anemia (MAHA) is a special type of hemolytic anemia in which the RBCs undergo mechanical shearing due to a problem within the blood vessels ("microangiopathy"). When microthrombi are the cause of a MAHA—resulting in platelet consumption and consequent thrombocytopenia—the patient is said to have a *thrombotic microangiopathy* (TMA). MAHA and TMA can be life-threatening and demand their own focused workup.

Common laboratory features of all MAHAs include:

- Anemia

- Positive hemolysis labs: Haptoglobin is very low (usually undetectable), whereas the LDH, indirect bilirubin, and corrected reticulocyte count are high.

- *Schistocytes* on peripheral blood smear (the hallmark of MAHA)

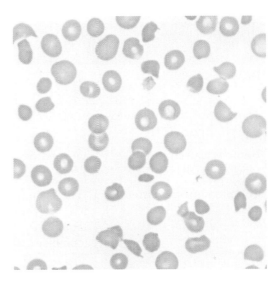

Figure 20.6 Schistocytes, the distorted helmet-like red blood cells seen here, are the laboratory hallmark of microangiopathic hemolytic anemia. You may also see so-called bite cells (just what they sound like, they look like someone or something took a bite out of the cells) and spherocytes. (From McClatchey KD. *Clinical Laboratory Medicine*. 2nd ed. Lippincott Williams & Wilkins; 2002.)

Disseminated Intravascular Coagulation

The prototypical example of MAHA is *DIC*, in which severe illness activates the coagulation system leading to the widespread formation of microthrombi and diffuse end-organ damage. The clotting is so profound that all hemostatic components—including the coagulation components and platelets—are soon used up. The clinical picture thus can be a mixed one, including thrombosis, bleeding, or both.

The lab is essential for confirming the diagnosis and establishing the severity of DIC. Lab results will be consistent with MAHA, along with some additional findings:

- Consumption of platelets and coagulation factors results in thrombocytopenia and a prolonged *prothrombin time (PT)* and *activated partial thromboplastin time (aPTT)*.

- *Fibrinogen*, which is converted to fibrin in the process of microthrombus formation, is usually low in DIC—often less than 100 mg/dL (normal range is 200-400 mg/dL). Because fibrinogen is also an acute-phase reactant, a normal result does not rule out DIC in the setting of active inflammation; a patient who is severely ill with a normal but falling fibrinogen may have DIC. It is reasonable to trend fibrinogen every few hours in such a patient.

- The *D-dimer* (see Chapter 15; normal value is <0.5 µg/mL), a fragment of dissolving clots, is high in patients with DIC. A normal D-dimer makes DIC unlikely.

Other Causes of Microangiopathic Hemolytic Anemia

There are several other causes of MAHA, most of which can usually be distinguished from one another based on the clinical picture. When the diagnosis is not clear, the lab can be helpful:

Table 20.2 Comparing Different Causes of Microangiopathic Hemolytic Anemia (MAHA)

MAHA	Distinguishing Laboratory Features	Other Clues
DIC	↑PT/PTT, ↓fibrinogen, ↑D-dimer	Bleeding and clotting Severe/critical illness
Thrombotic thrombocytopenic purpura (TTP)	↓ADAMTS13	Neurologic symptoms
Hemolytic uremic syndrome (HUS)	↑Cr, + stool Shiga toxin	Diarrhea (+/− bloody)
Complement-mediated TMA[a]	↑Cr, ↓complements (C3 and C4), +/− autoantibodies against complement factor H (CFH)	Underlying SLE or APS

(continued)

Table 20.2 Comparing Different Causes of Microangiopathic Hemolytic Anemia (MAHA) (*continued*)

MAHA	Distinguishing Laboratory Features	Other Clues
Malignant hypertension	↑Cr	↑↑Blood pressure
HELLP[b]	↑Transaminases (AST and ALT)	Patient is pregnant
Mechanical heart valve (causing RBC shearing)	Anemia and hemolysis are usually mild	New heart murmur

ALT, alanine aminotransferase; APS, antiphospholipid syndrome; AST, aspartate aminotransferase; DIC, disseminated intravascular coagulation; PT, prothrombin time; PTT, partial thromboplastin time; SLE, systemic lupus erythematosus; TMA, thrombotic microangiopathy.
[a]You may also hear this referred to as "atypical HUS." It can be caused by an inherited disorder of complement regulation or by an underlying autoimmune disorder.
[b]Hemolysis with elevated liver enzymes and low platelets.

The enzyme *ADAMTS13* normally regulates the interaction between von Willebrand factor (vWF; see page 391) and platelets. ADAMTS13 deficiency results in the unregulated formation of widespread platelet-vWF complexes (clots) and is thought to be central to the pathogenesis of TTP. This is a life-threatening disease that requires treatment with emergent plasmapheresis; it is prudent to send ADAMTS13 activity levels in any patient with MAHA of unclear etiology.

Liver Disease Can Mimic Microangiopathic Hemolytic Anemia

Severe liver disease is not a MAHA at all but can cause both bleeding and clotting along with thrombocytopenia, low fibrinogen, low haptoglobin, and a prolonged PT and aPTT (due to impaired hepatic synthesis of coagulation factors). All of these findings are also seen in DIC. How can the lab help us distinguish liver disease from DIC?

Schistocytes may point you in the direction of MAHA/DIC. Similarly, a clinical picture consistent with new or advanced liver disease may point toward the liver as the culprit. In cases of uncertainty, consider sending a *factor VIII activity level*. Because the liver does *not* produce factor VIII, we expect factor VIII activity to be normal in liver disease. On the other hand, factor VIII is consumed in DIC, where we expect levels to be low.

FLOW CYTOMETRY

This technique is a powerful tool for separating out different populations of cells by their distinguishing characteristics. It is most frequently performed on blood or bone marrow samples as part of the evaluation of hematologic malignancies (ie, lymphoma and leukemia) or immune disorders (eg, HIV, primary immunodeficiencies).

The principles involved are simple. Cells are directed one by one through a laser beam. The flow cytometer measures (1) the forward scatter of light, a measure of the *size of the cells*, and (2) the side scatter of light, a measure of the *granularity of the cells*, that is, the amount of stuff—proteins and organelles—in their cytoplasm. These measures alone are sufficient to distinguish many different populations of cells from one another. But that's not all.

The real strength of this technique comes from the use of fluorescent antibodies directed against molecules on the *surface* of cells and—following a procedure to make the cell membranes porous—against molecules in the *interior* of the cells. The laser light excites the fluorophores attached to these antibodies, and these in turn emit light that is picked up by various detectors. Many different fluorophores can be used, each of which emits light of a different color. The cytometer analyzes the various patterns of light that are emitted, allowing for the precise identification of the different cell types in the sample. This, for example, is how we can distinguish CD3, CD4, and CD8 T cells from each other or detect the immunophenotypic markers (ie, surface and interior antigens) that identify a particular hematologic malignancy.

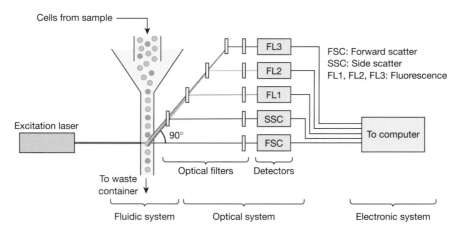

Figure 20.7 Flow cytometry. The cells are fed in a line past the excitation laser. Forward scatter, side scatter, and fluorescence are measured by detectors, and the information is fed to a computer that converts all the data into a series of graphs that yield the identities of the different types of cells in the sample.

SERUM PROTEIN ELECTROPHORESIS, URINE PROTEIN ELECTROPHORESIS, SERUM FREE LIGHT CHAINS, AND IMMUNOELECTROPHORESIS

Each of these tests is used primarily in the diagnosis of multiple myeloma as well as the related disorders Waldenstrom macroglobulinemia, monoclonal gammopathy of undetermined significance (MGUS), and less common disorders such as primary amyloidosis, light chain disease, heavy chain disease, and POEMS syndrome (polyneuropathy, organomegaly, endocrinopathy, monoclonal protein, and skin changes). What these disorders all have in common is excessive production of a single monoclonal immunoglobulin* or fragment of an immunoglobulin; they are therefore referred to as *monoclonal gammopathies*. All are characterized by the appearance of a narrow spike in the γ-globulin range on *serum protein electrophoresis (SPEP)* or *urine electrophoresis (UPEP)*.

There are four essential tests we will discuss:

- *SPEP*: Identify a monoclonal protein in the serum.

- *UPEP*: Identify a monoclonal protein in the urine.

- *Immunoelectrophoresis*: Identify the *type* of monoclonal protein (eg, antibody class, light chain, heavy chain) in the serum or urine.

- *Serum free light chains*: Detect monoclonal light chains in the serum that may be missed by the studies above.

The most common reasons to order these tests are to evaluate:

- An elevated *protein gap* (total protein minus the albumin; normal is ≤4 g/dL) on a comprehensive metabolic panel (CMP). The "gap" may be made up of regular old proteins like polyclonal antibodies and acute-phase reactants or, of interest here, a population of monoclonal antibodies.

- Other clinical signs of a monoclonal gammopathy (eg, unexplained bone pain, hypercalcemia, anemia, peripheral neuropathy)

 ## *Serum Protein Electrophoresis*

A blood sample is introduced into an agarose gel that is subjected to an electrical gradient. Driven through the gel matrix by the electrical field, the proteins in the sample are separated

---

*Some other diseases, notably chronic lymphocytic leukemia and lymphoma, can also produce a monoclonal immunoglobulin spike.

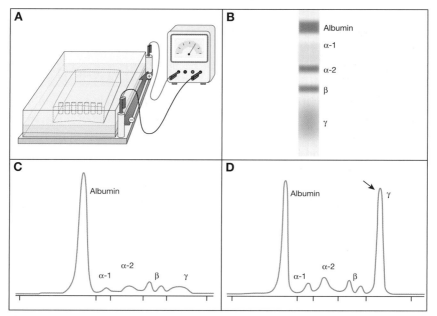

Figure 20.8 A. A typical setup for a serum protein electrophoresis (SPEP). (Courtesy of Soleil Nordic/Shutterstock.) B. After some time, the proteins separate out by charge and size. C. The results can then be graphed, revealing five basic categories of protein. Here is a normal SPEP. D. An SPEP of a patient with multiple myeloma showing a tall, abnormal spike in the γ-globulin range ("M spike").

out by size and electrical charge. Small proteins and more negatively charged proteins move more quickly.

Take a look at Figure 20.8C. A normal SPEP is dominated by the tall peak of albumin. The α and β peaks are rarely of clinical interest, reflecting the concentrations of many other circulating proteins that are best detected individually by other tests we discuss in this book. The γ region consists of circulating antibodies, and this is where the action is. A broad peak in the γ region reflects a *polyclonal gammopathy*, a nonspecific finding indicative of a generalized inflammatory reaction to infection, an autoimmune disorder, neoplasia, or sometimes liver disease. A sharp spike (aka M protein) in the γ region is the hallmark of a *monoclonal gammopathy*, and is never normal.

The amount of protein making up the M spike can be quantitated by gel *densitometry*—the lab will automatically do this for you—and is an important factor in differentiating malignancies such as multiple myeloma and Waldenstrom macroglobulinemia from MGUS, a benign condition that has the potential to progress to a more serious disorder, such as multiple myeloma. The M protein in MGUS, by definition, should be no greater than 3 g/dL. In patients with multiple myeloma, the size of the M protein can be used to follow disease progression and response to therapy.

Urine Protein Electrophoresis

A UPEP is run on a sample taken from a 24-hour urine collection and uses the same methodology as the SPEP.

In as many as 20% of patients with multiple myeloma, the M protein consists only of light chains.* These small molecules, called *Bence-Jones proteins*, are readily filtered by the kidneys and may not accumulate in the serum, but will appear in the urine. The UPEP may then be the only way to establish the diagnosis.

In addition to looking for Bence-Jones proteins, another reason for ordering this test is to assess the amount of immunoglobulin light chains in the urine of a patient with an established or highly suspected monoclonal gammopathy. These proteins can be toxic to the kidneys, and the risk of developing light chain nephropathy is correlated with the concentration of light chains in the urine.

 ## Immunoelectrophoresis (aka Immunofixation)

This test exposes the electrophoretic gel to labeled antibodies. Immunofixation can be performed following either SPEP or UPEP. This technique is used to identify the class of immunoglobulin that comprises the M protein: IgA, IgD, IgE, IgG, IgM, kappa light chain, lambda light chain, heavy chain, or antibody fragments. The identity of the M protein is important because the clinical manifestations, complications, and treatment may differ. For example, the manifestations and management of Waldenstrom macroglobulinemia, in which the M protein is an IgM molecule, are different from those of multiple myeloma.

 ## Serum Free Light Chains

This test can detect monoclonal light chains missed by an SPEP. It may even be more sensitive for the detection of light chains than a UPEP with immunofixation. Therefore, the serum free light chain assay is often used as part of the initial screening for a monoclonal gammopathy. This test will also tell you the relative amounts of the two types of light chains, kappa and lambda. A kappa-to-lambda ratio significantly outside the normal range of 0.26 to 1.65 suggests the selective production of one type of light chain, and can therefore clue you in to the presence of a monoclonal gammopathy.

Diagnosing Multiple Myeloma

A monoclonal spike on an SPEP or UPEP is just one piece of the diagnosis of multiple myeloma. The following three criteria are required, and the lab plays a key role in all of them:

- A monoclonal protein in the serum or urine

- Monoclonal plasma cells (≥10%) in the bone marrow or a biopsy-proven plasmacytoma

- Associated organ dysfunction: A serum calcium more than 10.5 mg/L, serum creatinine more than 2 mg/dL, hemoglobin less than 10.0 g/dL (or 2 g below normal), lytic bone lesions, or osteoporosis

Monoclonal Gammopathy of Undetermined Significance

MGUS is present in more than 3% of the population. Unlike the more serious plasma cell disorders—multiple myeloma and Waldenstrom macroglobulinemia—patients have no symptoms and fewer clonal plasma cells in the bone marrow (<10%). The monoclonal immunoglobulin can be IgM, less often IgG or IgA, rarely IgD or IgE, or just a kappa or lambda light chain. The risk of progression to frank malignancy is highest with IgM and IgA isotypes. The risk is also increased in patients when the levels of the other noninvolved immunoglobulin classes are suppressed. Once the diagnosis is made, patients should have repeat testing in 6 months to look for progression. If the M protein is stable, they should be tested again every few years.

INTRINSIC RED BLOOD CELL DISORDERS

These disorders can be divided into three categories. We'll discuss common examples of each:

- Disorders of hemoglobin (hemoglobinopathies)
  - Thalassemias (α and β)
  - Sickle cell disease (hemoglobin S)
  - Hemoglobin C and SC
- Disorders of the RBC membrane
  - Hereditary spherocytosis
- Enzymatic disorders
  - Glucose-6-phosphate dehydrogenase (G6PD) deficiency
  - Pyruvate kinase deficiency (PKD)

Diagnosis relies on examination of the peripheral blood smear and a few tests you should become familiar with.

 ## *Hemoglobinopathies*

One of your most powerful tools for diagnosing a hemoglobinopathy is *hemoglobin electrophoresis*. Like SPEP and UPEP (see page 375), hemoglobin electrophoresis allows you to identify types of protein—in this case, types of hemoglobin. The normal distribution of hemoglobins in adults is: Hb A, 96.5% to 98.5%; Hb A_2, 1.5% to 3.5%; and Hb F, less than 1%.

- Hemoglobin A consists of two α chains and two β chains and is normally by far the dominant hemoglobin.

- Hemoglobin A_2 is a normal variant of hemoglobin A and consists of two α chains and—instead of two β chains—two γ chains.

- Hemoglobin F is the dominant hemoglobin in the fetus—a tiny percentage of which can normally persist into adulthood; the most important difference from Hb A is a single-nucleotide substitution in the β chain that increases the affinity of the molecule for oxygen.

As we'll discuss, a hemoglobinopathy may throw off the proportions of each type of hemoglobin. Sometimes, entirely different types of hemoglobin may be seen.

An alternative to hemoglobin electrophoresis is *high-performance liquid chromatography (HPLC)*. Like electrophoresis, HPLC is a process for separating out various components of the blood. The sample is driven through a column containing solid absorbent material. The different components interact uniquely with the solid material, altering their various flow rates and allowing for separation.

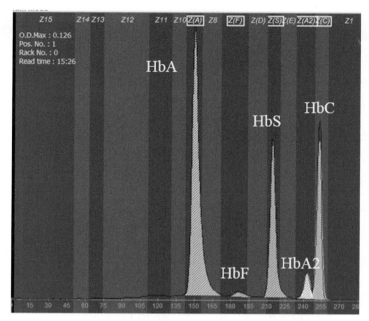

Figure 20.9 Hemoglobin electrophoresis. In addition to normal amounts of hemoglobin A, A₂, and F, this patient has hemoglobin S and hemoglobin C, which we will discuss. The *x* axis represents time, and the *y* axis represents the amount of hemoglobin present in the sample. A graph of high-performance liquid chromatography (HPLC) looks very much the same. (From Weksler B. *Wintrobe's Atlas of Clinical Hematology*. 2nd ed. Lippincott Williams & Wilkins; 2017.)

The Thalassemias

As we briefly discussed in Chapter 4 when we looked at the CBC, the thalassemias are inherited disorders in which the production of globin chains is defective, leading to a mismatch between the number of α and β chains. In adults, the diagnosis of thalassemia usually first enters into the differential diagnosis when you encounter a patient with a microcytic, hypochromic anemia. Iron deficiency must be ruled out; but if the iron studies are normal and the RBC count is high, then thalassemia is a leading possibility. The anemia is almost always mild, but the mean corpuscular volume (MCV) can be quite small, almost always less than 75 fL.

There Are Many Thalassemia Syndromes

Patients with a mutation in the *β-globin* gene (and there are hundreds of these mutations) have decreased β-globin production and are said to have β-thalassemia. Those with a mutation in the *α-globin* gene have decreased α-globin production and are said to have α-thalassemia. β-Thalassemia is by far the more common of the two.

The severity of thalassemia—alpha or beta—depends on the particular genetic mutation that causes an imbalance in the production of normal alpha and beta chains. Unpaired chains can precipitate, compromising erythropoeisis and hemoglobin production. A useful classification scheme for the thalassemias divides them into non-transfusion-dependent (mild) and transfusion-dependent (more severe) thalassemia.

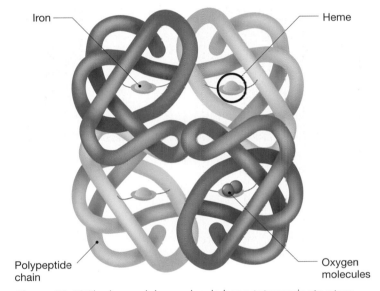

Iron   Heme

Polypeptide chain   Oxygen molecules

Figure 20.10 The hemoglobin molecule has a tetrameric structure consisting of two α and two β chains each of which contains a heme moiety. (Courtesy Designua/Shutterstock.)

The peripheral blood smear is likely to show microcytosis and may show *nucleated RBCs* and *target cells*. Target cells look just like what they sound like (see Figure 20.11). They are the result of an increased ratio of cellular membrane to volume, which in thalassemia is due to their decreased hemoglobin content.

Target Cells

Thalassemia is not the only cause of target cells. They can, for example, be present in obstructive liver disease, hemoglobin C disease, asplenia (functional, as can be seen in sickle cell disease; or surgical), and iron deficiency anemia.

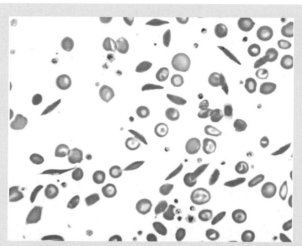

Figure 20.11 Target cells in a patient with sickle cell disease. (From Weksler B. *Wintrobe's Atlas of Clinical Hematology*. 2nd ed. Lippincott Williams & Wilkins; 2017.)

Once you suspect thalassemia, you should order a hemoglobin analysis performed either by electrophoresis or HPLC.

In β-thalassemia, both Hb A_2 and Hb F are increased. In α-thalassemia, the hemoglobin analysis will typically be normal; you will need to order genetic testing for diagnosis. Although still uncommonly used as the initial screen, genetic testing is becoming more common whenever either β- or α-thalassemia is suspected. DNA analysis can be performed on whole blood or prenatally on amniotic fluid or chorionic villus samples.

Hemoglobin S (Sickle Cell Disease)

Sickle cell disease is an inherited disorder caused by a single amino acid substitution—valine for glutamine—in the sixth position of the β-*globin* gene.

The hemoglobin molecule that results from this mutation, hemoglobin S, tends to form crystalline aggregates that distort the RBC when deoxygenated. As you can see from Figure 20.9, hemoglobin S can be detected by *hemoglobin electrophoresis* (or HPLC). However, the diagnosis is usually apparent from the clinical picture plus a *peripheral blood smear* that shows the sickle cells. Sickle cells are not seen in patients who are heterozygous for the disease (sickle cell trait). Genetic testing is used for prenatal diagnosis. Other tests you may have heard of, such as solubility testing, are rarely used anymore.

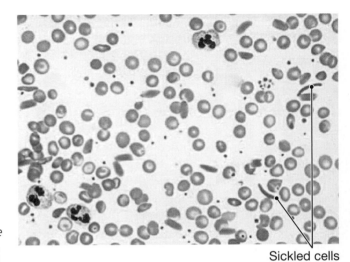

Sickled cells

Figure 20.12 Sickle cells in a patient with sickle cell anemia. (From McConnell TH. *The Nature of Disease Pathology for the Health Professions.* Lippincott Williams & Wilkins; 2007.)

Hemoglobin C and SC

Hemoglobin C is the result of another amino acid substitution at the same sixth position of the *β-globin* gene, although this time glutamic acid is replaced by lysine. Patients who are homozygous may have a mild or chronic anemia. Those who are heterozygous are generally asymptomatic. Hemoglobin C can also occur in conjunction with other hemoglobinopathies. Patients with SC disease, for example, have one S allele and one C allele, and tend to follow a much milder course than those with homozygous sickle cell (SS) disease.

Figure 20.13 Hemoglobin C crystals can sometimes be seen on the peripheral blood smear of patients with hemoglobin C disease. The typical crystal is rod-shaped (resembling, some say, the Washington Monument) and can distort the shape of the red blood cell. (Pereira I, George TI, Arber DA. *Atlas of Peripheral Blood.* Wolters Kluwer Health; 2011.)

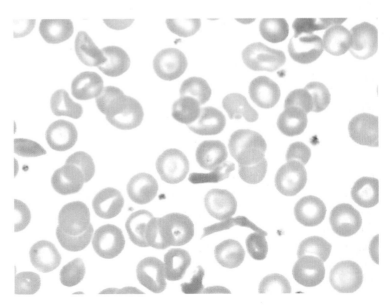

There are many other mutations in the globin chains that slightly alter the hemoglobin molecule (hemoglobin D, E, and so on, up the alphabet). These are generally benign unless present along with the sickle cell mutation.

 ## Disorders of the Red Blood Cell Membrane

Hereditary spherocytosis is caused by mutations in α- or β-spectrin, an RBC membrane protein. The result is that the RBCs appear spherical; the decreased surface-to-volume ratio causes an increased *mean corpuscular hemoglobin concentration*. Other laboratory findings may include anemia, reticulocytosis, and increased *osmotic fragility*. The last is rarely tested anymore, and today the definitive test is *flow cytometry*, which can directly identify cells with the abnormal membrane protein.

There are other disorders of the red cell membrane, both inherited (eg, elliptocytosis) and acquired (eg, jagged red cells called acanthocytes can be seen with liver disease, due to cholesterol deposition on the red cells). Again, the peripheral blood smear is the first step in diagnosis.

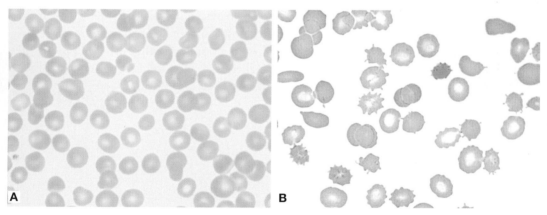

Figure 20.14 (A) Hereditary spherocytosis. Note the scattered small spherocytes that lack central pallor. (This image was originally published in The American Society of Hematology Image Bank. Scordino T. Spherocytes-hereditary spherocytosis. ASH Image Bank. 2016; 00060308. © The American Society of Hematology.) (B) Acanthocytes in a patient with liver disease. (Courtesy of Irma Pereira MT [ASCP] SH.)

 ## Enzyme Disorders

Glucose-6-Phosphate Dehydrogenase Deficiency

G6PD protects RBCs from oxidative damage by maintaining levels of nicotinamide adenine dinucleotide phosphate hydrogen (NADPH), a reducing agent. In patients with G6PD deficiency, sudden and rapid hemolysis can occur under oxidative stress. The most common precipitants are drugs (most often sulfonamides and antimalarials), high fevers, and the ingestion of fava beans. The predominant abnormal finding on a peripheral blood smear is the presence of denatured aggregates of hemoglobin called *Heinz bodies*. You may also see *bite cells*, which are produced by partial destruction of the RBCs in the spleen.

There are two major types of abnormal G6PD enzymes:

- The A form, seen mostly in African American males; this form is the milder of the two.

- The Mediterranean form, seen mostly in people from the Mediterranean and Middle Eastern regions; these patients have almost no detectable G6PD.

Suspect G6PD deficiency in patients with nonimmune-mediated hemolysis induced by oxidative stress. The diagnosis can then be established either by *genetic testing* or by measuring the ability of the patient's cells to reduce NADP to NADPH, that is, measuring G6PD activity. An RBC hemolysate created from the patient's blood is added to a sample containing NADP and glucose 6-phosphate, and spectroscopy is used to see how much NADPH is generated.* Point-of-care rapid detection tests are available for use in the field before starting certain medications (eg, the antimalarial primaquine) in regions where G6PD deficiency is particularly common.

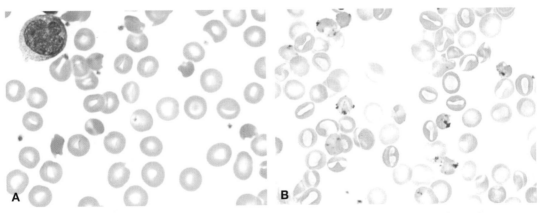

Figure 20.15 Blood smears from a patient with glucose-6-phosphate dehydrogenase (G6PD) deficiency. A. Bite cells. B. Heinz bodies (the purple splotches). (From Pereira I, George TI, Arber DA. *Atlas of Peripheral Blood: The Primary Diagnostic Tool.* Wolters Kluwer Health/Lippincott Williams & Wilkins; 2012.)

---

*NADP and NADPH absorb light at different wavelengths.

Pyruvate Kinase Deficiency

Pyruvate kinase (PK) is an intracellular enzyme that plays a key role in energy generation. In PKD, an autosomal recessive mutation of PK leads to diminished activity of the enzyme inside RBCs and can cause a hemolytic anemia. Testing is recommended for patients with unexplained hemolytic anemia in whom autoimmune hemolysis has been ruled out, especially if they are first degree relatives of patients with known PKD.

The first step in testing is to assess the *activity of PK* in the patient's RBCs. Before the standard test is run, the white blood cells and platelets are filtered out, because they contain different PK enzyme isoforms unaffected by the genetic mutation. A more rapid test assays PK activity in a hemolysate of RBCs without filtering out the white blood cells and platelets; this test is less sensitive but still very specific for the diagnosis when positive. The diagnosis can be confirmed with genetic testing.

TESTS OF HEMOSTASIS AND ABNORMAL BLEEDING

Bleeding from trauma is normal. *Excessive* bleeding from trauma—a subjective criterion but you know it when you see it—is not. And spontaneous bleeding, without any obvious cause, is always cause for concern.

There are two major reasons why someone might bleed spontaneously or excessively*:

- *A platelet problem* (primary hemostasis): This can occur as a result of:

  - Too few circulating platelets due to low production, sequestration, or destruction

  - Platelets that don't function properly, either due to an intrinsic problem or extrinsic factor (eg, antibody)

- *A coagulation factor problem* (secondary hemostasis): This can occur as a result of:

  - Inadequate circulating levels of one or more coagulation factors

  - One or more coagulation factors that don't function properly, either due to an intrinsic problem or extrinsic factor (eg, antibody)

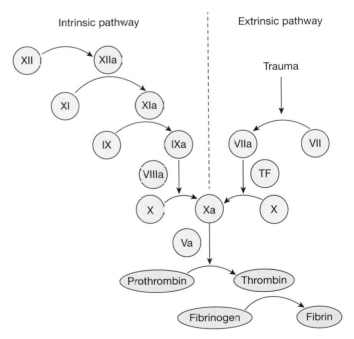

Figure 20.16 The coagulation cascade consists of intrinsic, extrinsic, and common pathways. The intrinsic pathway is activated by exposure of plasma to endothelial collagen and is called "intrinsic" because all the components are contained within the circulation. The extrinsic pathway is activated by tissue factors released by damaged cells surrounding the blood vessels (hence, extrinsic). The two pathways both generate factor Xa, which when acted upon by factor Va generates thrombin that in turn converts circulating fibrinogen to fibrin to form a stable clot.

---

*There is a third and that is a problem with the integrity and functioning of the vascular system itself. But this is not amenable to laboratory analysis, and while undeniably important in certain situations (eg, DIC), not a topic for a book about lab testing.

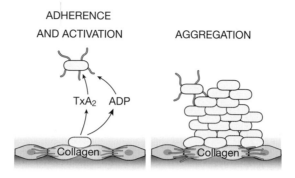

ADHERENCE
AND ACTIVATION   AGGREGATION

⬭ Platelet

Figure 20.17 The steps by which platelets act
to staunch bleeding: adherence, activation, and
aggregation. TxA2, thromboxane A2; ADP, adenosine
diphosphate

 ## Who Needs to Be Evaluated, and How?

Otherwise unexplained bleeding—particularly if unprovoked, excessive, or recurrent—is the
most common reason you might want to evaluate a patient for a coagulopathy. Remember
that this workup is unlikely to immediately change anything in the acute setting; someone
who is bleeding acutely and profusely requires aggressive intervention before you even start to
think about what lab tests to order.

When an abnormality of hemostasis is a possibility, you will of course first want to assess
the patient's hemoglobin. Checking for the severity of anemia will help you determine how
urgently you need to expedite your evaluation. The next step is to check for an abnormality
of the platelets and/or the coagulation cascade.

A Note of Caution: Checking the Hemoglobin in Acute Blood Loss

It is important to note that the hemoglobin can be normal with *acute* blood loss. This occurs
because both RBCs and plasma are lost in the bleed. It is only as the extracellular volume is re-
stored (by the body itself or with intravenous [IV] fluids) that the RBC population becomes diluted. The bone marrow can't churn out enough RBCs to keep up and the hemoglobin drops.

As a general rule, platelet disorders cause mucocutaneous bleeding or petechiae, whereas
coagulation disorders present with deep tissue hematomas such as muscle or joint bleeding.
Either can cause easy bruising. Von Willebrand disease (vWD), which we will discuss later,
can present with any of the above. Although these clues from the physical exam can help
guide your thinking, in almost all cases, whatever the presentation, you will probably need
the lab to figure out what is wrong.

Assessing the Platelets

The Platelet Count

Thrombocytopenia is the primary platelet-related cause of abnormal bleeding. As we discussed in Chapter 4, bleeding with minor trauma can occur when counts dip below 20,000/μL, and dangerous, spontaneous bleeding (eg, into the central nervous system [CNS] or gastrointestinal [GI] tract) can occur with counts below 10,000/μL. Counts as low as 50,000/μL are considered safe, even for many surgeries. However, once they dip below 50,000/μL, whenever possible they should be corrected before any major surgical procedure. The most common causes of thrombocytopenia are discussed in Chapter 4.

Platelet Function Testing

Platelets can be the cause of abnormal bleeding even without thrombocytopenia. Platelet dysfunction has a number of causes. The most common is *drug-induced;* common culprits include aspirin and the P2Y$_{12}$ receptor antagonists, such as ticagrelor and clopidogrel, which are used in the setting of acute coronary syndrome for the prevention of stent thrombosis. Platelet dysfunction is a major contributor to bleeding in patients with *uremia*.

Can we measure platelet dysfunction? Yes, but you will want to consult with your lab or a trusted hematologist to help guide you. The tests are many, varied, and not always as reliable as we would like. Of these, the *platelet function analyzer* has risen to the top of the heap. It utilizes a relatively simple process that measures the time it takes platelets, forced to move at high shear rates, to close off a tiny aperture within a membrane coated with collagen, epinephrine, or adenosine diphosphate (ADP), all of which are platelet agonists. Prolonged closure time indicates platelet dysfunction. Results are available in minutes. While not specific for any particular disorder, the test has good negative predictive value. A normal result pretty much rules out any underlying platelet dysfunction.

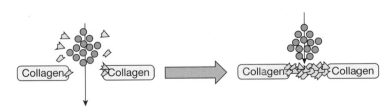

○ Unactivated platelet
△ Activated platelet

Figure 20.18 The platelet function analyzer at work.

Assessing the Coagulation Cascade

Two tests are all you need for an initial evaluation of the coagulation cascade. The *PT* and *aPTT* measure how long it takes to form a clot by converting prothrombin into thrombin.

Blood for testing the PT and aPTT must be collected in a tube containing an inhibitor of coagulation, usually sodium citrate. Without this, the blood would coagulate in the tube, making any measurements impossible. The tube must be adequately filled with blood so it is not overly diluted with the sodium citrate and must be thoroughly mixed by inverting the tube several times.

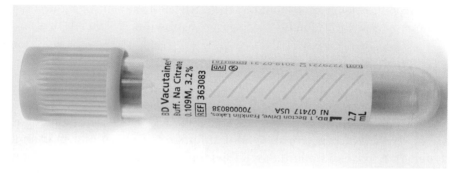

Figure 20.19 A typical tube for collecting blood to measure the prothrombin time international normalized ratio (PT INR) and activated partial thromboplastin time (aPTT). Note the light blue top.

Prothrombin Time and Prothrombin Time International Normalized Ratio

A commonly cited normal range for the PT is 11 to 13 seconds. However, you will usually hear health care providers talk about a patient's "PT INR" (prothrombin time international normalized ratio), or "INR" instead. The reason for using the PT INR is simple: the unadorned PT varies too much from lab to lab, so the PT INR was created to correct this problem by generating a number that is not dependent on the reagent and testing protocol of any one lab. The PT INR is a ratio and thus has no dimensions. A PT INR of 1 is normal, with a little wiggle room (~0.8 to 1.1).

The PT INR measures the activity of the extrinsic and common coagulation pathways. The synthesis of factor VII, the key protein in the extrinsic pathway, is dependent on vitamin K, so one of the main uses of the PT INR is to monitor the effects of warfarin, a vitamin K inhibitor (eg, a patient on warfarin for a DVT might have an "INR goal" of 2-3). An elevated PT INR can also be seen in patients with an endogenous vitamin K deficiency as can be seen in disorders of malabsorption and in severe liver disease.

How the Lab Runs the Test: The patient's blood is drawn into a tube containing sodium citrate that prevents clotting. The plasma is then separated out and added to a sample containing some tissue factor that can activate the extrinsic and common pathways. Calcium is then added to the sample, inactivating the sodium citrate, and the time to clot is measured. Clotting should take only a few seconds.

Activated Partial Thromboplastin Time

This is the other side of the coagulation coin. The aPTT measures the activity of the intrinsic and common pathways—in other words, all the coagulation factors except factor VII. Unlike the PT INR, this test comes with a value measured in seconds; 25 to 35 seconds is the usual normal range.

The intrinsic pathway contains multiple coagulation factors, and a deficiency of any of them can raise the aPTT. Heparin, which inhibits the intrinsic pathway, will raise the aPTT, and the aPTT is therefore used to monitor heparin therapy. Factor IX of the intrinsic pathway as well as factors II (prothrombin) and X of the common pathway are, like factor VII of the extrinsic pathway, vitamin K-dependent, but neither vitamin K deficiency nor warfarin therapy affects the aPTT nearly as much as they impact the PT INR. You typically correct a high PT INR with vitamin K; you correct an elevated aPTT with fresh frozen plasma.

Patients with an unexplained *isolated* elevation of the aPTT should be tested for:

- Hemophilia: *Hemophilia A* is due to a deficiency of factor VIII and *hemophilia B* to a deficiency of factor IX. Hemophilia A is the more common of the two. They are both due to x-linked recessive mutations, although as many as one-third of cases are the result of de novo mutations. Rarely, hemophilia results from autoantibodies that block the activity of factor VIII. Diagnosis of hemophilia A or B can be confirmed by demonstrating a *factor VIII* or *IX activity level*, respectively, below 40%, or by genetic testing.

- *von Willebrand disease* (discussed next)

How the Lab Runs the Test: As you might suspect, the test is run just like the PT, except a different activating substance is used—that is, one that activates the intrinsic and common pathways.

Von Willebrand Factor and Von Willebrand Disease

vWD affects about 1% of the population and is inherited in an autosomal dominant fashion. It can cause almost any type of bleeding. Typical presentations include epistaxis, menorrhagia, and bleeding from seemingly trivial wounds or dental work.

vWD can be due to either deficiency or dysfunction of vWF, the main function of which is to promote platelet adhesion to and aggregation on the vascular endothelium. vWF is also a major carrier of factor VIII. If there isn't a good amount of healthy vWF around, the half-life of factor VIII is greatly shortened and it will drop to low levels.

Expected laboratory findings in vWD include:

- Normal platelet count

- Normal PT INR

- Normal or slightly increased aPTT

Suspect vWD whenever there is unexplained excessive bleeding and initial coagulation studies are normal or show only a mildly elevated aPTT.

The evaluation should include measurement of *vWF antigen, vWF activity,* and *factor VIII activity.* With decreased amounts of vWF (type I disease), both the concentration and activity of vWF are decreased. With dysfunctional vWF (type 2 disease), only vWF activity is diminished. There is also type 3 disease, in which the concentration of vWF is severely reduced or even absent; this can lead to severe bleeding and fortunately is quite rare.

These tests are not perfectly reliable markers, however. The results can vary with stress, ongoing bleeding, inflammation, or hormonal cycling. If you suspect vWD and this panel is normal, repeat it.

 ## When All the Tests Are Abnormal

DIC is a profound, catastrophic complication of severe illness that involves activation of the entire hemostatic apparatus and notoriously leads to both bleeding and clotting. As a result of the widespread inflammation, the coagulation factors and platelets are all consumed, so the PT INR and aPTT are both prolonged, and the platelet count is low. Evaluation of the blood smear and additional lab tests—see page 372—will confirm the diagnosis.

HYPERCOAGULABLE DISORDERS

A patient with a hypercoagulable disorder (also called thrombophilia or hypercoagulability) has an excessive tendency to form blood clots (thromboses). A hypercoagulable disorder can be inherited or acquired.

Hypercoagulability can result from several different mechanisms:

- Deficiency of an anticoagulant
  - Protein C deficiency
  - Protein S deficiency
  - Antithrombin III deficiency
- Overactivity of a procoagulant
  - Prothrombin G20210A
- The presence of an inhibitor of one (or more) of the anticoagulant or fibrinolytic factors*
  - Antiphospholipid syndrome (APS)

Most patients with a blood clot (even a potentially serious one such as a deep venous thrombosis or pulmonary embolism) do *not* have a hypercoagulable disorder, but instead have some other risk factor for clotting such as immobility, medications (eg, estrogen), smoking, liver disease, or cancer. *Hypercoagulability testing should be reserved for patients with one or more thromboses in the absence of any clear risk factors or precipitating events.* Testing, therefore, might be warranted in a young otherwise healthy patient with an acute pulmonary embolism who is not on any medications. A family history of a hypercoagulable disorder or a strong family history of clotting may also prompt testing.

Testing is unlikely to change management in the acute setting and is almost never urgent. A patient with an acute pulmonary embolism, for example, should—in the absence of contraindications—be started on anticoagulation regardless of the presence of absence of an underlying hypercoagulable disorder. The results of hypercoagulability testing may play a role in subsequent management.

It is often appropriate to test for multiple hypercoagulable disorders at once. As is always the case with laboratory panels, if your institution or laboratory has a hypercoagulability panel, be sure to check what tests are included before ordering it—do not assume that the panel includes all of the tests that may be relevant to your patient.

Can patients who are already on an anticoagulant be tested for a hypercoagulable disorder? The answer depends on the clinical circumstances, the specific disorder, and—sometimes— the specific anticoagulant. We'll address this issue as we discuss each disorder.

---

*The mechanisms of hypercoagulability in APS also involve antibody-mediated proinflammatory effects.

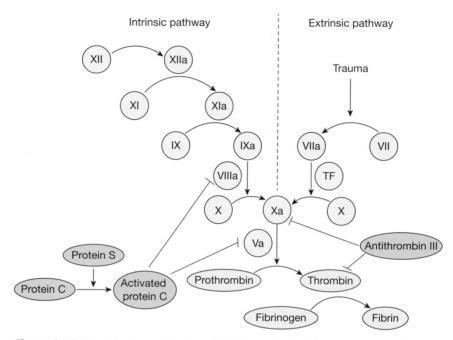

Figure 20.20 Protein C, protein S, and antithrombin III inhibit various steps in the coagulation cascade—they function as anticoagulants. A deficiency in (or resistance to) any one of them results in hypercoagulability. (From Abali EE, Cline SD, Franklin DS, Viselli SM. *Lippincott Illustrated Reviews: Biochemistry*. Wolters Kluwer Health; 2021.)

 ## Factor V Leiden

Factor V Leiden (FVL) is the most common inherited thrombophilia. An autosomal dominant mutation in factor V of the coagulation cascade renders its activated form (factor Va) resistant to inhibition by protein C, which normally acts as a natural anticoagulant by degrading factor Va. The result is a tendency to form clots.* Both genetic testing and a functional assay are available.

Factor V Leiden Genetic Testing

Most modern FVL genetic tests are performed by polymerase chain reaction (PCR), allowing for direct detection of the abnormal FVL variant. Sensitivity and specificity are excellent, with the added advantage that this test remains accurate even in patients taking an anticoagulant.

---

*In the absence of a personal history of thrombosis, anticoagulation is not indicated for individuals who are heterozygous and is controversial for patients who are homozygous.

Factor V Leiden Functional Assay (Activated Protein C Resistance)

Activated protein C is added to a sample of the patient's plasma. An aPTT is measured before and after adding the activated protein C; the smaller the increase in aPTT after adding the activated protein C, the higher the likelihood that the patient is resistant to protein C and has FVL. The result is typically reported as a ratio (aPTT without protein C to aPTT with protein C, or vice versa) and the normal range varies by laboratory. A positive result should be confirmed with FVL genetic testing.

This functional assay has two main advantages over genetic testing: it is inexpensive and it can pick up rare causes of protein C resistance besides FVL. However, unlike genetic testing, protein C resistance testing is susceptible to error due to the concomitant use of anticoagulants (false negatives) or the presence of a lupus anticoagulant (LA; false positives).

 ## *Protein C Deficiency*

Because protein C acts as an anticoagulant by inhibiting factor Va and VIIIa, a deficiency in protein C is associated with hypercoagulability. Like FVL, protein C deficiency is most often inherited in an autosomal dominant pattern and the majority of affected individuals are heterozygotes. Unlike FVL, protein C deficiency is quite rare.

Because protein C deficiency may be caused either by low levels of circulating protein C or by dysfunctional protein C, just measuring the concentration of protein C is not a sufficient diagnostic test. Most modern assays are functional tests—they are designed to detect low protein C activity regardless of whether the cause is protein C deficiency or dysfunction.

The methodology of the various available tests generally takes one of two forms:

1. Measure the degree of prolongation of clotting time (eg, PT, aPTT) in the presence of a protein C sample taken from the patient ("clot-based" assay).

2. Add a synthetic peptide to the patient's blood sample and measure the amount of protein C-mediated peptide cleavage. The term for this type of assay is *amidolytic,* which simply refers to any process involving cleavage of a peptide bond.

Genetic testing for protein C deficiency is used in research settings but is not available in routine clinical practice.

Results of any protein C activity assay may be reported as a concentration (eg, functional protein C level of 5 μg/mL; normal range varies significantly by assay) or as a percentage (eg, 80% expected protein C concentration; most affected individuals have <65%).

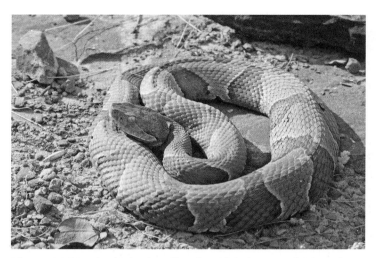

Figure 20.21 In both clot-based and amidolytic assays for protein C deficiency, the venom of *Agkistrodon contortrix* (the copperhead snake) is typically used to activate protein C before measuring its activity. (Courtesy Creeping Things/Shutterstock.)

Be wary of the following potential pitfalls:

- The use of anticoagulants (eg, heparin, direct thrombin inhibitors, factor Xa inhibitors) interferes with clot-based assays because these agents prolong the baseline PT and/or aPTT. This is one reason why many laboratories preferentially perform amidolytic assays.

- Protein C is activated by vitamin K in the liver. Therefore, patients on warfarin (a vitamin K antagonist) or with liver disease may have reduced protein C activity in the absence of any inherited deficiency. Under these circumstances, the results of both clot-based and amidolytic assays are affected.

- Levels of protein C are transiently elevated in the setting of acute thrombosis or, to a lesser extent, significant inflammation. It is therefore wise to delay protein C testing until at least 1 to 2 weeks after an acute thrombotic event and to avoid testing if possible during a severe or acute illness.

- Protein C activity gradually increases from birth through adolescence before reaching adult levels. Make sure your laboratory takes age into account when considering the lower limit of normal among pediatric patients.

Protein S Deficiency

Protein S is a cofactor ("helper molecule") for protein C and therefore functions primarily as an anticoagulant. The "S" stands for Seattle, the city in which protein S was discovered.* Like protein C** deficiency, protein S deficiency results in hypercoagulability, usually venous thromboembolism (VTE). It is rare and is inherited in an autosomal dominant pattern.

Testing is challenging for several reasons. First, protein S levels vary widely among the general population, even among those without any increased risk for thrombosis. Second, protein S exists in two forms in the bloodstream: free (the active form) and bound to a complement component called C4b-binding protein.

The most straightforward—and probably most accurate—approach to testing is to measure a *free protein S concentration*. Several assays are available, most of which are ELISAs using monoclonal antibodies to free protein S. Although protein S functional assays are available, most experts do not recommend their use because false positives are common in patients with protein C resistance (eg, FVL). Genetic testing is not available outside the research setting.

The lower limit of normal for free protein S varies by assay and by individual. In general, provided testing is done under the appropriate clinical circumstances (eg, recurrent thromboses, strong family history of clotting), it is reasonable to consider a free protein S less than 60 IU/dL to be strongly suggestive of protein S deficiency. The lower the clinical suspicion for protein S deficiency, the lower the cutoff should be.

Keep in mind the following potential pitfalls when sending free protein S testing:

- Dynamic changes in both total and free protein S throughout childhood necessitate adjusted cutoff values among pediatric patients. As with protein C testing, make sure your laboratory takes age into account. Birth sex should also be considered: men tend to have higher levels of both total and free protein S than women.

- There are several noninherited (ie, acquired) causes of protein S deficiency, although in many cases the clinical implications of these forms of protein S deficiency are not clear. For example, patients with advanced liver disease often have low total and/or free protein S due to impaired hepatic synthetic function. However, because synthesis of other anticoagulant enzymes and cofactors is also impaired, it is not clear to what extent the protein S deficiency itself contributes to the hypercoagulability seen in these patients. Other causes of acquired (often transient) protein S deficiency include pregnancy, oral hormonal contraceptives, hypertriglyceridemia, HIV, and nephrotic syndrome.

---

*Seattle is also known for the Space Needle, great coffee, and its grunge music scene.
**You didn't ask, but protein C got its name because it was the third protein eluted from a chromatograph of bovine plasma.

- C4b-binding protein is an acute-phase reactant. As a result, any acute inflammatory state (or, importantly, acute thrombosis) will produce elevated levels of C4b-binding protein, reducing free protein S concentration. For this reason, it is wise not to perform protein S testing until at least 1 to 2 weeks after an acute thrombotic event.

- Warfarin may lower free protein S levels. Other anticoagulants (eg, factor Xa inhibitors, heparin) do not seem to interfere with free protein S testing.

 ## *Antithrombin III Deficiency*

Antithrombin III (AT III) is an enzyme produced in the liver that functions as an endogenous anticoagulant by inhibiting several coagulation factors, most strongly Xa and thrombin (IIa). Heparin works by potentiating AT III. It makes sense, then, that there are two main reasons to check for AT III deficiency:

1. As part of a hypercoagulability workup

2. To determine the cause of heparin resistance in a patient who does not respond appropriately to heparin (ie, an aPTT does not increase as expected)

AT III deficiency can either be inherited (autosomal dominant) or acquired (eg, in patients with nephrotic syndrome, cirrhosis, or acute thrombosis).

Testing is done in a stepwise process:

- A *functional assay* is done to measure AT III activity: This involves adding heparin to a sample of the patient's blood and measuring its ability to inhibit either factor Xa or IIa, which depends on adequate baseline AT III activity. A result of at least 80% (of the control value) rules out AT III deficiency, whereas a result less than 80% should be followed by

- *AT III antigen quantification*: The normal range for AT III antigen concentration varies significantly by laboratory and specific assay—when done by immunoassay, a result less than 17 mg/dL is consistent with AT III deficiency.

Patients who have both reduced AT III activity and reduced AT III antigen are said to have "type 1" AT III deficiency, where AT III activity is low because of low circulating AT III. Those who have reduced AT III activity but normal AT III antigen have "type 2" AT III deficiency, where circulating levels of AT III are normal but the function of AT III is abnormal.

Some laboratories are able to perform genetic testing for inherited AT III deficiency. However, it is costly and often unnecessary because the testing algorithm works well. The clinical context is often sufficient for determining the reason for AT III deficiency (eg, strong family history of clotting supporting an inherited cause, or nephrotic syndrome supporting an acquired cause).

Be wary of the following pitfalls to AT III testing:

- AT III levels may be transiently low in patients who are pregnant or who are taking oral hormonal contraceptives.

- Consumption of AT III in acute thrombosis reduces its levels. Wait until at least 1 to 2 weeks after an acute thrombotic event to send AT III testing.

- Avoid AT III testing in any patient on a heparin product (eg enoxaparin, unfractionated heparin) because results are unreliable. Depending on how testing is done (factor Xa-based vs factor II-based functional assay), results may also be unreliable in patients on factor Xa inhibitors or direct thrombin inhibitors. Warfarin does not interfere with AT III testing.

- Both acute hepatitis and obstructive jaundice may increase AT III levels, leading to potential false-negative results of AT III testing.

 ## Prothrombin G20210A

This not-so-catchily named thrombophilia is the second most common inherited hypercoagulable disorder after FVL. Prothrombin, also called factor II, plays a key role in the final common pathway of the coagulation cascade. The G20210A mutation in prothrombin—inherited in an autosomal dominant pattern—causes overactivity of prothrombin largely by boosting its serum concentration. The result is hypercoagulability. Indications for testing are similar to those for other hypercoagulable disorders (eg, strong family history of clotting, recurrent unprovoked thrombotic events).

The G20210A point mutation can be detected by genetic testing. Acute illness, recent thrombosis, or anticoagulant use do not interfere with the results. Measurement of the prothrombin concentration itself is generally unhelpful, given its wide variation in the general population.

 ## Antiphospholipid Syndrome

Consider testing for APS in a patient with one or more otherwise unexplained arterial or venous thromboses or with late pregnancy losses (especially in the setting of preeclampsia or placental insufficiency). Other clinical characteristics that should raise suspicion for antiphospholipid antibody (aPL) positivity include livedo reticularis/racemosa and systemic lupus erythematosus (SLE). Common incidental laboratory findings that may prompt suspicion for APS include otherwise unexplained mild thrombocytopenia (in the range of ~100,000 platelets/µL), an increased aPTT, or a false-positive VDRL test for syphilis (see Chapter 14).

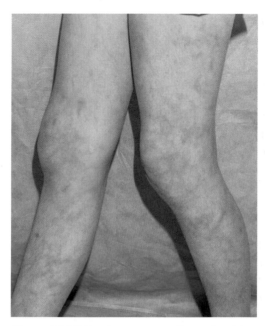

Figure 20.22 Livedo racemosa. (From Gru AA. *Pediatric Dermatopathology and Dermatology.* 12th ed. Wolters Kluwer; 2019.)

Antiphospholipid antibodies target various phospholipid-binding plasma proteins, ultimately resulting in hypercoagulability and inflammation. The three key tests that detect these antibodies* are:

- Lupus anticoagulant (LA)

- Anti-β-2-glycoprotein I (aβ2GPI)

- Anti-cardiolipin (aCL)

At least one positive aPL test is necessary but not sufficient to make the diagnosis of APS. All of the following are required for diagnosis:

- Either aβ2GPI or aCL in at least moderate titers (>40 ELISA units; see later) or a positive LA

- aPL positivity persisting over the span of at least 12 weeks, confirmed by repeat testing

- At least one clinical manifestation that is characteristic of APS (eg, otherwise unexplained thrombosis or late pregnancy loss)

---

*There are other antibodies that may be clinically significant (eg, confer risk of thrombosis) but that are not routinely tested for or included in APS criteria. Examples include anti-phosphatidylserine/prothrombin (aPS/PT) and anti-annexin A5. These may become more important in the near future.

Lupus Anticoagulant

Of all of the aPL tests, a positive LA is most strongly predictive of thrombosis and adverse pregnancy outcomes.

What does the term LA actually mean? LA is not a single antibody. Instead, it refers to any of a group of antibodies that prolong phospholipid-dependent clotting assays. The LA test measures phospholipid-dependent clotting; it is therefore a *functional* assay. A positive LA test means that one or more antibodies with LA activity are present.

These antibodies were originally detected in patients with lupus. The name LA is a bit of a misnomer, assigned after the first patients with antibodies with LA activity were found to have a prolonged aPTT and bleeding complications. We now know that LA positivity is more strongly associated with thrombosis than bleeding.

When you order LA testing, the lab initiates a stepwise coagulation-based functional assay:

1. Demonstrate a prolonged clotting time: A special phospholipid-dependent coagulation test is done using a modified aPTT and/or dilute Russel viper venom time (dRVVT; the venom is used to activate the coagulation cascade). If the result is negative (ie, normal), the patient is LA negative. If it is positive (ie, prolonged), the lab proceeds to step two.

2. Demonstrate the presence of an inhibitor: The patient's plasma is mixed with normal plasma. If this mixing corrects the prolonged coagulation time, then the patient must not have antibodies with LA activity. If mixing does *not* correct the prolonged coagulation time, then it is on to step three.

3. Demonstrate that the inhibitor is phospholipid dependent: Exogenous phospholipid is added to the sample. Correction of the prolonged coagulation time with addition of phospholipid confirms that the patient has antibodies with LA activity. Results are typically reported as either positive or negative.

Two positive LA results at least 12 weeks apart support a diagnosis of APS. Because of the strong association of LA with APS, some experts consider a single positive LA sufficient to diagnose a patient with APS in the setting of a compelling clinical presentation. Remember that APS can never be diagnosed without at least one otherwise unexplained clinical manifestation.

False-negative LA results may be seen in the setting of acute thrombosis. It is still reasonable to check LA at the time of thrombosis in a patient suspected of having APS in case it comes back positive; it will likely need to be repeated several weeks later anyway (either to confirm or rule out APS). Most LA assays are affected by the concomitant use of anticoagulants (particularly those that prolong the aPTT), although LA testing does not always have to be avoided in the setting of anticoagulation because adjustment of testing is sometimes possible. If you are considering LA testing in a patient on anticoagulation, we recommend discussing the approach and feasibility with your institution's laboratory.

Anti-cardiolipin and Anti-β-2-Glycoprotein I Antibodies

Send both of these tests along with LA when you suspect APS. For each, testing is done by ELISA, and both IgG and IgM isotypes are measured. The significance of IgA isotype positivity is not clear; we do not recommend making a diagnosis of APS based on the presence of aCL and/or aβ2GPI IgA positivity alone unless the clinical presentation is extremely compelling; even then, skepticism is appropriate.

For both aCL and aβ2GPI, IgG or IgM titers of at least 40 units, checked twice at least 12 weeks apart, support a diagnosis of APS in the appropriate clinical setting. IgG positivity is more strongly associated with APS than IgM positivity. For both IgG and IgM, the higher the titer above 40 units, the higher the specificity for APS.

Both aCL and aβ2GPI may be transiently positive either in the setting of an acute infection or—in some cases—for no apparent reason at all. For this reason, it is important that positive results be followed by repeat testing at least 12 weeks later. Results of aCL and aβ2GPI testing are not affected by the concurrent use of anticoagulation.

HEPARIN-INDUCED THROMBOCYTOPENIA

There are two types of heparin-induced thrombocytopenia (HIT):

- Type I HIT results from platelet aggregation associated with heparin exposure. It causes mild, clinically benign, and self-limited thrombocytopenia, almost always occurring within 1 to 2 days of heparin exposure.

- Type II HIT results from the production of autoantibodies against heparin-platelet factor four (PF4) complexes, leading to platelet activation and consumption. It causes thrombosis and, less commonly, bleeding. Onset is usually 5 to 10 days after heparin exposure. When clinicians refer to "HIT," they usually mean type II HIT—this is the type of HIT with significant clinical implications. Going forward, we will use the term HIT to mean type II HIT.

Consider the possibility of HIT in any patient with recent heparin exposure who has new otherwise unexplained thrombocytopenia, especially if accompanied by new clotting. The *"4 T" score* should be calculated and paired with your clinical judgment to help you establish your level of suspicion for HIT and decide whether testing is indicated:

Table 20.3 The 4T Score for Evaluating Heparin-Induced Thrombocytopenia (HIT)

4Ts Category	2 Points	1 Point	0 Points
Thrombocytopenia	Platelet count fall >50% and platelet nadir ≥20	Platelet count fall 30%-50% or platelet nadir 10-19	Platelet count fall <30% or platelet nadir <10
Timing of platelet count fall	Clear onset days 5-10 or platelet count fall ≤1 d (prior heparin exposure within 30 d)	Consistent with days 5-10 fall, but not clear (eg, missing platelet counts); onset after day 10; or fall ≤1 d (prior heparin exposure 30-100 d ago)	Platelet count fall ≤4 d without recent exposure
Thrombosis or other sequelae	New thrombosis (confirmed); skin necrosis; acute systemic reaction post-intravenous unfractionated heparin bolus	Progressive or recurrent thrombosis; non-necrotizing (erythematous) skin lesions; suspected thrombosis (not proven)	None
Other causes of thrombocytopenia	None apparent	Possible	Definite

A 4T score of ≤3 confers a low probability of HIT—testing is usually not indicated. The probability of HIT is at least intermediate (≥14%) in those with a 4T score of ≥4, most of whom should have further workup. Those patients with a 4T score of 3 to 4 are the trickiest—as always, consider the clinical scenario; remember that this tool is meant to be used in conjunction with your clinical judgment, not in place of it.

The risk of thrombosis in patients with HIT is very high (estimated at around 50%). Therefore, most experts agree that, if your suspicion for HIT is high enough that you are testing for it, you should stop all heparin products and initiate therapeutic anticoagulation with another agent (eg, argatroban) while results are pending.

The goal of laboratory testing for HIT is to identify the presence or absence of *anti-PF4-heparin antibodies* that activate platelets.

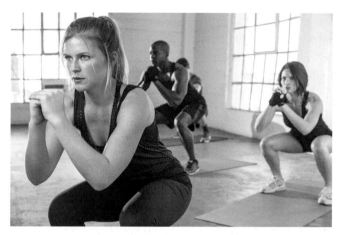

Figure 20.23 Do not confuse HIT (heparin-induced thrombocytopenia—an immune-mediated disorder of platelet activation and consumption) with HIIT (high-intensity interval training—a great way to get in shape). (Courtesy El Nariz/ Shutterstock.)

 ## Heparin-Induced Thrombocytopenia Enzyme-Linked Immunosorbent Assay

Testing for anti-PF4-heparin antibodies by ELISA is the initial screening test of choice. Sensitivity is excellent. Because the detection enzyme used in the immunoassay produces a characteristic color change, results are reported as an optical density (OD) at the detection enzyme's wavelength: the higher the OD, the higher the amount of detection enzyme present, the higher the amount of anti-PF4-heparin antibodies present in the patient's serum, and the higher the likelihood of HIT.

A negative result rules out HIT. Even a weakly positive result, including any OD less than 1, makes HIT very unlikely (<5%). When the OD reaches 1.4, the probability of HIT becomes more than 50%; when the OD reaches 2, the probability of HIT is about 90% and confirmatory testing (see later) may not be necessary depending on the clinical picture and/ or the 4T score.

Serotonin Release Assay

The serotonin release assay (SRA) establishes not only the presence of anti-PF4-heparin antibodies but confirms their ability to activate platelets; it is a "functional assay." This test takes longer than the HIT ELISA to come back—up to several days—but it is far more specific, and should be obtained as confirmatory testing in any patient with a positive HIT ELISA in whom any uncertainty remains about the diagnosis (in practice, this typically means most patients with a HIT ELISA OD between 1 and 2).

The SRA involves combining the patient's serum with heparin (usually unfractionated heparin, although low-molecular-weight heparin is occasionally used), then adding platelets radiolabeled with serotonin. Activation of the test platelets is indicated by release of the radiolabeled serotonin. Results are reported as positive or negative (ie, either serotonin release is seen or it is not). The SRA is considered to be the gold standard test for HIT, with a sensitivity and specificity both more than 95%. Its high cost and long turnaround time, however, necessitate the use of the HIT ELISA as an initial screening test.

 ## Heparin-Induced Platelet Activation

The heparin-induced platelet activation (HIPA) test is popular outside the United States as a confirmatory functional assay for HIT. Unlike the SRA, it does not require the use of radioactive material. Instead, the patient's serum is combined with platelet-rich plasma (from donors). The degree of platelet aggregation (used as a surrogate for platelet activation) is measured in the absence or presence of heparin in various concentrations. If significant platelet aggregation is seen in the presence of therapeutic concentrations of heparin but *not* in the absence of heparin, the result is reported as positive. Like the SRA, the HIPA has excellent sensitivity and specificity (both >95%).

BLOOD TYPING

All RBCs express antigens on their surface that can elicit an immune response. Of course, under normal circumstances, we don't make antibodies against our own RBCs. But these antigens play a critical role in blood and tissue transplantation.

Antigens that are controlled by a single gene or a set of linked genes are grouped together into what are called blood group systems. You undoubtedly know the ABO and Rh groups already. These are the most important and are responsible for the most dangerous reactions. However, there are many others. You may not be as familiar with their names—Duffy, Lewis, MNS, Kell, and Kidd among them—and you don't have to know anything about them other than that they can on rare occasions cause transfusion reactions.* The good news is that we can test for their presence as well.

Transfusion reactions occur when donor RBCs and recipient plasma are incompatible. What do we mean by incompatible? We all contain naturally occurring antibodies (isoagglutinins) to those antigens that are *not* present on our RBCs. Thus, people who have the type A blood group possess antibodies against type B, and vice versa. People who are type AB have no isoagglutinins (they are thus considered to be universal recipients) and those who are type O have antibodies against both the A and B antigens (they can only safely be transfused from donors who are also type O).

What Are These Antigens, Anyway?

The ABO antigens are polysaccharides and the Rh antigens are proteins. Do patients with type O blood have no surface antigens? No—they express the H antigen; the A and B antigens are created by tacking on an additional chemical group to the H antigen. Antibodies against the H antigen itself are very rare.

What is the purpose of these antigens? After all, they evolved long before humanity started transfusing blood from one person to another. The truth is that we actually don't know their physiologic function. Different illnesses and predispositions have been associated with the different blood types, but none of these convincingly explain their role in human biology.

A patient's blood type is obtained in anticipation of a transfusion of:

• RBCs

• Platelets, which express the ABO antigens but not the Rh antigen on their surface

• Plasma, which contains antibodies directed against the ABO antigens

Blood typing is also essential before organ or stem cell transplant.

---

*The more often a patient is transfused, the more antibodies to these RBC antigens may be produced, which can make finding compatible blood more complicated.

Testing Before Transfusion

Prior to possible transfusion, you will order a *type and screen*, establishing the recipient's ABO/Rh blood group (the *type* in your order) and the presence or absence of any antibodies present in the plasma against other, minor blood groups (the *screen* in your order).

Before high-risk procedures when multiple units of blood may be transfused, specific units of blood will be further tested against the recipient's blood in a process called *crossmatching.* The purpose of crossmatching is to check for the presence of recipient antibodies that may not have been caught by the type and screen. In this procedure, referred to as an indirect Coombs test, the recipient's serum and the donor's RBCs are mixed. They are then exposed to Coombs serum, which consists of rabbit anti-human immunoglobulin that reacts against both human antibodies and complement. If unexpected antibodies are present, the red cells will agglutinate. In patients with a normal type and screen, these antibodies are usually directed against one of the minor blood groups mentioned on the previous page.

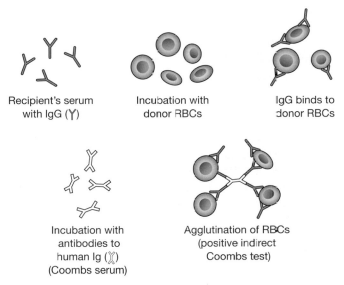

Figure 20.24 A positive indirect Coombs test, in which the patient's serum contains antibodies that react to the donor's red blood cells.

Additional Testing

Prior to transfusion, donor blood products are tested for more than just blood type. Laboratory testing usually includes screening for hepatitis B and C, HIV, West Nile virus, T-cell lymphotropic virus I and II, syphilis, and—in some areas of the United States and abroad—serologic evidence of infection with Babesia, Zika, and *Trypanosoma cruzi.*

 Rh Antigen in Pregnancy and Childbirth

Pregnant females who are Rh negative (strictly speaking, negative for the RhD antigen—there are many Rh antigens but it is almost always the D antigen that really matters) are at risk of becoming sensitized to the Rh antigen during delivery (or from feto-maternal hemorrhage prior to delivery) of an Rh positive baby. The mother develops antibodies against Rh, and—to make matters worse—these are IgG antibodies that can cross the placenta. A subsequent pregnancy therefore poses a risk to an Rh positive fetus. Among the most feared complications is hemolytic disease of the fetus and newborn (HDFN).

Current guidelines recommend that females undergo testing for the RhD antigen and RhD antibodies at their first prenatal visit. If they are RhD antigen negative, the antibody screen is repeated at 28 weeks of gestation and at delivery. Fortunately, sensitization to RhD can be prevented by giving anti-D immune globulin to women at risk.

TUMOR LYSIS SYNDROME

The sudden, massive lysis of tumor cells and the resulting release of their intracellular contents can be clinically devastating. Most cases occur with hematologic malignancies. The release of intracellular nucleotides can result in hyperuricemia, and the release of potassium and phosphate (the latter also causing hypocalcemia) can cause lethal cardiac arrhythmias. All of these laboratory abnormalities can contribute to the development of acute renal failure.

The most common cause of tumor lysis syndrome is the initiation of cytotoxic chemotherapy, usually within 12 to 72 hours. However, rapidly proliferating tumors can cause a similar picture spontaneously even without chemotherapy.

There are specific criteria, the Cairo-Bishop criteria, for diagnosing tumor lysis syndrome. When renal failure, a cardiac arrhythmia, or seizures develop in a patient with a rapidly dividing cancer or treatment-sensitive tumor following the initiation of therapy, the diagnosis of tumor lysis syndrome can be made by documenting at least two of the following if they occur between 3 and 7 days after starting cytotoxic therapy:

- Hyperuricemia (uric acid ≥8 mg/dL, or 25% increase from baseline)

- Hyperkalemia (potassium ≥6 mEq/L, or 25% increase from baseline)

- Hyperphosphatemia (phosphorus ≥4.5 mg/dL in adults, ≥5.5 mg/dL in children, or 25% increase from baseline)

- Hypocalcemia (calcium ≤7 mg/dL, or 25% decrease from baseline)

CANCER SCREENING

The detection of cancer in its earliest stages, when curative treatment is theoretically possible, remains the Holy Grail of oncology. In this chapter, we will look at some of the more commonly used (and misused) laboratory screens for cancer and briefly discuss some exciting new lab tests peering over the horizon.

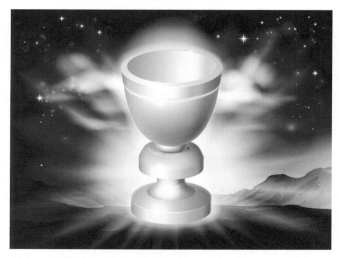

Figure 20.25 (Courtesy Christos Georghiou/Shutterstock.)

What Makes a Good Screening Test?

Whether we are talking about lab tests, imaging studies, the history, or the physical exam, the same principles apply when asking what makes for a good screening test. For a test to be a useful screen for cancer, we must as a bare minimum consider the following factors:

- How common is the cancer you are looking for? The prevalence of the disease in the population you are screening affects a test's positive predictive value and is a major determinant of how useful that test may be.

- How sensitive and specific is the test for a particular cancer? In other words, what are the rates of false negatives and false positives?

- Does identifying the cancer early actually make a difference? Is there treatment that is effective in the early stages of the cancer that would be ineffective later? If there is no such treatment, or if treatment later in the course would be just as efficacious, there is no advantage to detecting the cancer early in its course.

- A test is only helpful if patients are willing to undergo it. This may seem obvious, but what's the value of a test that is so burdensome and unpleasant that no one will go through with it?

These are big questions. After all, we are talking about ordering a test on asymptomatic individuals who believe that they are perfectly healthy, a test that may in the blink of an eye change their whole view of themselves and impact their plans for the future. The result of a positive test—which may be a true positive or a false positive—may cause tremendous patient anxiety and lead to a battery of additional tests, some of which may be invasive and carry significant procedural risks. You may also be condemning your patient to a lifetime of ongoing monitoring.

Keeping these questions in mind, there are a few laboratory tests for cancer screening that are particularly useful:

- **Human papillomavirus (HPV) and Pap testing**: Regular screening for cervical cancer or lesions that may progress to cervical cancer reduces cancer incidence and cancer-related mortality. Cervical specimens are tested for high-risk strains of HPV and may also be examined under the microscope for cytologic abnormalities (ie, dysplasia). The guidelines for interpretation and follow-up of results are complex but not complicated; the World Health Organization, the American Cancer Society, and the National Institutes of Health among many others all offer clear and effective guidelines that you should become familiar with.

- **BRCA1/2 genetic testing**: These genetic mutations substantially increase the risk of a number of cancers, most notably of the breast and ovary. Current recommendations are to consider screening anyone with a personal or family history of breast, ovarian, tubal, or peritoneal cancer or who have a high-risk ancestry (predominantly Ashkenazi

Jewish). Those deemed at high risk should be referred for genetic counseling prior to BRCA1/2 testing. Those who then test positive should be engaged in a thoughtful discussion about the pros and cons of intensive, regular monitoring and the possibility of initiating risk-lowering medications or undergoing prophylactic mastectomy and/or oophorectomy.

- **Fecal immunochemical testing (FIT)**: Annual FIT screening is an acceptable alternative to colonoscopy as a screen for colon cancer. FIT is more accurate than the original hemoccult tests and can be combined with testing for DNA mutations associated with colon cancer. Stool samples can be collected at home and then sent to the lab for testing. If FIT testing is positive, the patient should be referred for colonoscopy.

Unlike the tests above, the search for *serum tumor markers* of cancer has not been nearly as successful. Nevertheless, several of these come up often in discussion with patients and colleagues. They include:

- Prostate-specific antigen (PSA)

- Carcinoembryonic antigen (CEA)

- Cancer antigen 125 (CA 125)

- Cancer antigen 19-9 (CA 19-9)

- Cancer antigen 15-3 (CA 15-3)

 Prostate-Specific Antigen

As many as 11% of men in the United States will be given a diagnosis of prostate cancer at some point in their lives. Most often the pathway to this diagnosis begins with a *prostate-specific antigen (PSA)*, a simple blood test that can be run as a screening test in an asymptomatic patient. So this is a good thing, right? Not necessarily.

Most prostate cancers are not aggressive and never become clinically significant; so identifying an early-stage prostate cancer is, for many men, a classic example of overdiagnosis—that is, making a correct diagnosis which nevertheless contributes nothing to the patient's overall health outcomes. For men at average risk, regular PSA screening conveys little to no benefit in terms of overall mortality. In addition, many patients with an elevated PSA turn out not to have prostate cancer at all. Instead, they may prove to have benign prostatic hyperplasia (BPH) or prostatitis. The PSA test is just not very specific for cancer. It can even be elevated by manipulation of the prostate gland, such as from a rectal exam or a long bike ride. Normal values are typically cited as less than 4 ng/mL, but what is considered normal increases with age, and many experts consider any value less than 6.5 ng/mL normal in males over the age of 70.

Many experts and most guidelines recommend discussing the pros and cons with your patient starting at age 55 until age 70 as long as the patient's life expectancy is at least 10 years. The discussion should begin earlier in men at increased risk; this category includes Black males as well as men who are *BRCA1* or *BRCA2* positive.

If your patient opts for testing, the PSA should be repeated every 1 to 2 years. Should the PSA increase by more than 30% (the rapidity with which the PSA increases is called *PSA velocity*), it is reasonable to consult urology to decide on next steps. It is also recommended that urology should be consulted if the PSA exceeds 7 ng/mL.

Efforts to make the PSA more specific for the detection of aggressive, clinically significant tumors have not turned out to be as successful as hoped. We already mentioned the PSA velocity, and although it may be useful in selected patients, there are no compelling data supporting its routine use.

Another approach has been to measure *the ratio of free, unbound PSA to the total PSA*. PSA is a glycoprotein made by the prostate, some of which circulates bound to protein and some of which circulates free. The ratio of free PSA to total PSA is higher with benign disease than with malignancy; a ratio less than 25% is associated with a higher risk of cancer. However, there is no evidence that this test helps identify aggressive tumors that require treatment.

The one noncontroversial use of the PSA is in monitoring patients with prostate cancer who are undergoing treatment. The PSA should decline to undetectable levels if the tumor has been eradicated; any bump in the PSA requires investigation for recurrence.

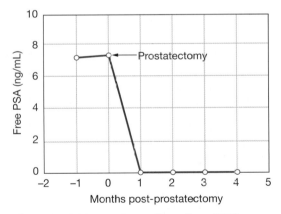

Figure 20.26 Prostate-specific antigen (PSA) should become undetectable with successful treatment of prostate cancer. (From Bishop ML, Fody EP, Schoeff LE. *Clinical Chemistry*. 7th ed. Wolters Kluwer Health; 2013.)

Carcinoembryonic Antigen

Carcinoembryonic antigen (CEA) is another glycoprotein, this one produced by the epithelial cells of the GI tract. Normal values are less than 2.5 ng/mL in nonsmokers and less than 5.0 ng/mL in smokers. Initially, it was hoped that the CEA might be useful for the detection of early-stage colorectal cancer. However, many patients with colon cancer have a normal CEA, especially if they have localized disease. Conversely, CEA is elevated in many other malignancies as well as in liver disease (it is metabolized by the liver) and renal failure. For these reasons, a CEA is not recommended as a screening tool for colorectal cancer (or any other malignancy) in asymptomatic individuals. The CEA is, however, used to monitor response to therapy.

 Cancer Antigen 125

Originally touted as a screen for ovarian cancer, Cancer antigen 125 (CA 125) is far too nonspecific to be useful as a screening tool in asymptomatic women at average risk. It can be used to monitor response to therapy.

 Cancer Antigen 15-3

Cancer antigen 15-3 (CA 15-3) is associated with breast cancer but should not be used for screening asymptomatic patients.

 Cancer Antigen 19-9

A high cancer antigen 19-9 (CA 19-9) is associated with pancreatic cancer. However, the CA 19-9 has a low specificity: it can also be elevated in patients with other malignancies of the GI tract and in those with pancreatitis. It is not recommended for use as a screening tool. Overall, an elevated CA 19-9 has a positive predictive value for pancreatic cancer of less than 1% in the asymptomatic population.

Other Tumor Markers for Monitoring Disease

Although most of the serum tumor markers above are not useful for screening, we have indicated that they can sometimes be useful for monitoring response to therapy. There are others that can also serve this function. Among those you may have heard of are:

- **α-Fetoprotein, β-human chorionic gonadotropin (β-hCG), and LDH** for testicular germ cell tumors

- **Calcitonin** for medullary thyroid tumors

Carcinoid Syndrome and 5'-HIAA

One tumor marker stands out as being useful in actually confirming a diagnosis of a specific malignancy. One of the potential causes of otherwise unexplained diarrhea and/or flushing is a neuroendocrine tumor that secretes *5-hydroxyindoleacetic acid (5'-HIAA)*, a breakdown product of serotonin; you may know this entity better as *carcinoid syndrome*. These tumors usually arise in the GI tract or lungs. The diagnosis can be made by finding elevated levels of 5'-HIAA in a 24-hour urine collection. Not all carcinoid tumors secrete 5'-HIAA, but an elevated level, should you find one, is highly specific. We need hardly point out, however, that the vast majority of patients with diarrhea or flushing do not have carcinoid syndrome.

 Cell-Free DNA

Our publisher has asked us to keep the size of this book within manageable limits, so we can only touch on one of the more exciting developments in the laboratory diagnosis of cancer. Cell-free DNA (cfDNA) technology is based on the observation—reported as early as 1971—that all cells, and particularly cancer cells, release minute amounts of DNA fragments into the circulation. These fragments can be detected and analyzed in a routine blood sample. The amount of detectable cfDNA depends on the tumor burden, cancer type, and a multitude of other host and tumor-specific factors. These DNA fragments can be analyzed for mutations, copy-number alterations, gene fusions, methylation, and other alterations that are seen with malignant transformation.

cfDNA is already proving helpful in diagnosing lung cancers and CNS tumors (a sample of cerebrospinal fluid [CSF] can also be subjected to the same analysis) in situations where a mass has been identified on imaging and it is inadvisable to obtain an actual biopsy or when a biopsy has been interpreted as indeterminate. It is also being used to identify mutations that may confer resistance to particular therapies.

Can this technique be used as a screen for cancer in asymptomatic persons? The answer is not yet clear. cfDNA testing is already being offered to the public for this purpose, but false-positive rates are very high. In people with risk factors for cancer, the data are a little more promising: about 6 out of 10 positive signals turn out to uncover a previously unsuspected malignancy.

Importantly, we also do not yet know if early detection of tumors by this technique will improve mortality. In other words, if these tumors could be successfully treated later on when they are symptomatic, then there is no real benefit to early detection.

Patients with a positive cfDNA test need to follow up with their clinicians for further blood tests and imaging in order to confirm the type and location of the malignancy. The cancers that have been detected by cfDNA technology include lymphomas, hematologic malignancies, and many solid tumors, almost all at an early stage.

At present, cfDNA technology is still in its infancy as a screening modality. It is not intended to supplant current screening procedures (eg, mammography, FIT testing) but rather should be offered—if at all—only as an adjunct.

Cancer of Unknown Primary: Tumor Markers

Patients with cancer of unknown primary pose a diagnostic challenge. Most commonly these are adenocarcinomas in which a biopsy is inconclusive as to their site of origin. The leading possibilities include cancer of the lungs, pancreas, kidneys, liver, and biliary tract. Treatment options vary greatly among these different malignancies, so it is incumbent upon the clinical team to do everything in their power to identify the tissue of origin.

The laboratory can be helpful here. Although it rarely points to a specific diagnosis, it can help guide subsequent steps.

The initial workup includes a very thorough history and physical examination, imaging as appropriate (typically a mammogram in females and a computed tomography (CT) of the chest, abdomen, and pelvis in both men and women), and the following blood tests:

- CBC

- CMP

- Urinalysis

- PSA (in males)

Other tumor markers are rarely helpful in helping to localize the primary tumor. They are often elevated in patients with cancer of unknown primary, but their lack of specificity limits their utility.

If this initial evaluation is not fruitful, immunohistochemical staining and genetic analysis of the biopsy specimen will often—although not always—provide an answer.

THE PORPHYRIAS

Porphyrins are a particular class of pigmented ring structures (that's all the chemistry we are going to give you). Chlorophyll is one, but we don't run into many human disorders related to impaired photosynthesis. Heme, a key component of hemoglobin, is another. The porphyrias are disorders of impaired heme synthesis, and because the enzymatic pathway is a complicated one, there are many porphyrias. Each causes the accumulation of different precursors, depending on where the problem lies in the heme biosynthetic pathway.

The major manifestations vary from one type of porphyria to another and can include abdominal pain, central and peripheral neurologic symptoms, psychiatric symptoms, and skin manifestations. Based on the predominant symptomatology, the porphyrias are grouped into three basic types: neurovisceral, chronic blistering cutaneous, and acute nonblistering cutaneous.

 ## Neurovisceral Porphyrias

The most common of these porphyrias is *acute intermittent porphyria (AIP)*. It is an inherited deficiency of the enzyme porphobilinogen deaminase, and its major symptom is abdominal pain; skin manifestations are not seen. You should consider screening for AIP in patients 15 to 50 years of age with recurrent attacks of abdominal pain that are unexplained by any other etiology. The attacks can be initiated by any of a variety of stressors and are believed to be caused by the accumulation of porphyrin precursors in the circulation. Measurement of one of these precursors, porphobilinogen (PBG), is the screening test of choice for AIP. PBG should be measured in a random urine sample along with a spot urine creatinine. A normal PBG/creatinine ratio rules out AIP, while a ratio greater than 10 mg/g is highly specific for the presence of AIP or another neurovisceral porphyria. The diagnosis can be nailed down by measuring the levels of other porphyrin precursors in the urine, plasma, and/or stool—expect both PBG and Δ-aminolevulinic acid (ALA) to be disproportionately elevated in patients with AIP—followed by genetic testing for confirmation.

 ## Chronic Blistering Cutaneous Porphyrias

The most common of these is *porphyria cutanea tarda* (PCT). This photosensitive disorder typically presents with blistering lesions on the dorsum of the hands along with skin fragility. The leading cause is hepatitis C, but other liver diseases—such as alcoholic liver disease and hemochromatosis—can also be responsible. Unlike AIP and other less common porphyrias, PCT is caused by an *acquired* enzyme inhibitor. The screening tests of choice are either a *plasma or urine porphyrin level*. Both are very sensitive. Positive results should be followed by porphyrin fractionation; highly carboxylated porphyrins including uroporphyrin are characteristically elevated in PCT.

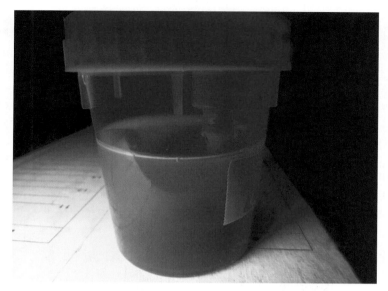

Figure 20.27 The urine of a patient with porphyria cutanea tarda (PCT) glows pink under a Wood lamp. (From Handler NS, Handler MZ, Stephany MP, Handler GA, Schwartz RA. Porphyria cutanea tarda: an intriguing genetic disease and marker. *International Journal of Dermatology* 2017;56(6):e106-e117.)

Examination of the urine under fluorescent light can also be a helpful diagnostic test. The urine appears red or brown under normal light, but glows a dramatic pink or red under a Wood lamp. This, in fact, used to be the only way to make the diagnosis of PCT prior to our ability to identify the specific biochemical abnormalities in the lab.

 ## Acute Nonblistering Cutaneous Porphyrias

This is the rarest type of porphyria. *Erythropoietic protoporphyria* (EPP) is the most well-known example and results from a deficiency of the enzyme ferrochelatase, responsible for combining iron and protoporphyrin to create heme. It causes a painful photosensitive skin reaction without blisters. The screening test of choice is to measure the *erythrocyte total protoporphyrin*. Normal levels are less than 70 μmol/mol heme. A normal result rules out EPP; an elevated result warrants further testing with protoporphyrin fractionation—in EPP, metal-free protoporphyrin constitutes at least 85% of the patient's erythrocyte protoporphyrin (the other 0%-15% is made up of zinc protoporphyrin). Genetic testing can further confirm the diagnosis.

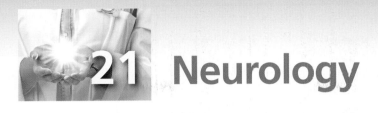

21 Neurology

THE LABORATORY IN NEUROLOGIC DISEASE

In Chapter 10, we reviewed how analysis of the cerebrospinal fluid (CSF) can aid in the diagnosis of central nervous system (CNS) hemorrhage, infection, inflammation, and malignancy. In this section, we will focus on a few of the other more common CSF tests that can be useful, as well as some blood tests specific to neurologic disease.

 ### *Cerebrospinal Fluid Oligoclonal Bands*

Almost all patients with *multiple sclerosis* (MS) have antibodies in the CSF, detectable with electrophoresis, that are not present in their serum. We call them oligoclonal bands because they literally show up as bands on immunofixation (see Figure 21.1). Only 2% to 3% of patients with MS will *not* have these oligoclonal bands, so their absence, while not ruling out the diagnosis of MS, makes it highly unlikely. The CSF of patients with *neuromyelitis optica spectrum disorder*, the most common mimic of MS, usually does not show oligoclonal bands.

The presence of oligoclonal bands in the CNS is not specific for MS. They can also occur in a wide range of other conditions such as *neurosarcoidosis, Lyme disease of the CNS, herpes simplex virus 1 encephalitis, HIV,* and *neurosyphilis.* The presence of oligoclonal bands, therefore, cannot be used alone to establish the diagnosis of MS but is just one criterion that can be incorporated into the diagnostic process.

Another helpful CSF tool in patients with suspected MS is an assessment of the *immunoglobulin G (IgG) synthesis rate*, a measure of how fast IgG is being made in the CSF. The rate is elevated in MS.

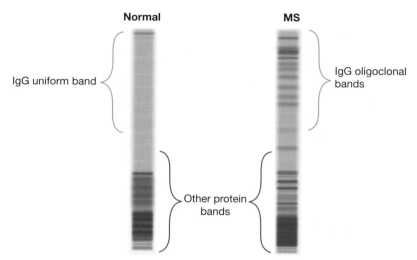

Figure 21.1 An example of oligoclonal bands on electrophoresis from a patient with multiple sclerosis (MS). (From Thaler AI, Thaler MS. *The Only Neurology Book You'll Ever Need*. Lippincott Williams & Wilkins; 2021.)

Cerebrospinal Fluid 14-3-3 Protein

The 14-3-3 protein, present in all the body's cells, appears to play a role in the ability of B cells to switch from producing one type of immunoglobulin to another. Increased levels in the CSF are associated with *Creutzfeldt-Jakob disease (CJD)*. Although this test is highly sensitive (>90%) and thus useful for ruling out the disease, it is not specific for CJD. The specificity most often cited is approximately 80%. This may sound like a reasonable specificity, but for a disease as uncommon as CJD, it means that most positive tests will actually be false positives. The 14-3-3 protein can also be elevated with other causes of CNS neuronal injury, such as stroke or malignancy. At best, this test can modestly increase the likelihood of the diagnosis in a patient with suspected CJD; it should never be relied upon alone.

Other Cerebrospinal Fluid Markers

Many different types of paraneoplastic and autoimmune encephalitis are now diagnosed and even defined by specific antibodies. The majority of these can be reliably detected in the serum, but a handful are best tested for in the CSF. Probably the best-known example is the detection of *antibodies against the NMDA* receptor* in the CSF, a finding that is highly sensitive and specific for the aptly named *anti-NMDA receptor encephalitis*. There are also extended panels to screen for autoimmune or paraneoplastic encephalitis, which can detect multiple antibodies in the CSF and serum. If an antibody is found in the serum but not in the CSF, consider the possibility of a false positive.

CSF biomarkers should soon prove helpful in the diagnosis of many other neurologic disorders, including Alzheimer dementia.

At present, some of the most widely used CSF laboratory tests are for specific infections. Two particularly important examples include neurosyphilis and CNS Lyme disease (see Chapter 14).

Autoantibodies in Myasthenia Gravis

Myasthenia gravis is a muscle disease characterized by muscle fatigability (weakness that worsens with use) with a predilection for the ocular muscles. Approximately 80% of patients have *autoantibodies directed against postsynaptic acetylcholine receptors (AChR)* detectable in their serum. Of those who do not, about one-third will have *muscle-specific tyrosine kinase (MuSK) antibodies*. In seronegative patients, that is, those with neither of these autoantibodies, there are tests for other, less common autoantibodies.

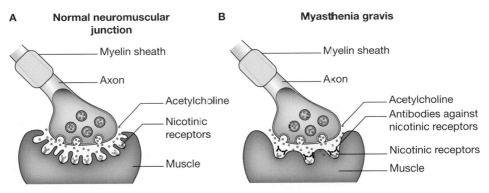

Figure 21.2 Nerve transmission across the synapse to a muscle cell is blocked by acetylcholine receptor (AChR) antibodies. (From Thaler AI, Thaler MS. *The Only Neurology Book You'll Ever Need.* Lippincott Williams & Wilkins; 2021.)

One important note about AChR antibodies: they should be used only for diagnosis. They do not vary predictably with disease activity, severity, or therapy.

---

*N-methyl-D-aspartate; the receptor plays an important role in excitatory transmission in the CNS.

Genetic Markers of Alzheimer Disease

The genetics of late-onset Alzheimer disease are complex and still being evaluated. One important association we do know about is with the *APOE* gene, which is involved in lipid metabolism. One allele of this gene, APOE-ε4, has been closely associated with late-onset Alzheimer disease, the most common form of the disease. The ε4 allele is present in approximately 14% of the general population. Heterozygotes have a 3-fold increased risk of developing Alzheimer disease, and homozygotes have a 10 to 14 times increased risk.

Routine testing for APOE-ε4 is not recommended for screening the general population. It is also not recommended for diagnosis; the test is neither specific nor sensitive for Alzheimer disease. Thirty to fifty percent of patients with Alzheimer disease do not have the allele. Nevertheless, family members of patients with Alzheimer disease may request the test to assess their risk. Genetic counseling is advised before you go ahead with testing. When testing is ordered, it can be run on either whole blood or a buccal smear.

Early-onset Alzheimer disease, occurring in persons under the age of 65, is far less common than late-onset disease. It has a strong genetic component. Many cases are associated with autosomal dominant mutations in *amyloid precursor protein (APP)* or *presenilin 1*, which converts APP to β-amyloid. Genetic testing should be considered to confirm the diagnosis when suspected, as well as to inform family members who wish to understand their risk.

Concussion

In the United States alone, about one million people are seen in emergency rooms for traumatic brain injuries (TBIs) every year. The major concern is to determine who is at risk for a bleed and would benefit from a CT scan, and who is not. There are decision tools to help in this determination, but we now have a blood test, still under investigation and as of this writing not yet widely available, that appears to be a useful adjunct. It must be performed within 12 hours of the injury and has only been studied in patients with mild TBI. It looks for two biomarkers that correlate with serious brain injury: (1) *ubiquitin C-terminal hydrolase L1*, an enzyme found in neurons, and (2) *glial fibrillary acidic protein*, present in astrocytes. While false-positive results are common—more than half of patients with a positive test will prove to have a normal CT scan—the negative predictive value is very high, exceeding 99%. A negative result may therefore spare many patients a head CT.

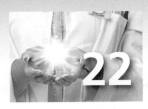# 22 Rheumatology

AUTOIMMUNE DISORDERS: PRINCIPLES OF TESTING

It is easy to become overwhelmed by the vast array of labs that fall under the umbrella of autoimmune testing. How—and when—do you go about working up a patient for a possible autoimmune disease? We will try to demystify this process by providing you with some guiding principles.

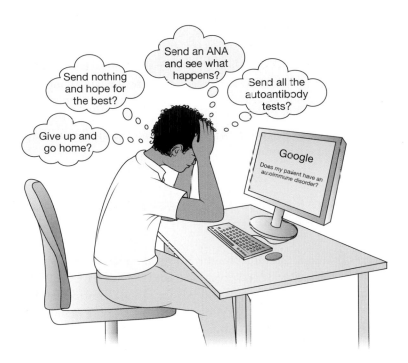

Figure 22.1

Autoimmune disorders comprise a very heterogeneous group (consider the difference between celiac disease, which can be controlled with a gluten-free diet, and rheumatoid arthritis, which decidedly cannot). So why lump them together? Autoimmune disorders tend to share a few key features:

- They are not very common. Even rheumatoid arthritis, one of the most common autoimmune disorders, has a worldwide prevalence of only about 0.5%. Compare that to the prevalence of osteoarthritis, estimated at more than 5%.

- An immune response gone awry results in the formation of *autoantibodies* (more on this later) directed against normal bodily constituents such as proteins or nucleic acids. Autoantibody testing plays an important role in the workup of many autoimmune disorders.

- Multiple organs can be affected.

- Symptoms can be vague, nonspecific, and highly variable both in quality and time course.

- Chronic or recurrent inflammation is common.

- Having one autoimmune disease often increases the risk of having another.

- There is usually a significant genetic component to risk (inherited susceptibility).

We can take advantage of these common features to tailor a widely applicable approach to testing for and monitoring autoimmune disorders.

 ## Have a Good Reason to Suspect an Autoimmune Disorder Before Testing

Common things are common,* and uncommon things are not. Your elderly patient with hip and knee pain that worsens with activity is far more likely to have osteoarthritis than rheumatoid arthritis or lupus. It is wasteful and unwise to start hunting for underlying autoimmune disease in a patient with a very low pretest probability. At the very least, you should have one or more specific autoimmune diseases in mind. Some health care providers mistakenly use the antinuclear antibody (ANA) test as an "autoimmunity screen," often leading to false positives and further unnecessary testing (see page 436). Similarly, if you send off an autoimmune panel without knowing what exactly is in the panel or what specific disease(s) you are looking for, you will likely end up confused about what to do with the results.

---

*As is this tired expression.

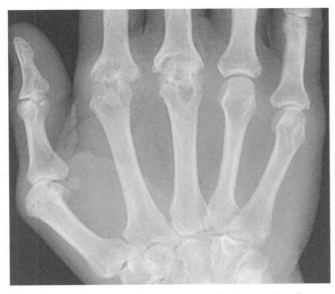

Figure 22.2 Imaging results may prompt further workup for autoimmune disease. This hard x-ray, for example, shows erosions and severe joint space narrowing of the second and third metacarpophalangeal joints that are highly suggestive of rheumatoid arthritis. This patient needs further laboratory workup. (From Ballantyne JC, Fishman SM, Rathmell JP. *Bonica's Management of Pain*. 5th ed. Wolters Kluwer Health; 2019.)

Test results that suggest ongoing acute or chronic inflammation may, in the right clinical context, prompt an evaluation for a possible underlying autoimmune disease. These can include:

- An elevated erythrocyte sedimentation rate (ESR) and/or C-reactive protein (CRP). We discuss these further on page 463.

- An elevated ferritin

- Almost any alteration in the complete blood count (CBC). Anemia, thrombocytopenia or thrombocytosis, and leukopenia or leukocytosis are common features of these diseases.

None of these findings, however, are specific for an autoimmune disorder.

Acute Phase Reactants

The CRP and ferritin are examples of acute phase reactants, meaning proteins whose levels increase in the setting of acute or chronic inflammation (the ESR, on the other hand, is not an actual protein—more on this on page 463). Other examples of acute phase reactants include procalcitonin (see page 208), hepcidin (important in iron regulation and storage), fibrinogen (important in hemostasis), multiple clotting factors, and serum amy-loid A. There are many more. The roles of these proteins in the inflammatory response are highly variable, ranging from recognizing and eliminating pathogens to protecting against the formation of reactive oxygen species.

There are also negative acute phase reactants—that is, proteins whose levels *decrease* in the setting of inflammation. Examples include albumin and transferrin.

Lab results consistent with an acute phase reaction (ie, an increase in acute phase reactants, or a decrease in negative acute phase reactants) are nonspecific and only indicate ongoing inflammation. Whereas these labs can support a clinical picture suggestive of autoimmune disease, an acute phase reaction is also commonly seen in infection, trauma, and malignancy.

 ## *What We Measure*

Immunoglobulins (Antibodies)

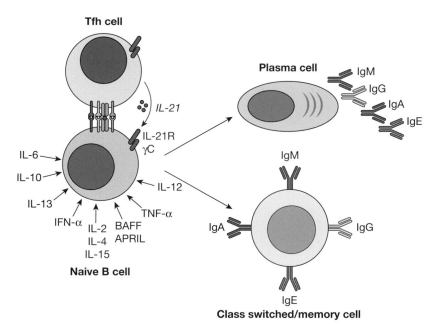

Figure 22.3 Small molecules called cytokines can induce B cells to differentiate into plasma cells or memory cells that are able to recognize and respond to a specific antigen upon reexposure. The plasma cells can secrete a wide variety of immunoglobulins, proteins that bind and fight off foreign invaders. We commonly refer to immunoglobulins as antibodies. Measuring levels of specific antibodies can give us a much more granular picture of the immune system than measuring just the basic cell types that are present. IFN-α, interferon alpha; Ig, immunoglobulin; IL, interleukin; TNF-α, tumor necrosis factor alpha.

Immunoglobulins (antibodies) come in five basic classes, each with its own structure and functional niche:

- Immunoglobulin (Ig)A: found in secretions in the respiratory, gastrointestinal (GI), and genitourinary (GU) tracts

- IgM: relatively unspecialized "first responder" antibodies

- IgG: a jack of all trades, the major immunoglobulin of the secondary (target-specific) immune response; particularly good at enhancing phagocytosis of pathogens and at interacting with the complement system (see page 430)

- IgE: important in allergic reactions and in fighting off parasites

- IgD: the least important immunoglobulin for our purposes; its precise function remains unclear

In autoimmune disorders—in which the normal regulation of the immune system has gone awry—some immunoglobulin levels may be too high and others may be too low. As a result, it can be helpful to directly measure total levels of IgA, IgM, IgG, and IgE (IgD is generally not measured). For example, elevated levels of total IgA are commonly found in IgA nephropathy and IgA vasculitis. Conversely, low IgA levels are associated with several other conditions, notably celiac disease.

Some autoimmune disorders are associated with abnormalities in specific antibody *sub*classes; for example, elevated levels of IgG4 correlate with disease activity in the conveniently named IgG4-related disease.

Autoantibodies, Self-Antigens, and Immune Complexes: Through a complex series of interactions with other immune cells, populations of B cells can evolve—over a period of days—to produce antibodies with a strong binding affinity for a specific antigen or set of antigens. This is great when it goes right—this basic process forms the backbone for how we fight infections and how vaccines work. But when this process goes wrong and we mistakenly make antibodies directed against normal bodily constituents (eg, proteins and nucleic acids), autoimmune disease can ensue. These self-attacking antibodies are called *autoantibodies*. Autoantibodies (eg, anti–thyroid peroxidase in Hashimoto thyroiditis and anti–double-stranded DNA [anti-dsDNA] in lupus) are what most of us think of when we think about testing for autoimmune disorders.

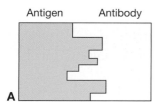

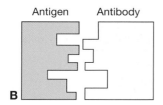

Figure 22.4 A specific antibody—one that binds a particular antigen very tightly (A)—is one likely to do its job effectively. A poor fit, seen in (B), limits the antibody affinity and renders it relatively ineffective. Specific antibodies directed against our own normal bodily constituents (autoantibodies) can be dangerous. However, not all autoantibodies are necessarily harmful. Many are thought merely to be markers for, rather than causes of, autoimmune disease—that is, by-products of the larger underlying pathophysiologic process.

The antigen that the autoantibodies target is called a *self-antigen* or *auto-antigen*. We typically don't measure self-antigens because they are normal components of healthy patients (eg, we check for anti-dsDNA antibodies but not for dsDNA; everyone, hopefully, has dsDNA in their cells!).

An *immune complex* is formed when an autoantibody binds to a self-antigen. Immune complexes can circulate in the blood (measured with blood testing) or deposit in tissues (measured with tissue biopsy).

Two Secrets of Autoantibody Testing: These really aren't secrets, but too often they are forgotten in the rush to diagnosis.

1. *Look for patterns. Do not rely on a single result.*

   Many autoimmune diseases are associated with specific autoantibodies, and we will discuss them. But remember that the key word here is *associated*. Although certain autoantibodies may point more toward one autoimmune disease than another, it is common for different autoimmune diseases to share autoantibodies (eg, a positive ANA is often found not only in lupus but also in scleroderma, Sjögren syndrome, rheumatoid arthritis, and even in many perfectly healthy patients). Your job, then, is to put each result in the context of the clinical picture and the laboratory data already obtained. For example, your patient with a strongly positive ANA along with a malar rash and cytopenias is likely to have lupus. Hopefully, this approach— considering what you already know and incorporating new results into your analysis—should sound familiar. It is nothing more than Bayesian thinking, our old friend from Chapter 1.

Table 22.1 Autoimmune Disorders and Associated Positive Autoantibody Tests

Autoimmune Disorder	Associated Positive Autoantibody Tests
Systemic lupus erythematosus	ANA, dsDNA, Smith, U1-RNP, SSA, SSB, histone, antiphospholipid antibodies
Drug-induced lupus	ANA, histone, SSA
Antiphospholipid antibody syndrome	Lupus anticoagulant, β-2 glycoprotein, cardiolipin
Scleroderma	ANA, Scl-70, centromere, RNA polymerase III, U3-RNP (fibrillarin), PM-Scl
Sjögren syndrome	SSA, SSB, RF, ANA
Rheumatoid arthritis	RF, CCP, ANA
Idiopathic inflammatory myositis (eg, polymyositis, antisynthetase syndrome)	Antisynthetase antibodies (eg, Jo-1, EJ, OJ), Mi-2, SAE1, SRP, HMG-CoA reductase, NXP2, TIF1γ, MDA-5, PM-Scl, U3-RNP, SSA
ANCA-associated vasculitis	c-ANCA/PR3, p-ANCA/MPO

ANA, antinuclear antibody; ANCA, antineutrophil cytoplasmic antibody; c-ANCA, cytoplasmic ANCA; CCP, cyclic citrullinated peptide; dsDNA, double-stranded DNA; HMG-CoA, 3-hydroxy-3-methylglutaryl coenzyme A; MPO, myeloperoxidase; p-ANCA, perinuclear ANCA; PR3, proteinase 3; RF, rheumatoid factor; RNP, ribo-nucleoprotein; SRP, signal recognition particle; SSA, Sjögren syndrome A; SSB, Sjögren syndrome B. It's good to know these associations. But remember that they really are just associations—take a look at all of the overlap. Knowing the approximate sensitivity and specificity of each test for each disease is very important. We will discuss these antibody-disease relationships in more depth later in this chapter (when we will also deconstruct the alphabet soup of antibody acronyms—most actually stand for something). For now, it's ok if your eyes have glazed over. This should be helpful as a quick reference later on.

2. *How abnormal matters a lot.*

It is not uncommon for healthy people to have low levels of circulating autoantibodies. Similarly, diseases besides autoimmune disorders, such as many infections, can cause transient or mild elevations in various autoantibodies. So when the results of an autoantibody test come back positive or abnormal, pay close attention to *how* abnormal—markedly abnormal results are much more likely to indicate the presence of the autoimmune disorder(s) of interest.

Titers

It is relatively easy to determine whether a particular number is "markedly abnormal." For example, the upper limit of normal for the liver enzyme aspartate aminotransferase (AST) is 35 U/L. We can confidently say that an AST of 10,000 U/L is markedly abnormal—it is hundreds of times higher than the upper limit of normal. But the results of many antibody tests are reported as *titers* expressed as ratios rather than numbers. What does that mean?

Many antibody tests employ a method called *serial dilution*. When the result of the test is positive—that is, when the lab tech detects antibodies—the sample is then diluted over and over until the tech can no longer detect the antibodies. *The antibody titer is the highest level of dilution at which antibodies can still be detected in the sample.* Titers are usually reported as ratios, such as 1:640 or 1/640. Think of this as a fraction representing how concentrated the final solution is compared to the original. The higher the second (or bottom) number in the ratio, the more diluted the final solution and the more antibodies must be present (in other words, you can detect the antibodies even when you add a lot of diluent). For reference, a commonly reported "low-level" ANA titer is 1:80. A titer of 1:320 is moderately high, and a titer of 1:1280 is generally considered markedly elevated.

Complement

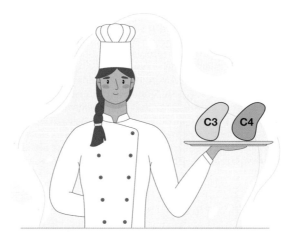

Figure 22.5 Complements of the chef. (Adapted from OWLISKO DESIGN/Shutterstock.)

Complement, or the complement system, refers to a group of proteins that literally complement the antibody response, helping to destroy or sequester the perceived threat. The complement proteins are made in the liver and all conveniently start with a capital C.

The most commonly measured complement proteins are *C3* and *C4*. Levels increase with inflammation (complements are acute phase reactants) and decrease when they are used up and deposited in tissues. The finding of an elevated C3 and/or C4 is a nonspecific indicator of ongoing inflammation, whereas a low C3 and/or C4 usually indicates either impaired liver synthetic function or active immune complex deposition (as, for example, can occur with lupus nephritis or cryoglobulinemic vasculitis).

The *CH50* is a measure of a patient's overall complement capacity or function. In order to measure CH50, serial dilutions are performed on the patient's serum, to which antibody-coated red blood cells (RBCs) are added. The CH50 is the highest level of serum dilution at which the patient's complement system is still able to lyse 50% of the antibody-coated RBCs. Therefore, the higher the CH50 (normal range: 150-250 units/mL), the higher the functional capacity of the patient's complement system. An abnormally low number indicates a deficiency in one or more components of the complement system (includes C1 through C9). The most common use of this test is in the workup of immunodeficiency (eg, a patient with recurrent infections) rather than autoimmune disease.

Cytokines

Cytokines are a diverse group of small proteins secreted by various immune cells that modulate the inflammatory response and assist in communication between immune cells. Their effects are wide ranging and can be either pro- or anti-inflammatory. Examples include the *interleukins (IL-1, IL-2,* etc; there are many), *tumor necrosis factor (TNF)* α, and *transforming growth factor (TGF)* β.

Although cytokines have become important therapeutic targets of modern immunomodulatory medications, the cytokines themselves are rarely measured in practice—doing so seems to have little clinical utility (this could change in the future).

The Human Leukocyte Antigen System*

Human leukocyte antigen (HLA) genes code for cell surface proteins. Many of these proteins are involved in recognizing foreign antigens and presenting them to immune cells.

Different people have different HLA proteins—you may have HLA-B51 but I may have HLA-B52. Why do we care? There are many reasons, but for the purposes of immunologic testing it is sufficient to recognize that certain HLAs are associated with specific autoimmune disorders. For example, HLA-B27 is strongly associated with spondyloarthritis, particularly ankylosing spondylitis (AS; see page 446). Thus, checking for certain HLAs (*HLA typing*) can help determine the likelihood of a given associated disease. The stronger the association, the higher the diagnostic utility of testing for a given HLA type. In most cases, the HLA-disease association isn't strong enough for HLA typing to provide much diagnostic utility—for example, notice that many of the diseases in Table 22.2 share predisposing HLAs.

Think of specific HLAs as risk factors. Perhaps even more so than most other tests, HLA typing should not be done alone as a diagnostic test for an autoimmune disorder, just as screening for tobacco use should not be done alone as a diagnostic test for emphysema. Instead, use HLA typing in conjunction with other labs and diagnostic studies.

---

*The HLA system is also referred to as the major histocompatibility complex (MHC). We will stick with the simpler term, HLA.

Human Leukocyte Antigen Typing in Transplant Medicine

It is standard practice to perform HLA typing on both donor and recipient tissues prior to a potential organ or bone marrow transplant. A close match between donor and recipient HLAs reduces the risk of organ rejection and graft-versus-host disease (GVHD).

Table 22.2 Diseases and Associated HLAs

Disease	HLA(s)
Spondyloarthritis	B27
Rheumatoid arthritis	DR4, DR1
Systemic lupus erythematosus	DR2, DR3
Celiac disease	DQ2, DQ8
Type 1 diabetes	DR3
Hashimoto thyroiditis	DR5, DR3
Behçet syndrome	B51
Abacavir hypersensitivity[a]	B57:01
Allopurinol hypersensitivity[a]	B58:01

HLA, human leukocyte antigen.
[a]Yes, certain HLAs can predispose patients to severe hypersensitivity reactions to particular medications. In the case of allopurinol hypersensitivity, patients of Han Chinese, Thai, and Korean descent and African Americans are at particularly high risk of carrying HLA B58:01 and should be tested for it before being started on allopurinol. It is standard practice for all patients to be tested for HLA-B57:01 before being started on the antiretroviral drug abacavir.

 ## How We Measure

Enzyme-linked immunosorbent assay (ELISA) and immunofluorescence (IF) are two of the most widely applied methods of testing in the world of autoimmune disorders. Understanding the basics of how these tests work will help you to properly interpret their results.

Enzyme-Linked Immunosorbent Assay

We've already described this type of testing in Chapter 14. The only difference here is that the target antigen is not a protein on the surface of a pathogen, but rather an autoantibody. The process, however, is otherwise the same.

Immunofluorescence

IF works similarly to ELISA. The first step is to make an antibody to the protein of interest and add that antibody to the patient's sample. But instead of linking the antibody to an enzyme, you link the antibody to a fluorescent dye that will light up under the microscope if the patient has the target protein (ie, the autoantibody of interest).

One big advantage of IF is that the fluorescent dye lights up exactly where the target protein is located. This method of testing therefore allows you to visualize how the autoantibody (or immune complex) is distributed in space. This distribution is called the *IF pattern*. Different IF patterns correspond to different diseases:

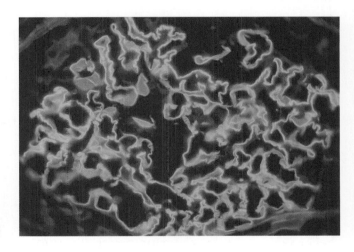

Figure 22.6 Linear immunofluorescence for immunoglobulin G is seen along the glomerular basement membrane in Goodpasture disease. (From Rubin R. Strayer DS, Rubin E, eds. *Rubin's Pathology: Clinicopathologic Foundations of Medicine*. 6th ed. Lippincott Williams & Wilkins; 2012.)

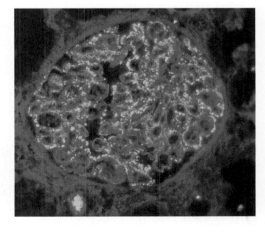

Figure 22.7 Granular immunofluorescence of the glomerulus is indicative of immune complex deposition. This pattern is seen in lupus nephritis and post-streptococcal glomerulonephritis. (From Rubin R, Strayer D, Rubin E, eds. *Rubin's Pathology: Clinicopathologic Foundations of Medicine*. 6th ed. Lippincott Williams & Wilkins; 2012.)

Once You Make the Diagnosis: Concepts in Autoimmune Disease Monitoring

Suppose you diagnose your patient with systemic lupus erythematosus (SLE). What next? How do you know what tests to send at subsequent visits? You can use the following principles to guide your thinking when it comes to autoimmune disease monitoring.

End Organ Damage

Any given autoimmune disease may affect one or nearly all of our organs. When monitoring a patient with an established (or highly likely) autoimmune disorder, you should use the lab to check for end organ damage. In order to do this, all you need to know is which organs are likely to be affected by the patient's disease. Don't forget that the medications used to treat the patient's disease can cause end organ damage of their own.

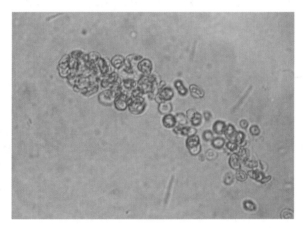

Figure 22.8 Red blood cell casts in the urine may indicate glomerulonephritis, one sign of active autoimmune disease (eg, lupus nephritis) that you may not pick up on history or exam. For this reason, periodic urinalysis is an important part of monitoring patients with lupus. (From Rennke HG, Denker BM. *Renal Pathophysiology: The Essentials*. 4th ed. Wolters Kluwer; 2014.)

Disease Activity

Although some autoimmune disorders can present with a single isolated episode, a chronic or relapsing-remitting course is more the rule than the exception. The term *disease activity* refers to a snapshot of how bad the patient's disease is *right now*. Is the patient currently having a disease flare? Is the disease worsening despite treatment? Beyond the obvious clinical signs and symptoms (eg, joint swelling, fevers), how can you tell when a patient's autoimmune disorder is acting up? Various tests can be helpful:

Erythrocyte Sedimentation Rate and C-Reactive Protein: Not all autoimmune diseases cause inflammation, but for those that do, the ESR and CRP provide useful measures of disease activity. It is common practice to trend the ESR and/or CRP over time for patients with known autoimmune disorders; an upswing in inflammatory markers *may* indicate active or uncontrolled disease. These labs are less helpful in patients with an underlying malignancy, infection, severe tissue injury, or ischemia, all of which also commonly cause significant inflammation. However, even in a patient with a chronically elevated ESR or CRP, changes over time can still be clues to changes in disease activity. See page 463 for more on the ESR and CRP.

Trending Complement Levels: We recommend checking C3 and C4 when you are concerned for active immune complex deposition—examples include lupus nephritis and cryoglobulinemic vasculitis. If checking for nonspecific inflammation is your goal, complement levels are unlikely to add additional diagnostic information beyond what you can learn from the ESR and CRP.

Trending Autoantibody Levels: Autoantibodies tend to be more helpful as diagnostic tools than as measures of disease activity. Fluctuations, when they occur, do not have any clear clinical implications. There are two main exceptions to this rule:

- Anti-dsDNA antibody levels correlate well with renal disease activity in most patients with lupus (see page 438).

- In some—but not all—patients with antineutrophil cytoplasmic antibody (ANCA)-associated vasculitis, ANCA titers correlate with disease activity (see page 456).

ANTINUCLEAR ANTIBODIES

Antinuclear antibodies (ANAs) are exactly what they sound like: antibodies to nuclear antigens. Because *the ANA test* is ordered as a single test, it is tempting to think of it as a single antibody. However, just as there are many nuclear antigens, there are many antinuclear antibodies. It makes sense, then, that the ANA can be positive in multiple different diseases, each of which is associated with a different combination of antinuclear antibodies.

An ANA should not be ordered in patients with nonspecific symptoms unless you have reason to suspect an underlying autoimmune disorder. Too often an ANA is ordered as part of a shotgun approach to a patient with ill-defined symptoms in the hope that it will come back negative and thus be reassuring. However, frequently the test will come back with a low titer that is impossible to interpret, leading you down a rabbit's hole of needless testing and creating understandable anxiety in your patient.

Consider ordering an ANA if you are suspicious for one or more of the following diseases:

Table 22.3 ANA Positivity Rate in Autoimmune Diseases

Disease	Percent With Positive ANA[a]
Lupus (SLE or drug-induced lupus)	95-100
Mixed connective tissue disease	95-100
Scleroderma (limited or diffuse)	95
Autoimmune hepatitis	70
Polymyositis or dermatomyositis	60
Sjögren syndrome	60
Primary biliary cirrhosis	60
Autoimmune thyroiditis[b]	50
Graves' disease	50
Antiphospholipid antibody syndrome	40-50
Rheumatoid arthritis	40-50
Primary sclerosing cholangitis	40-50

ANA, antinuclear antibody; SLE, systemic lupus erythematosus; TG, thyroglobulin; TPO, thyroid peroxidase; TSH, thyroid-stimulating hormone.
[a]The titer at which ANA is considered positive varies significantly by lab. Many labs use 1:80 as a cutoff.
[b]Even "euthyroid" patients (ie, with a normal TSH) who happen to have circulating anti-TPO or anti-TG antibodies (see Chapter 19) may have an associated positive ANA. Consider sending these thyroid antibody tests in a patient with an otherwise unexplained positive ANA.

The higher the *sensitivity* of ANA for the disease(s) of interest, the higher its clinical utility. For example, a patient with a negative ANA almost certainly does not have lupus or mixed connective tissue disease (MCTD), and is very unlikely to have scleroderma. On the other hand, a negative ANA does not rule out any of the other diseases mentioned earlier. ANA is *not specific* and cannot be used alone to make any diagnosis.

ANA is most commonly measured by an immunofluorescence assay (IFA; see page 433 for more on IF), allowing for the determination of:

1. *Titer*

   The titer tells you how positive the result is. Many healthy people without any clinical evidence of autoimmune disease have low titers of circulating antinuclear antibodies: about 20% to 30% have a titer of 1:40, and about 5% have a titer as high as 1:160. For this reason, clinical context is extremely important in interpreting an ANA, especially if it is only weakly positive.

2. *Pattern*

   The pattern describes the antibody distribution inside the cell. Different ANA patterns correlate (albeit sometimes weakly) with different specific antinuclear antibodies and therefore with different autoimmune diseases. Here are some examples:

Table 22.4 ANA Patterns in Autoimmune Diseases

ANA Pattern	Antibodies	Diseases
Homogeneous	dsDNA	Lupus
	Histone	Drug-induced lupus
Speckled	SSA/Ro and SSB/La	Sjögren syndrome Lupus Scleroderma
	U1-RNP	MCTD
	Smith	Lupus
	Mi-2	Dermatomyositis
Nucleolar	Topoisomerase I (Scl-70)	Diffuse scleroderma
	RNA polymerase III	Diffuse scleroderma
	Fibrillarin (U3-RNP)	Diffuse scleroderma
Centromere	Centromere (CENP)	Limited scleroderma

ANA, antinuclear antibody; CENP, centromere protein; dsDNA, double-stranded DNA; MCTD, mixed connective tissue disease; RNP, ribonucleoprotein; SSA, Sjögren syndrome A; SSB, Sjögren syndrome B.

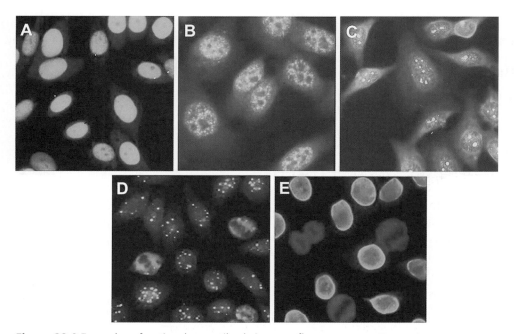

Figure 22.9 Examples of antinuclear antibody immunofluorescence patterns. A: Homogeneous, B: speckled, C: nucleolar, D: multiple nuclear dots, E: rim like. (From Terziroli Beretta-Piccoli B, Mieli-Vergani G, Vergani D. Autoimmune hepatitis: Serum autoantibodies in clinical practice. *Clin Rev Allergy Immunol* 2022;63:124-137. doi: 10.1007/s12016-021-08888-9. Provided by the Springer Nature SharedIt content-sharing initiative.)

Depending on the disease(s) of interest, follow up a positive ANA by testing directly for specific autoantibodies ("sub-serologies"). It is at this point that many patients are referred to a rheumatologist.

There are over 100 antinuclear antibodies, only a few of which we routinely test for. As a result, many patients with a positive ANA will have negative testing for specific autoantibodies (sub-serologies) even in the presence of one or more ANA-associated autoimmune diseases. In other words, sub-serology testing tends to be insensitive. The big advantage of sub-serology testing is that it can be very specific.

Here are the most commonly ordered and clinically relevant antinuclear antibodies.

Anti–Double-Stranded DNA

This test is less sensitive but much more specific than the ANA for the diagnosis of SLE. If your suspicion for SLE is moderate to high, order an anti-dsDNA. A positive result in this setting makes SLE very likely. After the diagnosis of SLE has been confirmed, dsDNA should be checked periodically, because levels tend to correlate with disease activity.

There are several commonly used methods for measuring anti-dsDNA antibodies, the most specific of which is an immunofluorescence assay using the unicellular *Crithidia luciliae* organism (which contains a giant mitochondrion with an isolated circle of dsDNA) as a substrate. If you have a patient with a positive anti-dsDNA test by another method (eg, ELISA) and the clinical picture is not otherwise compelling for SLE, consider resending the anti-dsDNA by *Crithidia* assay.

Anti-histone

Associated with drug-induced lupus (estimates of sensitivity range from 75% to 95%), anti-histone antibodies are also commonly seen in SLE (ie, idiopathic). Although the presence of anti-histone antibodies can be used to support a diagnosis of drug-induced lupus, this test alone cannot reliably rule in or rule out the diagnosis.

Anti-SSA/Ro and Anti-SSB/La

Both of these autoantibodies are associated with Sjögren syndrome. Anti-SSA/Ro is more sensitive than anti-SSB/La (75% vs 45%). Neither is specific; both can be found in patients with SLE, rheumatoid arthritis, MCTD, diffuse scleroderma, polymyositis, and primary biliary cirrhosis. It is particularly important to check anti-SSA/Ro in pregnant patients whom you suspect of having one of the disorders above because circulating antibodies are associated with congenital heart block in the fetus.

> ### Why Are These Sjögren Antibody Names so Complicated?
>
> They aren't really, once you get to know them. SSA simply stands for Sjögren syndrome A and SSB for, well, you get the idea. Ro and La are the names of two types of RNA-associated proteins that are the targets of these autoantibodies. SSA is associated with antibodies to Ro proteins, SSB with antibodies to La proteins. That's all there is to it.

Anti-U1-Ribonucleoprotein (U1-RNP)

Ribonucleoproteins (RNPs) live up to their name: they consist of proteins bound to RNA. Patients with MCTD uniformly have antibodies to U1-RNP, making this test very sensitive for MCTD (it is an exception to the "sub-serologies are insensitive" rule). Anti-U1-RNP positivity is also seen in some patients with SLE, diffuse scleroderma, and, less commonly, Sjögren syndrome.

Anti-Smith (Sm)

The Smith antigen was named after Stephanie Smith, in whom this SLE-associated nuclear antigen was first discovered in the mid-20th century. It binds RNPs (one of which is U1-RNP) to form structures called small nuclear ribonucleoproteins (snRNPs). Some assays detect antibodies to Smith or U1-RNP individually, whereas others detect antibodies to the Smith/RNP complex (ie, snRNP). When you see that Smith/RNP is positive, look for the results of the anti-Smith assay (typically run along with Smith/RNP) to help determine whether the patient is positive for anti-Smith, anti-U1-RNP, or both.

Anti-Smith antibodies are insensitive but highly specific for SLE (even more specific than anti-dsDNA). Order this test when your clinical suspicion for SLE is moderate to high. A positive result confirms the diagnosis.

Anti-Mi-2

Mi-2 is a protein involved in transcription regulation in the nucleus. Anti-Mi-2 antibodies are insensitive but highly specific for dermatomyositis. We discuss testing for dermatomyositis and polymyositis further on page 450.

Anti-topoisomerase I (Anti-Scl-70)

Topoisomerase I is an enzyme that helps to maintain the structure and stability of DNA. Although insensitive, anti-topoisomerase I (aka Scl-70) antibodies are highly specific for scleroderma. They are associated with diffuse skin involvement and with the development of scleroderma-associated interstitial lung disease.

Anti-centromere

This test is also highly specific for scleroderma. Send anti-centromere antibodies if you suspect any form of scleroderma (limited or diffuse). A positive result predicts more limited skin and visceral organ involvement and a better overall prognosis. Although anti-centromere positivity is associated with an increased risk of pulmonary hypertension, these patients rarely develop interstitial lung disease, the other major pulmonary complication of scleroderma.

Anti-centromere antibodies are also positive in a minority of patients with primary biliary cirrhosis.

Anti-RNA Polymerase III

The presence of anti-RNA polymerase III antibodies in a patient with scleroderma indicates a high risk of severe disease including renal, musculoskeletal, and pulmonary complications. This test should be part of the workup of any patient with confirmed or highly suspected scleroderma.

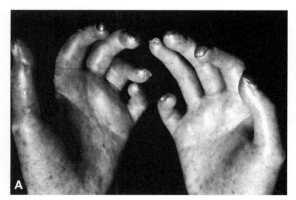
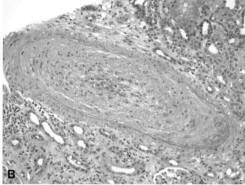

Figure 22.10 Anti-RNA polymerase III antibodies are associated with severe disease in scleroderma. A. Severe sclerodactyly with ulcerations and telangiectasias. (From McConnell TH, Paulson VA, Valasek MA. *The Nature of Disease: Pathology for the Health Professions.* 2nd ed. Wolters Kluwer Health/ Lippincott Williams & Wilkins; 2014.) B. Renal biopsy in a patient with scleroderma renal crisis. (From Ahn W, Radhakrishnan J. *Pocket Nephrology.* Lippincott Williams & Wilkins; 2019.)

Extractable Nuclear Antigens

Some of the tests we've just reviewed are often grouped together in an *extractable nuclear antigen (ENA) panel*, commonly ordered as a follow-up test after a positive ANA. The name refers to a method of extracting antigens from cells using saline.

Since the advent of the ENA panel, some of the presumed nuclear antigens included in the panel have since been found to be components of the cytoplasm rather than the nucleus. The misnomer, however, seems to have stuck. As a result, many modern ENA panels include both antinuclear antibodies *and* some anti-cytoplasmic antibodies. The most common example of an included anti-cytoplasmic antibody is *anti-Jo-1*, an antibody associated with myositis (including dermatomyositis and polymyositis).

It is reasonable to order an ENA panel in a patient with a clinically significant positive ANA and/or high pretest probability of connective tissue disease (eg, SLE, Sjögren syndrome, scleroderma), but it is good practice to check which antibodies are included first and make sure they are relevant to the disease(s) you are considering. Conversely, do not assume that an ENA panel includes all the ANA sub-serologies of interest—you will likely need to order some tests separately (dsDNA, for example, is not included in an ENA panel). The most common version of the panel includes anti-SSA, anti-SSB, anti-Smith, and anti-U1-RNP antibodies.

RHEUMATOID FACTOR AND ANTI–CYCLIC CITRULLINATED PEPTIDE ANTIBODIES

Rheumatoid factor (RF) and anti–cyclic citrullinated peptide (anti-CCP) antibodies are frequently ordered together in the evaluation of rheumatoid arthritis.

Rheumatoid Factor

RF is an autoantibody directed against one's own IgG (an antibody to an antibody). RF comes in a few forms, or isotypes: IgM RF, IgA RF, IgE RF, and, perhaps confusingly, IgG RF (IgG against IgG). IgM RF is the most common isotype and is what most widely available assays test for when you order an RF.

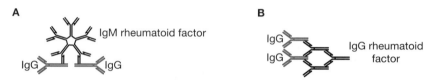

Figure 22.11 A. IgM rheumatoid factor. Because it is a pentamer with 10 antigen binding sites, a single IgM molecule can bind several target IgG antibodies. B. IgG rheumatoid factor. On the other hand, it takes more than one IgG, with just two antigen binding sites, to join the target IgG molecules. In both cases, these aggregates can fix complement and initiate an inflammatory response. IgG, immunoglobulin G; IgM, immunoglobulin M.

The upper limit of normal varies by lab, but is most commonly around 14 IU/mL.

It is tempting, if only because of its name, to think that there is a one-to-one association between RF and rheumatoid arthritis. This is not the case. The sensitivity and specificity of an elevated RF for rheumatoid arthritis are about 70% and 85%, respectively. Clinically, this means that *RF cannot reliably rule in or rule out rheumatoid arthritis by itself.* An elevated RF may be seen whenever there is chronic stimulation of the immune system, such as with many infectious diseases and especially in the following autoimmune diseases:

Table 22.5 Rheumatoid Factor Positivity Rate in Autoimmune Diseases

Autoimmune Disease	Percent Rheumatoid Factor Positive
Rheumatoid arthritis	70
Sjögren syndrome	85[a]
Cryoglobulinemia	~70 (estimates vary)

Table 22.5 Rheumatoid Factor Positivity Rate in Autoimmune Diseases (*continued*)

Autoimmune Disease	Percent Rheumatoid Factor Positive
MCTD	55
Scleroderma	25
SLE	25
Sarcoidosis	15

MCTD, mixed connective tissue disease; SLE, systemic lupus erythematosus.
[a]Yes, you read that right. The sensitivity of RF for Sjögren syndrome may actually be better than for rheumatoid arthritis.

The higher the RF above the upper limit of normal, the higher the likelihood that the patient has one of the above autoimmune disorders, and the higher the likelihood that a patient with rheumatoid arthritis has aggressive disease.

Many *non-rheumatic* diseases also cause chronic immune stimulation, so mild-to-moderate elevations in RF may be seen in these cases as well; examples include *chronic lung diseases*, *hepatitis B*, *hepatitis C* (among whom a majority of patients will have detectable RF), other chronic infections, and many malignancies. *Infective endocarditis* is the most notable non-autoimmune cause of a positive RF; a positive RF is among the minor criteria for the diagnosis of infective endocarditis, and titers can be quite high.

A small percent of otherwise healthy, asymptomatic patients have a positive RF. Although these patients are at increased risk of developing rheumatoid arthritis compared to the general population, it is not at all clear what to do with such a result. We do not recommend checking RF in the absence of signs or symptoms of rheumatoid arthritis or another autoimmune disease.

Following fluctuations in the RF in patients already diagnosed with rheumatoid arthritis is not beneficial. The correlation between RF levels and disease activity is poor at best. The ESR and CRP are more helpful for this purpose as they tend to rise and fall concurrently with disease activity.

Bottom line: RF is not sensitive or specific enough for it to be used alone as a screening or confirmatory test for rheumatoid arthritis. It can, however, be combined with the rest of your data to help sway your diagnostic thinking in one direction or another, particularly when rheumatoid arthritis, Sjögren syndrome, or cryoglobulinemia is in the differential diagnosis. You should also consider sending an RF along with other testing if you are suspicious for any of the other autoimmune disorders in Table 22.5. When RF is high, pay close attention to *how* high; mild-to-moderate elevations are common with many chronic diseases and in some perfectly healthy individuals, whereas marked elevations are more likely to reflect underlying rheumatoid arthritis, another autoimmune disease in Table 22.5, or endocarditis.

Anti–Cyclic Citrullinated Peptide Antibodies

Anti-CCP antibodies target a category of proteins present in the joints. The upper limit of normal is 20 units. A result more than 60 units is considered strongly positive.

What Are Citrullinated Peptides?

Citrullination is a post-translational modification of proteins containing the amino acid arginine. In this process, arginine is converted to citrulline, thereby altering the charge, structure, and function of the affected protein. Why does the body do this? The reason is not well understood, but it appears that citrullination may be involved in immune function, the maintenance of skin integrity, and neurologic function.

The sensitivity of anti-CCP for rheumatoid arthritis is 75%, similar to that of RF. However, *anti-CCP is a more specific test for rheumatoid arthritis (95%) than RF (85%).* As with RF, a high titer of anti-CCP at the time of diagnosis predicts more aggressive disease.

Bottom line: Order anti-CCP along with RF in any patient in whom you have at least moderate clinical suspicion for rheumatoid arthritis. A positive anti-CCP in this context has excellent positive predictive value for rheumatoid arthritis. A negative anti-CCP does not rule out rheumatoid arthritis. Should you always order both tests when you suspect the diagnosis of rheumatoid arthritis? In most cases, yes, since patients may be positive for one and not for the other.

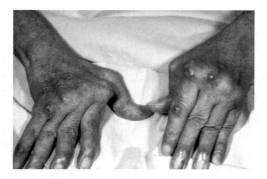

Figure 22.12 An example of severe deforming rheumatoid arthritis, seen most often in patients with high-titer RF and/or anti-CCP. The 30% of patients with clinically diagnosed RA who are negative for both RF and CCP are said to have "seronegative RA." This seronegative group may be at lower risk for aggressive joint disease or extra-articular complications. CCP, cyclic citrullinated peptide; RA, rheumatoid arthritis; RF, rheumatoid factor. (From Acosta WR, Roach SS. *Pharmacology for Health Professionals.* 2nd ed. Wolters Kluwer/ Lippincott Williams & Wilkins Health; 2013.)

HLA-B27 AND SPONDYLOARTHRITIS

The spondyloarthritides (formerly referred to as the seronegative spondyloarthropathies) are a group of autoimmune inflammatory arthritides that share a few key features:

- Negative test for RF (this is the "seronegative" part in the old name)

- Axial joint involvement (eg, the spine and sacroiliac joints) and/or asymmetric peripheral oligoarthritis

- Characteristic extra-articular features including dactylitis, uveitis, enthesitis (inflammation where the tendons and ligaments attach to the bones), skin involvement (especially psoriasis), and GU or GI involvement

- Association with *HLA-B27*; this is where the lab comes in.

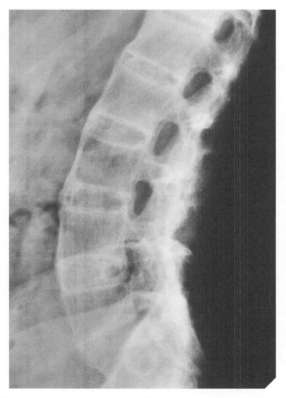

Figure 22.13 The fused lumbar vertebrae of this patient with advanced ankylosing spondylitis create the typical "bamboo spine" appearance. (From Greenspan A. *Orthopedic Imaging*. 5th ed. Lippincott Williams & Wilkins; 2011.)

The four classic* spondyloarthritides are

- *Psoriatic arthritis*

- *Ankylosing spondylitis (AS)*

- *Inflammatory bowel disease–associated arthritis*

- *Reactive arthritis*

The *HLA-B27* antigen is associated with all of the spondyloarthritides, most strongly with AS. HLA-B27 is present in approximately 90% of self-identifying white patients with AS and in approximately 65% of self-identifying non-white patients with AS. However, HLA-B27 is also fairly common in the general population, with an overall prevalence of 5% to 10%. This means that, by itself, HLA-B27 is neither sensitive nor specific for spondyloarthritis. So how should we use this test?

Consider sending HLA-B27 when you are concerned about spondyloarthritis, but only as part of a larger diagnostic workup that includes a thorough history, exam, and imaging of joints that are suspected to be involved, such as the sacroiliac joints or spine. If you are on the fence about whether a patient may have spondyloarthritis, HLA-B27 can help push you in one direction or another, but it should not be used by itself to definitively establish or rule out spondyloarthritis.

Do not send HLA-B27 on every patient with low back pain. In the vast majority of patients, muscular strain or degenerative spinal disease is a far more likely culprit than spondyloarthritis. Only send an HLA-B27 in a patient with low back pain if you have some other reason to suspect a spondyloarthritis (eg, prolonged morning stiffness, family history of spondyloarthritis, other painful or swollen joints, or characteristic extra-articular features).

Role of the Lab in Diagnosing Reactive Arthritis

Reactive arthritis most commonly presents as an asymmetric oligoarticular arthritis with or without accompanying extra-articular symptoms (eg, fevers, urethritis, uveitis, oral ulcers, GI distress) about 1 to 4 weeks after a GU or GI bacterial infection. The most common antecedent infections are *Chlamydia*, *Campylobacter*, *Salmonella*, *Shigella*, and *Yersinia*. If there are any red, hot joints, *arthrocentesis* is an important first diagnostic step, which will help rule out septic or crystalline arthritis and confirm inflammatory synovial fluid (see Chapter 13).

Importantly, reactive arthritis, like the other seronegative spondyloarthropathies, is a clinical diagnosis—the role of the laboratory is very limited. Patients with arthritis and ongoing symptoms of an underlying infection should be tested for those infections. However, infectious signs and symptoms have often resolved by the time the patient develops arthritis, in which case testing for the infecting organism may not be helpful. HLA-B27 can be checked but is neither sensitive nor specific. HLA-B27 positivity in a patient with established reactive arthritis may be an indicator of more aggressive disease.

---

*Newer, more nuanced criteria classify spondyloarthritis based on the pattern of joint involvement (axial vs peripheral), extra-articular features, and radiographic findings. For the purposes of this chapter, we will stick with the traditional terms.

CRYSTALLINE ARTHRITIS: GOUT AND PSEUDOGOUT

Gout and pseudogout are referred to as crystalline arthritides because each is caused by deposition of crystals in the joints—monosodium urate crystals in gout, and calcium pyrophosphate crystals in pseudogout. Crystalline arthritis most often presents as an acute monoarticular arthritis, but can progress to relapsing-remitting polyarticular arthritis if the disease goes untreated. Pseudogout, named for its tendency to mimic the acute-onset, exquisitely painful monoarticular arthritis of gout, is actually just one of many ways in which calcium pyrophosphate deposition disease (CPPD) can present.

You should have a high level of suspicion for crystalline arthritis in patients with inflammation of any characteristic joint, such as the first metatarsophalangeal joint in gout or the knee in pseudogout.

Arthrocentesis demonstrating monosodium urate (gout) or calcium pyrophosphate (pseudogout) crystals allows for the definitive diagnosis of crystalline arthritis (see Chapter 13). The role of the lab is otherwise limited.

 ## *Uric Acid and Gout*

A patient's serum uric acid must reach a concentration of at least 6.8 mg/dL ("hyperuricemia") in order to precipitate in the joints and cause gout. However, measuring the uric acid is of limited utility in the diagnosis of gout for two important reasons:

- Hyperuricemia (~20% prevalence among U.S. adults) is much more common than gout (~4% prevalence among U.S. adults). In other words, most patients with hyperuricemia do not have gout.

- The uric acid may be high, normal, or low in the setting of an acute gout flare (in other words, false negatives abound). Measuring the uric acid is therefore unhelpful for the diagnosis of gout during an acute flare.

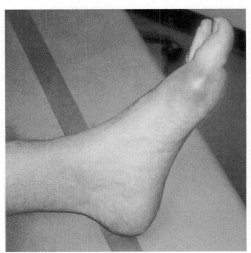

Figure 22.14 Acute inflammatory arthritis of the first metatarsophalangeal joint (podagra) commonly seen in gout. (From Berg D, Worzala K. *Atlas of adult physical diagnosis.* Lippincott Williams & Wilkins; 2006.)

So when should you check uric acid, and how should you use the result?

- *Diagnosis*: Check the uric acid at a time when the patient does *not* appear to be experiencing an acute flare. A uric acid more than 6.8 mg/dL supports a diagnosis of gout, but only in the setting of compelling clinical evidence or a positive arthrocentesis.

- *Monitoring*: Check the uric acid periodically, every few weeks to months, in patients with known gout who are on urate-lowering therapy. The target uric acid level is less than 6.0 mg/dL (<5.0 mg/dL if the patient has tophi). However, not all patients with gout require therapy—namely, those who do not have tophi, joint erosions, or frequent flares. Regular monitoring of uric acid in patients with a history of gout who do not qualify for urate-lowering therapy is controversial and may not be necessary.

Because renal insufficiency is a significant risk factor for gout, a basic metabolic panel (BMP) or comprehensive metabolic panel (CMP) should also be part of the evaluation of any patient with suspected gout.

 ## *Pseudogout (Calcium Pyrophosphate Deposition Disease)*

Aside from arthrocentesis, laboratory testing is generally unhelpful for the initial diagnosis of pseudogout.

Pseudogout is common with normal aging, so once the diagnosis is made in patients over 50, further evaluation may not be needed. Younger patients are more likely to have predisposing electrolyte derangements or metabolic conditions. Examples include *hemochromatosis*, *hyperparathyroidism*, *hypomagnesemia*, and *hypophosphatasia* (an inherited disorder affecting calcium and phosphate homeostasis). Consider sending the following labs to look for predisposing factors:

- Calcium, phosphorous, and magnesium

- Parathyroid hormone (PTH)

- Alkaline phosphatase (ALP; rule out hypophosphatasia)

- Iron studies (rule out hemochromatosis)

Some clinicians screen all patients with newly diagnosed pseudogout—including those over 50—for hyperparathyroidism given its relatively high overall prevalence.

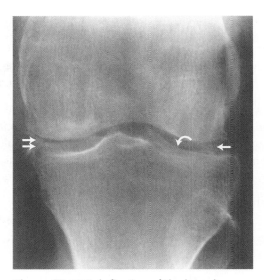

Figure 22.15 Calcification of the lateral meniscus (single arrow), medial meniscus (double arrows), and articular cartilage (curved arrow; also called chondrocalcinosis) of the left knee of a patient with calcium pyrophosphate deposition disease. These findings are common in patients with CPPD disease even in the absence of an acute flare. (From Erkonen WE, Smith WL. *Radiology 101: The Basics and Fundamentals of Imaging*. 4th ed. Lippincott Williams & Wilkins; 2013.)

MUSCLE ENZYMES AND MYOSITIS

Some Helpful Definitions Before We Get Started

Table 22.6 Myopathy, Myositis, and Myalgia

Term	Definition	Examples
Myopathy[a]	Muscle problem	Steroid myopathy Hypothyroid myopathy
Myositis	Inflammatory muscle problem	Polymyositis Dermatomyositis
Myalgia	Muscle pain	Myalgias from a viral infection

[a]Although myopathy technically refers to any muscle problem, we most often use this term to refer to noninflammatory muscle pathology. Frustratingly, some diseases are referred to as "inflammatory myopathies," which really just means myositis.

 Creatine Kinase

Creatine kinase (CK), an enzyme involved in energy storage and utilization, is present in disproportionately high concentrations in skeletal muscle. It comes in three forms, by far the most predominant of which is CK-MM, which constitutes over 99% of skeletal muscle CK. Much smaller amounts of CK are found in the heart (CK-MB; see Chapter 15) and brain (CK-BB). Any time skeletal muscle cells are damaged, CK can leak into the circulation. Thus, an elevated serum CK serves as a marker for skeletal muscle injury. A normal CK ranges from 30 to 170 U/L.

Common causes of an elevated CK include:

- *Infections*: Many viruses, bacteria, fungi, and parasites have been implicated. Influenza is the most common infectious cause of myositis.

- *Idiopathic inflammatory myopathies*: for example, polymyositis, dermatomyositis

- Muscle ischemia

- Severe electrolyte derangements

- *Medications/drugs:* statins, cocaine, antipsychotics (neuroleptic malignant syndrome), inhaled anesthetics (malignant hyperthermia), and many others

- Hypothyroidism

- *Congenital or metabolic disorders:* for example, Duchenne and Becker muscular dystrophies

- Strenuous exercise

- *Rhabdomyolysis:* acute, severe, and diffuse muscle damage and necrosis that may be due to trauma, seizures, severe infections, or other overwhelming metabolic demands

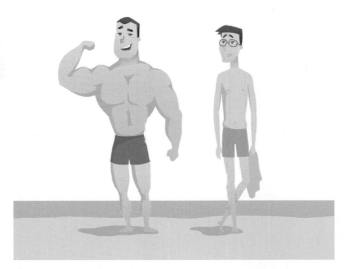

Figure 22.16 CK correlates with muscle mass in healthy patients. The patient on the left is likely to have a higher baseline CK (perhaps around 150 U/L) than the patient on the right (perhaps around 50 U/L). Patients who are very emaciated or cachectic may have a CK that is below the lower limit of normal (30 U/L) and those who are very muscular may have a CK that is slightly above the upper limit of normal. No amount of muscle can fully explain a CK more than 500 U/L. CK, creatine kinase. (Courtesy Boyko.Pictures/Shutterstock.)

There are many conditions that cause muscle pain (myalgias) and/or weakness that do *not* produce an elevated CK, such as fibromyalgia, steroid myopathy, and polymyalgia rheumatica. It makes sense, then, to check a CK level in a patient with muscle pain or weakness in order to differentiate between diseases that are associated with frank muscle damage and those that are not. A normal or low CK is a sensitive finding that makes significant muscle injury or inflammation very unlikely.

An elevated CK should always prompt the question, *"how* elevated?"

- An elevated CK less than 500 U/L is a common finding in many noninflammatory conditions (eg, hypothyroid myopathy, viral illnesses, recent strenuous exercise).

- A CK more than 1,000 U/L is more indicative of significant muscle damage and/or associated inflammation; examples include dermatomyositis or polymyositis, drug- or toxin-induced myositis, and trauma.

- A CK more than 5,000 U/L is indicative of rhabdomyolysis. The risk of myoglobin-induced kidney injury sharply increases at this threshold.

Rhabdomyolysis

Although the classic presentation of rhabdomyolysis includes muscle pain, weakness, and dark urine, many patients have very little pain or no pain at all. If the history supports the possibility of rhabdomyolysis (eg, a recent crush injury or recent cocaine use), you should have a very low threshold to check a CK level. This is a quick, simple, and cheap test that very well may change management.

Other laboratory findings that may be seen in rhabdomyolysis include:

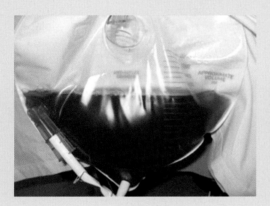

Figure 22.17 The dark "tea-colored" urine (indicative of myoglobinuria) seen in a patient with rhabdomyolysis. (From Yao FSF, Hemmings HC, Vinod Malhotra, Fong J. *Yao & Artusio's Anesthesiology: Problem-Oriented Patient Management.* 9th ed. Wolters Kluwer; 2021.)

- Elevated white blood cell count

- Elevated acute phase reactants (eg, CRP, ferritin, complements)

- Elevated potassium and phosphate with a low calcium

- Elevated creatinine (ie, acute kidney injury)

- Elevated uric acid

- Metabolic acidosis (normal or high anion gap)

- Myoglobinuria

You can remember many of these lab abnormalities by picturing the muscle cells breaking open and releasing their intracellular contents (eg, potassium, phosphate, uric acid, myoglobin).

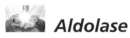

Aldolase

Like the CK, aldolase is an enzyme primarily found in skeletal muscle. However, it is both less sensitive and less specific for muscle injury than CK. For these reasons, aldolase is not routinely ordered in patients with suspected muscle damage or inflammation. However, the sensitivity of both tests together may be slightly higher than that of CK alone, so you may opt to order an aldolase along with CK in patients in whom you have a high suspicion for myositis.

The normal range of the serum aldolase is 1.0 to 7.5 U/L, with slight variation depending on the laboratory.

Other Muscle Enzymes

You may on occasion hear some clinicians refer to lactate dehydrogenase (LDH), aspartate aminotransferase (AST), and alanine aminotransferase (ALT) as "muscle enzymes." All three of these enzymes are present in muscle cells. However, like aldolase, they are less sensitive and specific for muscle injury than the CK. This is at least in part because the LDH, AST, and ALT are all found in significant concentrations in numerous tissues (AST and ALT predominantly in the liver; LDH throughout the body). As a result, they are rarely helpful in the diagnosis of muscle disorders. But because these enzymes are found in muscles, expect levels to be mildly to moderately elevated in the setting of muscle damage. Thus, patients with rhabdomyolysis and an elevated AST and ALT do not necessarily need further workup for liver disease—their transaminases may improve as the muscle injury resolves.

Myositis-Specific Autoantibodies

Patients with *idiopathic inflammatory myopathies* have traditionally been categorized as having polymyositis or dermatomyositis.* The hallmarks of these diseases include proximal muscle weakness, muscle enzyme elevations, and, in the case of dermatomyositis, characteristic skin manifestations (eg, heliotrope rash over the eyes, Gottron papules over the knuckles). Although the terms *polymyositis* and *dermatomyositis* are still widely used, several myositis-specific autoantibodies have emerged as more accurately predictive of the disease phenotype and the clinical course in patients with idiopathic inflammatory myopathies. The targets of these autoantibodies are various

---

*Other idiopathic inflammatory myopathies include inclusion body myositis (associated with antibodies against cytosolic 5'-nucleotidase 1A), antisynthetase syndrome (associated with antisynthetase antibodies), and immune-mediated necrotizing myopathy (associated with signal recognition particle [SRP] and 3-hydroxy-3-methylglutaryl coenzyme A [HMG-CoA] reductase antibodies).

intracellular antigens. Sending myositis-specific autoantibodies along with a CK is a reasonable next step in a patient with a confirmed or highly suspected idiopathic inflammatory myopathy. Most labs offer a panel of the most common of these autoantibodies. Results usually take at least a few days to come back.

Table 22.7 Examples of Myositis-Specific Autoantibodies

Myositis-Specific Autoantibody (Anti-)	Typical Clinical Features
Mi-2	"Shawl" sign rash (see Figure 22.18) Good response to immunosuppression
MDA-5	Limited or no weakness ("amyopathic") Rapidly progressive interstitial lung disease Poor prognosis
TIF-1γ	Strong association with cancer
NXP2	Ulcerations and subcutaneous calcifications Muscle enzymes may be normal Association with cancer
SRP	Acute-onset, severe myositis Myocarditis Poor response to immunosuppression
HMG-CoA reductase	Severe myositis (CK often >5,000 U/L) Strong association with statin exposure
Antisynthetase antibodies: Jo-1, PL-7, PL-12, EJ, OJ, KS, Zo, Ha, Mas, lysyl	Mechanic's hands (see Figure 22.19) Early interstitial lung disease Arthritis

CK, creatine kinase; HMG-CoA, 3-hydroxy-3-methylglutaryl coenzyme A.

These autoantibodies tend to be much more specific than they are sensitive. So, for example, a positive anti-Mi-2 in a patient with characteristic manifestations of dermatomyositis confirms the diagnosis. A negative anti-Mi-2 in the same patient, however, does not rule out dermatomyositis.

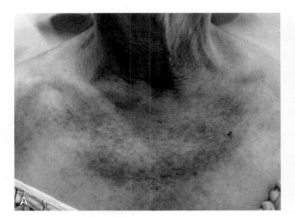
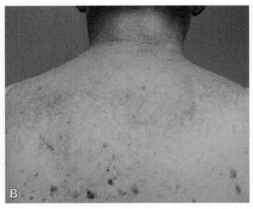

Figure 22.18 A and B. The "shawl" sign—an erythematous rash over the upper back and chest—is a common finding in patients with anti-Mi-2 positive dermatomyositis. (A: From Bennett R, Bradley K, Salem I, et al. A case of paraneoplastic anti-TIF1-γ antibody-positive dermatomyositis presenting with generalized edema and associated with aortic aneurysm. *Dermato*. 2023;3(4):232-240. B: From Council LM, Sheinbein DM, Cornelius LA, Mo L. *The Washington Manual of Dermatology Diagnostics*. Wolters Kluwer; 2016.)

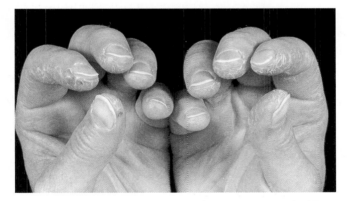

Figure 22.19 Antisynthetase antibodies are associated with the development of so-called antisynthetase syndrome. Common signs include myositis, interstitial lung disease, and—most specifically—cracking and fissuring of the lateral and palmar surfaces of the fingers ("mechanic's hands"). (From Koopman WJ, Moreland LW. *Arthritis and Allied Conditions: A Textbook of Rheumatology*. 15th ed. Lippincott Williams & Wilkins; 2005.)

VASCULITIS-ASSOCIATED ANTIBODIES

Many infections and autoimmune disorders (eg, syphilis, rheumatoid arthritis) can cause vasculitis. In these cases, the laboratory workup of vasculitis simply entails testing for the suspected underlying disease(s). There are a few important vasculitides, however, that warrant their own special diagnostic laboratory testing.

 Antineutrophil Cytoplasmic Antibodies

It's in the name: ANCAs are antibodies to proteins located in the cytoplasm of neutrophils. The most common target antigens are proteinase 3 (PR3) and myeloperoxidase (MPO).

ANCAs are often found in the aptly named ANCA-associated vasculitides, which include *granulomatosis with polyangiitis (GPA), eosinophilic granulomatosis with polyangiitis (eGPA),* and *microscopic polyangiitis (MPA).* The classic presentation of ANCA-associated vasculitis is a so-called *pulmonary-renal syndrome* involving both lung inflammation (often manifesting as hemoptysis) and glomerulonephritis. Multiple other organs may be affected, and associated arthritis is common. Rarely, some medications (eg, hydralazine and minocycline) and toxins (eg, levamisole-laced cocaine) may cause an ANCA-associated vasculitis that tends to present more nonspecifically with constitutional symptoms and arthralgias.

ANCA testing can be done in two ways:

1. Immunofluorescence

   • When fluorescence is seen throughout the *c*ytoplasm, the pattern is called *c*-ANCA. This pattern is most closely associated with GPA.

   • When fluorescence is seen around the nucleus (*p*erinuclear), the pattern is called *p*-ANCA. This pattern is most associated with eGPA and MPA. It may also be seen in drug-induced ANCA-associated vasculitis.

   • Other ANCA patterns are called *atypical ANCA* and are nonspecific.

2. ELISA

   • This tests directly for *anti-PR3* and *anti-MPO* antibodies.

   • Anti-PR3 antibodies usually correlate with a c-ANCA pattern.

   • Anti-MPO antibodies usually correlate with a p-ANCA pattern.

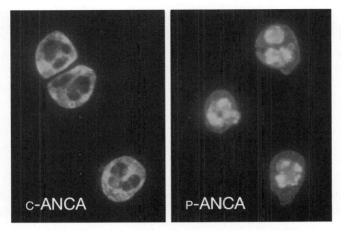

Figure 22.20 The c-ANCA pattern and anti-PR3 antibodies are associated with GPA. The p-ANCA pattern and anti-MPO antibodies are associated with eGPA and MPA. c-ANCA, cytoplasmic antineutrophil cytoplasmic antibody; eGPA, eosinophilic granulomatosis with polyangiitis; GPA, granulomatosis with polyangiitis; MPA, microscopic polyangiitis; MPO, myeloperoxidase; p-ANCA, perinuclear antineutrophil cytoplasmic antibody. (From Jennette JC, Olson JL, Schwartz MM, Silva FG. *Heptinstall's Pathology of the Kidney.* 6th ed. Lippincott Williams & Wilkins; 2007.)

If you are concerned about ANCA-associated vasculitis, send ANCA IFA as well as anti-PR3 and anti-MPO antibodies. Sending these tests together increases both the sensitivity and specificity for ANCA-associated vasculitis.

About 10% to 15% of patients with GPA or MPA, and nearly half of patients with eGPA, have completely negative ANCA testing. This means that ANCA testing is not sensitive enough to rule out ANCA-associated vasculitis —especially eGPA—by itself.

What about false positives? Positive ANCAs—usually p-ANCA or atypical ANCA—may occasionally be seen in other diseases such as rheumatoid arthritis, lupus, Sjögren syndrome, inflammatory bowel disease, primary sclerosing cholangitis (PSC), cystic fibrosis, HIV infection, parvovirus B19, Epstein-Barr virus, and tuberculosis. One clue that a patient might have one of these non-vasculitic causes of positive ANCAs is a discordant or "mismatched" result—for example, a positive c-ANCA but a negative anti-PR3, or a positive p-ANCA but a negative anti-MPO. Although c-ANCA has overall good specificity for GPA (about 90%), a positive c-ANCA, sometimes even with corresponding high-titer anti-PR3 antibodies, may be seen in endocarditis in cases of long-standing untreated disease.

Wonky Labs in Endocarditis

Endocarditis has come up several times in this chapter on autoimmune disorders. This is no coincidence. Endocarditis can affect nearly any organ via hematogenous spread (the heart, after all, pumps blood to the entire body). Not only does this mean it can mimic the symptomatology and end organ damage of many systemic autoimmune disorders, but it also tends to induce a robust immune response that can easily become pathologic in and of itself, especially if the infection goes undiagnosed and untreated for a long time. Here's a summary of the various immune phenomena and related labs you may see in a patient with infective endocarditis:

- Positive RF

- Glomerulonephritis caused by immune complex deposition in the kidneys resulting in hypocomplementemia (low C3 and C4), elevated creatinine, and cells and/or protein in the urine

- ANCA positivity, usually c-ANCA with anti-PR3 antibodies. ANCAs in endocarditis typically don't cause vasculitis; in the rare instances when they do, the treatment is still to treat the endocarditis, not to give immunosuppression.

- Cryoglobulinemia resulting from the formation of immune complexes (see next section). As with ANCAs, treat the endocarditis, not the cryoglobulins.

 Cryoglobulins

Cryoglobulins are antibodies (immunoglobulins) or antibody-containing complexes that precipitate out of the blood at cold temperatures (<37 °C) and dissolve again with rewarming. Many of these antibodies tend to have RF activity—that is, binding affinity for one's own IgG. This is why RF is so often positive in cryoglobulinemia (see Table 22.5).

Any patient with circulating cryoglobulins is said to have cryoglobulinemia. If the cryoglobulins consist of multiple types of antibodies (polyclonal immunoglobulins), the patient is said to have *mixed cryoglobulinemia*. This is by far the most common type of cryoglobulinemia; it may be idiopathic but often is associated with underlying hepatitis C infection or autoimmune disease (Sjögren syndrome, lupus, and rheumatoid arthritis are the most common culprits). Much less commonly, the cryoglobulins may consist of a single population of monoclonal antibodies; this so-called t*ype I cryoglobulinemia* is strongly associated with the monoclonal gammopathies (eg, multiple myeloma) and B-cell malignancies (eg, chronic lymphocytic leukemia [CLL]).

Cryoglobulinemia can be asymptomatic, but immune complex deposition in blood vessels can lead to cryoglobulinemic vasculitis. Signs and symptoms of cryoglobulinemic vasculitis that should prompt consideration of cryoglobulin testing include purpura, arthralgias, weakness (these first three symptoms together are known as "Meltzer triad"), peripheral neuropathy, and glomerulonephritis. Your threshold for testing should be much lower in patients with any of the related diseases mentioned above.

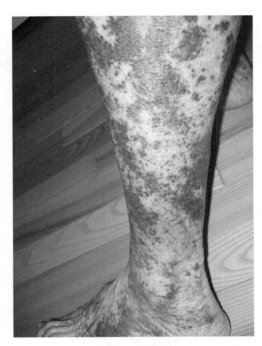

Figure 22.21 Confluent palpable purpura in a patient with mixed cryoglobulinemia. This disease is strongly associated with hepatitis C. (From Marder VJ, Aird WC, Bennett JS, Schulman S, White GC. *Hemostasis and Thrombosis: Basic Principles and Clinical Practice.* 6th ed. Wolters Kluwer/Lippincott Williams & Wilkins Health; 2013.)

Testing for cryoglobulins involves allowing a blood sample to clot at 37 °C, then removing the serum for transfer to the lab where it will be cooled and observed for the precipitation of cryoglobulins over several days. The presence of cryoglobulins is confirmed when they redissolve upon rewarming the sample.

There is significant variability in how labs report the results of cryoglobulin testing. Usually, the report of any positive result includes a cryoglobulin type (eg, monoclonal vs polyclonal, and IgM vs IgG vs IgA) and amount. The amount may be given in concentration, "cryocrit" (see Figure 22.22), or both. *A cryocrit more than 1% or a cryoglobulin concentration more than 50 µg/mL is generally considered to be clinically significant and confirms the diagnosis of cryoglobulinemic vasculitis in the appropriate clinical context.* Patients with type I cryoglobulinemia tend to have particularly elevated levels of circulating cryoglobulins and usually have a cryocrit more than 5%.

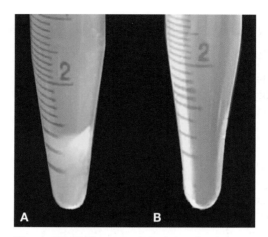

Figure 22.22 The cryocrit is determined by measuring the height of the column of cryoglobulins after centrifugation at 4 °C. Cryoglobulins redissolve upon rewarming of the solution. (From Chen YP, Cheng H, Rui HL, Dong HR. Cryoglobulinemic vasculitis and glomerulonephritis: concerns in clinical practice. *Chin Med J.* 2019;132(14):1723-1732.)

Sample mishandling is common because of the precise cooling and rewarming process that is required for proper cryoglobulin testing. As a result, false negatives are common. If you have a high level of suspicion for cryoglobulinemic vasculitis despite a negative result, consider retesting (and/or contacting the lab).

When Cryoglobulin Testing Comes Back Positive: Next Steps

If your patient has a known diagnosis of an associated condition (eg, a patient with known multiple myeloma tests positive for type I cryoglobulinemia; or a patient with known hepatitis C tests positive for mixed cryoglobulinemia), your diagnostic work may be done. However, any patient with otherwise unexplained cryoglobulinemia should be evaluated further for an associated underlying condition. Depending on cryoglobulin type (mixed vs type I) and clinical presentation, consider additional testing for the following:

- Hepatitis C (by far the most common underlying condition in patients with mixed cryoglobulinemia)

- Sjögren syndrome

- Lupus

- Rheumatoid arthritis

- Monoclonal gammopathy (eg, multiple myeloma, Waldenstrom macroglobulinemia)

- B-cell malignancy (eg, CLL, B-cell lymphomas)

  Always send complement levels to check for complement consumption from active immune complex deposition, especially in mixed cryoglobulinemia. A low C4 in particular correlates very well with disease activity.

 ## Anti–Glomerular Basement Membrane Antibodies

Anti–glomerular basement membrane (GBM) antibodies are directed against a collagen component found in the GBM of the kidneys *and*—less obviously—in the alveolar basement membrane of the lungs. The associated pulmonary-renal syndrome is known as *Goodpasture* (or *anti-GBM*) *disease* and presents most commonly with rapidly progressive glomerulonephritis with or without hemoptysis. Either or both of these findings should prompt consideration of anti-GBM testing.

Serologic anti-GBM testing is usually done by ELISA. The upper limit of normal varies by lab, but a result more than 2 U is generally considered abnormal. A positive anti-GBM ELISA is confirmed with a western blot; this combination has very good specificity and confirms anti-GBM disease in the appropriate clinical context. Sensitivity varies significantly by lab and technique. Biopsy (renal > lung) is the gold standard test for diagnosis and should be considered in any patient with a negative anti-GBM ELISA in whom you have high suspicion for anti-GBM disease.

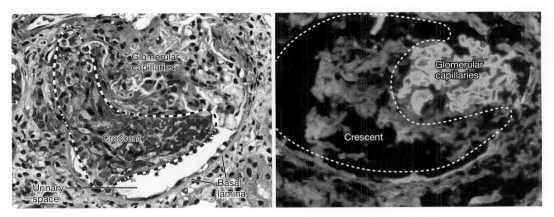

Figure 22.23 Definitive diagnosis of anti-GBM disease can be made by biopsy with immunofluorescence staining demonstrating linear IgG anti-GBM deposition. The crescents highlighted here represent collections of inflammatory and epithelial cells. In the setting of high clinical suspicion for anti-GBM disease, negative serum anti-GBM testing should usually be followed by biopsy. Positive serum anti-GBM testing may be enough to confirm the diagnosis without the need for biopsy. GBM, glomerular basement membrane; IgG, immunoglobulin G. (From Jennette JC, Olson JL, Silva FB, D'Agati VD. *Heptinstall's Pathology of the Kidney.* 7th ed. Wolters Kluwer; 2015.)

For reasons that are not fully understood, a significant minority (some estimates are as high as 50%) of patients with anti-GBM disease may also test positive for ANCAs, particularly p-ANCA/anti-MPO. Some of these patients have an "overlap syndrome" with features of both anti-GBM disease and ANCA-associated vasculitis. We recommend sending ANCA testing in any patient found to have anti-GBM disease. Although the implications for prognosis and treatment are not entirely clear, most experts agree it is helpful to know if a patient with anti-GBM antibodies also has ANCA positivity, and vice versa. As the clinical picture evolves, this knowledge may impact treatment decisions going forward.

 ## Anti-C1q Antibodies

Antibodies against the complement component C1q (anti-C1q) have been found to be associated with *hypocomplementemic urticarial vasculitis* (HUV), a small-vessel vasculitis that presents with recurrent hives (often lasting more than 24 hours), arthralgias, ocular inflammation, obstructive pulmonary disease, and recurrent angioedema. Elevated anti-C1q levels are highly specific for HUV in the appropriate clinical context. Sensitivity, however, is not as impressive (about 60%), so negative anti-C1q antibodies should not be used to rule out HUV.

Low levels of the C1q antigen itself are a more sensitive finding; we recommend sending both anti-C1q and C1q antigen levels in any patient with suspected HUV.

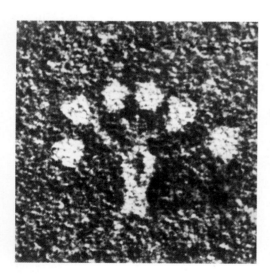

Figure 22.24 Magnified electron micrograph (500,000×) of C1q. Some experts also check anti-C1q levels in patients with suspected lupus nephritis as titer levels have been found to correlate with renal disease activity. Because the normal range of anti-C1q has not been well established (and varies significantly by lab), trending levels over time is most helpful. (From Schaechter M, Dirita VJ, Dermody T, Engleberg NC. *Schaechter's Mechanisms of Microbial Disease.* 5th ed. Wolters Kluwer Health/Lippincott Williams & Wilkins; 2013.)

ERYTHROCYTE SEDIMENTATION RATE AND C-REACTIVE PROTEIN

We refer to the ESR and CRP as *inflammatory markers* because they measure inflammation, a common sign of infection, malignancy, tissue injury, and many autoimmune disorders. By themselves, ESR and CRP are neither sensitive nor specific for autoimmune disease.

There are two main reasons to check an ESR and a CRP:

1. Differentiate an inflammatory condition from a noninflammatory condition. Common examples include osteomyelitis versus osteonecrosis, or giant cell arteritis versus temporomandibular joint dysfunction.

2. Monitor disease activity or response to treatment in a patient with an established inflammatory disease. This practice is most common in patients with autoimmune diseases and serious infections. The trend in ESR and CRP does not always line up with the trend in the clinical exam. You'll need to step back and look at all the data together to decide on the next steps.

 ## *Erythrocyte Sedimentation Rate*

The ESR is not actually a protein or any kind of molecule. *The ESR is the rate at which RBCs fall in the patient's plasma when suspended vertically.*

In inflammatory states, RBCs tend to flatten out and stick together, which causes them to fall to the bottom of the tube faster. Why does this happen? The cell membranes of RBCs are negatively charged and therefore tend to repel each other. During inflammation, various proteins, notably fibrinogen, coat the RBCs, reducing their negative charge and thereby allowing them to stack together and fall more quickly. A higher ESR indicates a faster rate of falling, which correlates with more inflammation.

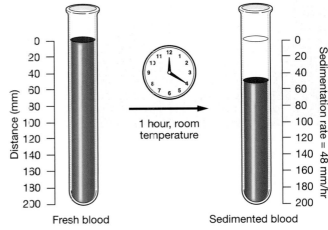

Figure 22.25 The farther the red blood cells fall in 1 hour, the higher the erythrocyte sedimentation rate. (From Rhoades R, Bell DR. *Medical Physiology: Principles for Clinical Medicine.* 4th ed. Lippincott Williams & Wilkins; 2013.)

A commonly used normal range for the ESR is 0 to 15 mm/hr in males and 0 to 20 mm/hr in females. However, for reasons that are incompletely understood, the ESR tends to increase slightly as we get older even in the absence of underlying inflammatory disease. We can account for this normal age-related increase in the ESR by defining the upper limit of normal as:

Males: ESR upper limit of normal (mm/hr) = (age in years)/2

Females: ESR upper limit of normal (mm/hr) = (age in years + 10)/2

So, for example, we consider an ESR of 44 mm/hr in an 80-year-old female to be normal ([80+10]/2 = 45 mm/hr = ESR upper limit of normal).

There are a few other conditions, none of which we conventionally think of as inflammatory conditions, that can cause elevations in the ESR:

- Anemia

- Chronic kidney disease

- Hypoalbuminemia

- Obesity

- Pregnancy

- Macrocytosis

- Hypergammaglobulinemia; for example, recent use of intravenous immunoglobulin (IVIG)

A false-positive ESR caused by lab error is rare. If this does happen, it is usually due to a high room temperature or mishandling of the test tube. Repeat the test if you suspect lab error.

When the Erythrocyte Sedimentation Rate Is Really High

A profoundly elevated ESR to more than 100 mm/hr should almost always be taken seriously; it cannot be chalked up to old age, obesity, anemia, or pregnancy. The most common causes of an ESR more than 100 include the following:

- Acute or severe infection (often bacterial)

- Malignancy

- Chronic kidney disease

- Autoimmune inflammatory disease (especially vasculitis)

Occasionally, the ESR may be normal (ie, <~20 mm/hr) in the presence of significant inflammation. Causes of a false-negative ESR tend to be those that increase plasma viscosity and include:

- Diseases that distort the normal RBC shape (eg, sickle cell disease or spherocytosis; picture the oddly shaped RBCs getting in each other's way as they try to fall to the bottom of the tube)

- Polycythemia (primary or secondary)

- Extreme leukocytosis

- Extreme elevations in bile salt levels

- Hypofibrinogenemia

- Severe cachexia

- Rarely, lab error (clotting of sample, low room temperature)

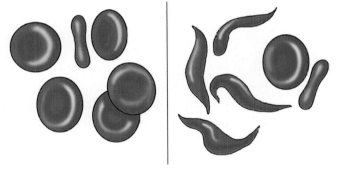

Figure 22.26 The irregular sickle-shaped red blood cells on the right are more likely to get in each other's way—lowering the rate of fall and hence the erythrocyte sedimentation rate—than the smooth, regular red blood cells on the left. (From Wilkins EM, Wyche CJ. *Clinical Practice of the Dental Hygienist*. 11th ed. Wolters Kluwer Health/Lippincott Williams & Wilkins; 2013.)

 ## C-Reactive Protein

Unlike the ESR, the CRP is actually a protein that we measure directly. It is produced by the liver. The CRP is an acute phase reactant—hence an indicator of inflammation—and has many functions in the immune response, including recognizing and eliminating pathogens and clearing away damaged cells.

A commonly used upper limit of normal for CRP is 0.8 mg/dL. However, the exact upper limit varies significantly depending on the lab. About 80% of healthy people have a CRP less than 0.3 mg/dL. A CRP between 0.3 and 1 mg/dL may indicate either low-grade inflammation or a normal result, depending on the patient. Consider a CRP more than 1 mg/dL abnormal—that is, a sign of clinically significant inflammation.

C-Reactive Protein: Common Pitfalls

1. Different units of measurement

   The normal values cited above are given in mg/dL. These are the units we will use. However, some labs report CRP in mg/L, moving the decimal point over one place to the right. A CRP of 3 mg/dL is the same as a CRP of 30 mg/L. So, using the normal ranges, a CRP more than 10 mg/L (>1 mg/dL) is abnormal. When interpreting the results of a CRP, always glance at the lab's listed units and normal range (if the latter is given).

2. CRP versus "high-sensitivity" CRP

   Many modern labs measure a "high-sensitivity" CRP (or "hs-CRP") using a modified assay designed to be more precise at lower levels (CRP < 1 mg/dL). *hs-CRP is exactly the same protein as regular old CRP and should be interpreted in exactly the same way.* It is unclear whether any small differences in low CRP levels that may be detected by these assays are clinically significant.

The CRP tends to increase slightly with age, but less so than the ESR.

Mild elevations in CRP—values between 0.3 and 1 mg/dL associated with "low-level inflammation"—commonly occur in metabolic syndrome, diabetes, atherosclerosis, obesity, obstructive sleep apnea, and hypertension.

The higher the CRP above 10 mg/dL, the stronger the association with infection (particularly bacterial infection).

We recommend that you order an ESR and a CRP together. Interpreting these results together allows you to better account for the multiple possible (noninflammatory) factors that can influence each lab test individually. Of the two tests, the ESR is much more prone to influence from noninflammatory confounding factors. In most patients with an active or flaring inflammatory disease, expect both the ESR and CRP to be elevated.

When the Erythrocyte Sedimentation Rate and C-Reactive Protein Don't Agree

Discordance between the ESR and CRP occurs frequently, often without any obvious reason. This phenomenon is particularly common in a few specific scenarios:

1. Inpatient or short-term monitoring: The CRP tends to rise and fall more rapidly than the ESR. This usually doesn't make a difference in the outpatient setting, where you may be checking these labs only every few weeks to months. But, in the inpatient setting,

where labs may be drawn every day, you may find that the trend in the ESR tends to lag behind the trend in the CRP by 1 day or even more.

2. Lupus: A disproportionately elevated ESR with a normal or only mildly elevated CRP is commonly seen in clinically active lupus.

3. The presence of confounding factors: As discussed earlier, many noninflammatory factors may influence either the ESR or CRP. For example, a patient with extreme baseline leukocytosis from underlying CLL is likely to have a low or normal ESR (see page 465) even in the presence of inflammation; the CRP, on the other hand, is affected much less (or not at all) by the severe leukocytosis and may be elevated.

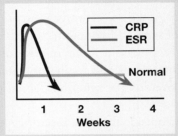

Figure 22.27 Typical patterns in the rise and fall of CRP and ESR, following an acute infection. CRP, C-reactive protein; ESR, erythrocyte sedimentation rate. (From Staheli LT. *Fundamentals of Pediatric Orthopedics.* 5th ed. Wolters Kluwer Health, 2015. Based on Unkila-Kallio, 1993.)

23 Toxicology and Therapeutic Drug Monitoring

TOXICOLOGY

Has your patient been poisoned? And if so, with what? Any *toxidrome*, a term sometimes used to describe the collection of signs and symptoms suggestive of a toxic ingestion or medication overdose, should prompt consideration of urine or serum toxicology testing. Classic examples are altered mental status, low respiratory rate, absent bowel sounds, and pinpoint pupils after an opioid overdose; or agitation, aggression, and nystagmus after phencyclidine use.

Toxicology is commonly used outside the clinical setting—in forensic medicine, competitive sports, and the legal system—but our focus will be on the use of these tests for clinical diagnosis and management.

 ### *Urine Toxicology Panel*

The urine toxicology panel combines tests for several common drugs (both illicit and prescription) and is by far the most widely used toxicology screen in medicine. Advantages include its convenience and noninvasiveness, rapid results (within minutes to hours), and the ability to detect many substances for days to weeks after they were last ingested. Although there is variation among labs as to which tests are included, the panel usually includes all or most of the drugs in Table 23.1.

Most drugs can be detected in the urine well after the signs and symptoms of acute intoxication have resolved. A positive result indicates that the patient used the drug within the detection time, not necessarily that he or she is currently intoxicated.

Results are usually calculated quantitatively (ie, as a concentration) but reported qualitatively (ie, as positive or negative). The threshold concentration at which each drug is reported as "positive" varies significantly among laboratories. In general, the cutoff values for clinical use are lower (fewer false negatives) than those for nonclinical/medicolegal use (fewer false positives).

Table 23.1 Drugs Commonly Included in a Urine Toxicology Screening Panel

Drug	Urine Detection Time[a]	May Cause False Positives	May Be Missed (False Negatives)
Amphetamines	2-3 d	Antihistamines Decongestants Bupropion β-Blockers	3,4-Methylenedioxy-methamphetamine (MDMA)[b] Methamphetamine
Barbiturates	Short acting: 2 d Long acting: 2 wk	Phenytoin Ibuprofen, naproxen	Rare
Benzodiaze-pines	Short acting: 3 d Long acting: 3 wk	Rare	Midazolam Lorazepam Alprazolam
Cocaine	2-3 d	Rare	Rare
Marijuana	1-6 wk	Hemp-containing foods Ibuprofen, naproxen Proton pump inhibitors Efavirenz	Synthetic cannabinoids
Opiates/opioids	Short acting: 2 d Long acting: 1 wk	Poppy seeds Fluoroquinolones	Synthetic/semisyn-thetic opioids[c]
Phencyclidine	1-2 wk	Antihistamines Dextromethorphan Tramadol	Rare

[a]Refers to the *typical* amount of time since the last use that the drug can still be detected in the urine. Detection time can vary significantly depending on factors such as drug dose and frequency, duration of use, and patient metabolism.
[b]The amphetamine screen may detect MDMA that has been used in large doses. Specific urine and serum tests for MDMA exist.
[c]Common examples of synthetic or semisynthetic opioids include fentanyl, meperidine, methadone, tramadol, hydrocodone, hydromorphone, oxycodone, oxymorphone, and buprenorphine. Assays that detect many of these drugs are widely available and are routinely added to many urine drug screen panels. Always check to see which opioids your lab tests for. You may need to add on specific tests manually.

Most components of the urine toxicology panel are prone to significant rates of both false positives and false negatives.

- Any substance with a chemical structure similar to the drug of interest may produce a false positive. Confirmatory tests exist but usually take several days to come back, and as a result, have limited clinical utility. Clinical context, then, is the most important factor in determining whether a positive result is a true positive.

- False negatives may occur after ingestion of a drug whose chemical structure (or that of its metabolites) differs from that of other drugs in the same class in such a way as to render it unreactive with the testing assay. You may need to send separate specific tests if you are concerned about the use of one or more drugs commonly missed on the urine toxicology screen. Other causes of false negatives—for any drug—include a highly dilute urine or sample adulteration (the addition of substances that destroy the drug in question or otherwise interfere with the testing).

Remember that there are many drugs that a routine urine toxicology screen does *not* test for at all—for example, hallucinogenic mushrooms, synthetic cathinones ("bath salts"), lysergic acid diethylamide (LSD), and many more. Do not rule out substance abuse in a patient based on a negative urine toxicology screen alone.

The Poppy Seed Defense

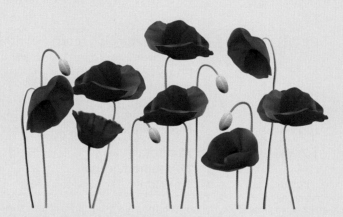

Figure 23.1 The seeds of poppies may cause false-positive results for opiates on urine toxicology screening. (Courtesy ecco/Shutterstock.)

Poppy seeds contain several opioid alkaloids and are a potential cause of false-positive testing for opiates (morphine or codeine) on urine toxicology screening. Historically, this issue was significant enough that the federal workplace testing guidelines increased the positivity threshold for morphine from 300 to 2,000 ng/mL in 1998. Although this change has made a false positive less likely (for morphine in particular), most data suggest that false positives from poppy seed consumption may still occur, even up to one day after consumption of as little as a single poppy seed roll or a single teaspoon of raw poppy seeds. The precise false-positive rate is not well established. Salivary testing has been proposed as an alternative, but similar issues with false positives have been reported.

If a patient tests positive for opiates on a urine toxicology screen and endorses a recent history (within ~24 hours) of poppy seed consumption, consider retesting in 1 to 2 days.

Additional Toxicology Testing

There are several substances that require specific blood and/or urine tests in cases of suspected ingestion or overdose. We will highlight a few of the most important and commonly tested.

Lead

Consider lead poisoning in patients with unexplained subacute neuropsychiatric symptoms, arthralgias, and/or abdominal pain in the setting of a possible exposure (eg, lead paint in the home). The most common clue on routine lab work is a microcytic anemia with *basophilic stippling* of the red blood cells. Even in the absence of signs or symptoms suggestive of lead toxicity, patients with known high-risk exposures or occupations (eg, welders) may warrant regular monitoring.

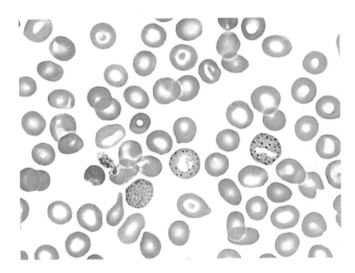

Figure 23.2 Basophilic stippling can be seen in several red blood cells. (From Pereira I, George TI, Arber DA. *Atlas of Peripheral Blood: The Primary Diagnostic Tool*. Wolters Kluwer Health/Lippincott Williams & Wilkins; 2012.)

The normal range for the venous lead level is less than 5 µg/dL in children and less than 10 µg/dL in adults. An elevated lead level in any patient should prompt further discussion about reducing environmental exposure. Above 10 µg/dL, higher blood lead levels tend to correlate with more severe symptoms and poorer prognosis. Any combination of symptoms attributable to lead toxicity or a blood lead level greater than 40 µg/dL is typically an indication for chelation therapy.

Erythrocyte Protoporphyrin: The "Hemoglobin A1c for Lead"

How do you approach the diagnosis of recent—but not ongoing—lead poisoning? This may come up in a patient with end-organ damage and suspected recent lead exposure who has a normal or only borderline-elevated blood lead level. Consider the analogy of blood glucose and hemoglobin A1c: if you can regard the blood lead level to be analogous to the blood glucose, you need a "hemoglobin A1c for lead." *Erythrocyte protoporphyrin* can be used in this way.

High concentrations of lead inhibit hemoglobin synthesis. As a result, hemoglobin precursors—including protoporphyrin—accumulate inside red blood cells. Elevated levels of protoporphyrin can, therefore, be found for up to 4 months following exposure to toxic levels of lead, the approximate lifetime of a typical red blood cell. Erythrocyte protoporphyrin is usually measured as zinc protoporphyrin (ZPP; free protoporphyrin is elevated, too, but measuring it doesn't add helpful information). A ZPP above 35 μg/dL is consistent with significant lead exposure in the last 3 to 4 months. But be careful! Elevations in ZPP are also seen in iron deficiency anemia, sickle cell disease, and porphyria.

Mercury

Mercury comes in several forms. *Organic mercury*—mercury combined with carbon compounds—can be found in contaminated seafood and constitutes the vast majority of mercury most of us come in contact with. *Elemental mercury*, the silver, odorless liquid you probably think of when you think of mercury, can be found in old thermometers, light bulbs, mined ores/rocks, and some dental fillings. *Mercury salts*, such as mercurous chloride and mercuric oxide, can be found in some disinfectants and cosmetic skin creams.

Exposure to any form of mercury can lead to mercury poisoning and cause a wide range of acute or chronic symptoms depending on the nature and extent of the exposure. Manifestations may range from subtle neuropsychiatric symptoms, such as insomnia or mild tremor, to renal disease, severe gastroenteritis, or acute respiratory failure. The term *acrodynia* refers to a syndrome specific for mercury poisoning seen almost exclusively in children that manifests as rash (often involving the palms and soles; desquamation is a late feature), peripheral edema, fever, photophobia, and irritability.

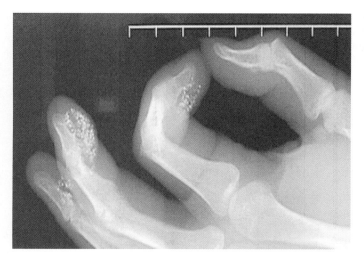

Figure 23.3 Subcutaneous mercury deposits in a patient who deliberately injected mercury into his fingers. Deliberate self-poisoning with mercury—in the form of pills or subcutaneous injection—has historically been used as a spiritual or folk remedy for many illnesses including syphilis and parasitic infections. Don't do this. (From Wolfson AB, Cloutier RL, Hendey GW, Ling LJ, Schaider LJ, Rosen CL. *Harwood-Nuss' Clinical Practice of Emergency Medicine.* 6th ed. Wolters Kluwer; 2014.)

Given the number of possible sources of mercury exposure in our environment, one would think that mercury toxicity is common. This, however, is not the case, at least in part because the amount of mercury we are exposed to on a routine basis (even if, for example, we have several mercury-containing dental fillings) is thought to be well below the threshold for clinical toxicity.

It is reasonable to consider testing for mercury toxicity in a patient with one or more relevant exposures and compatible clinical signs or symptoms. However, remember that *"common things are common."* Do not anchor on mercury poisoning when much more common etiologies remain on the differential diagnosis.

The two most useful tests for mercury toxicity are a *24-hour urine mercury* and *whole blood mercury*. It is reasonable to order both whenever mercury toxicity is suspected, but it is important to note that there are a few key differences in the utility of these two tests.

- *24-hour urine mercury* is most useful for cases of suspected *low-grade or chronic mercury toxicity* because levels are more reflective of long-term exposure than whole blood mercury. The upper limit of normal is controversial—50 µg/24 hr is a common estimation—as is the extent to which urine mercury concentration correlates with the severity of symptoms. Importantly, organic mercury (eg, from contaminated seafood) is not readily excreted in the urine, so blood testing must be used when organic mercury poisoning is suspected.

- *Whole blood mercury* is most useful for suspected *acute* mercury toxicity. Redistribution of mercury throughout the body makes whole blood mercury less and less reflective of the total body mercury burden over time. As with the 24-hour urine mercury, the upper limit of normal for whole blood mercury is controversial, with estimates ranging from 10 to 50 µg/L.

Because mercury accumulates in hair over the course of one's lifetime, a hair sample should theoretically be more representative of an individual's lifetime mercury exposure than a blood or urine sample. However, measurement of hair mercury concentration is prone to errors in specimen collection and analysis, and correlation with symptoms tends to be poor. Additionally, contamination of hair from environmental mercury that is never absorbed into the body (and thus is presumably clinically irrelevant) makes interpretation of hair mercury concentrations challenging.

The Heavy Metal Panel

Lead and mercury are only two of many heavy metals that can cause toxicity to humans. Other examples include arsenic, cadmium, chromium, thallium, aluminum, copper, nickel, selenium, cobalt, and many more. The heavy metals tend to share risk factors for exposure (eg, mining) and symptoms of toxicity (eg, neuropsychiatric and gastrointestinal [GI] symptoms). As a result, various panels have been developed that test blood levels of many heavy metals at once.

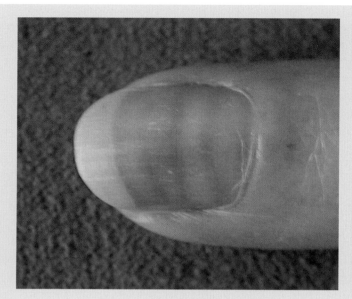

Figure 23.4 The transverse lines in this patient's nail bed are called "Mees lines" and are a feature common to poisoning with many heavy metals, usually arsenic or thallium. However, even this seemingly "heavy metal-specific" sign can be seen in other clinical scenarios including repeated hand/nail trauma, infection (mostly as a postinfectious phenomenon), and the use of certain medications (eg, systemic retinoids). (From Orient JM. *Sapira's Art & Science of Bedside Diagnosis*. 5th ed. Wolters Kluwer; 2018.)

Be judicious about whether or not to order a heavy metal panel. Small serum concentrations of some heavy metals can be normal findings in healthy individuals (eg, a venous arsenic concentration up to around 20 to 30 µg/L is considered normal; with some other heavy metals, the normal range is not at all well established). In addition, an elevated concentration of one or more heavy metals does not mean that the patient's presentation—which may include only nonspecific symptoms such as GI distress and brain fog—is necessarily attributable to heavy metal poisoning.

Acetaminophen

Acetaminophen overdose is by far the most common cause of acute liver failure in the United States. In cases of suspected acetaminophen poisoning, check an *acetaminophen level with a venous blood sample*. A urine screen exists but, because it is not quantitative, is generally not clinically useful.

Provided it has been at least 4 hours since the last dose of acetaminophen, a serum concentration greater than or equal to 150 µg/mL indicates potential toxicity. If it has not yet been 4 hours since the presumed acetaminophen ingestion, peak levels may not have been reached and a level should be rechecked at 4 hours.

It may be helpful to consult the *Rumack-Matthew nomogram* after obtaining an acetaminophen concentration; plotting acetaminophen concentration and time since ingestion on this graph roughly predicts the probability of liver injury and may help guide whether *N*-acetylcysteine (NAC; the antidote commonly used to prevent or mitigate liver damage due to acetaminophen poisoning) needs to be initiated or continued. This nomogram can only be used after a single acute ingestion. It is not applicable when the patient has repeatedly been taking supratherapeutic doses of acetaminophen. In the latter circumstance, clinical factors weigh heavily on the decision to hospitalize the patient and start NAC (eg, symptoms compatible with toxicity, underlying liver disease, amount and frequency of ingestion, liver enzyme abnormalities at presentation). In clinical practice, the threshold for initiating treatment with NAC in any case of suspected acetaminophen overdose (regardless of initial acetaminophen concentration) is extremely low given the minimal risks associated with NAC.

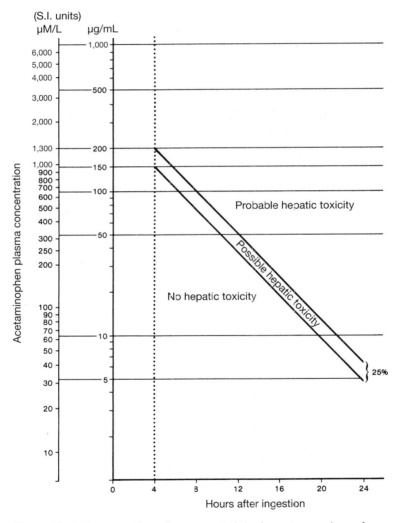

Figure 23.5 After a confirmed or suspected single acute overdose of acetaminophen, plot the acetaminophen concentration and time since ingestion on the Rumack-Matthew nomogram to help determine the patient's prognosis and need for *N*-acetylcysteine (NAC). (Reproduced with permission from Rumack BH. Acetaminophen overdose in children and adolescents. *Pediatr Clin North Am*. 1986;33:691-701.)

Ethanol

The most commonly ordered ethanol test is a *blood ethanol level*, which remains positive up to 12 hours after the most recent ingestion. A result less than 10 mg/dL is considered negative.

Most people begin to feel symptoms of alcohol intoxication such as decreased inhibition at a blood ethanol level of around 50 mg/dL. At around 150 to 200 mg/dL, significant behavioral and personality changes, unstable gait, and confusion are usually apparent. Chronic alcohol users and those with alcohol dependence may not develop symptoms until concentrations reach higher levels because of the downregulation of γ-aminobutyric acid (GABA) receptors. A blood ethanol level is rarely necessary to diagnose acute alcohol intoxication in the appropriate clinical context. However, this test can be helpful in the evaluation of suspected alcohol withdrawal (eg, GI distress, agitation, tremor, and headache after recent alcohol cessation). Those who withdraw from alcohol at higher blood ethanol concentrations tend to have a more severe course of withdrawal.

What tests can you check if you want to determine if your patient has ingested ethanol recently but not in the past 12 hours (ie, over the past few days or weeks)? This may come up in any setting where chemical confirmation of sobriety is required, such as in the workup of a potential candidate for liver transplantation. Two are widely used:

- *Urine ethylglucuronide (EtG)* is an ethanol metabolite that persists in the urine for 1 to 3 days after the most recent ingestion. Sensitivity and specificity are both very good.

- *Serum phosphatidylethanol (PEth)* is a phospholipid formed only when ethanol is present. The phospholipid hangs around a lot longer than the ethanol—PEth may be positive up to several weeks after the most recent ingestion. The degree of elevation correlates well with the total amount of alcohol intake. Sensitivity and specificity are excellent.

THERAPEUTIC DRUG MONITORING

Therapeutic drug monitoring refers to measuring the concentration of a medication in the blood, usually in the setting of chronic use. Most medications do not require therapeutic drug monitoring—appropriate dosing is based on generally accepted guidelines and the patient's clinical response.

Medications that require regular monitoring tend to be:

- Those that are variably metabolized by different individuals

- Those that have a narrow therapeutic window (a small range of blood concentrations within which the medication is both effective and safe)

If the drug level is too high or too low, the dosage is adjusted accordingly so as to avoid toxicity or ineffectiveness, respectively.

Timing is important when it comes to therapeutic drug monitoring. Drug levels are generally checked either at the drug's *peak* level (the highest concentration; the time to achieve peak levels varies by medication) or at its *trough* level (the lowest concentration; this is the most common timing for testing) in order to standardize the expected normal concentration range. A trough will typically be drawn just before the next dose of the medication, whereas a peak will be drawn at variable times depending on the medication's pharmacokinetics.

Occasionally, random levels may be checked—usually, this occurs in the setting of suspected acute or severe toxicity. In these cases, it is important to take into account when the patient last took the medication to help determine an approximate "therapeutic" or "normal" expected concentration.

A few common examples of medications that typically require therapeutic drug monitoring are provided in Table 23.2.

Do not interpret a report of a normal drug level to mean that the patient must be tolerating the drug well. Drugs can have side effects even at normal or therapeutic blood concentrations.

Table 23.2 Therapeutic Trough Levels for Some Common Medications

Medication	Therapeutic Trough Level
Vancomycin	10-20 µg/mL[a]
Lithium	0.6-1.2 mEq/L
Tacrolimus	5-15 ng/mL[a]
Digoxin	0.8-2.0 ng/mL
Carbamazepine	5-12 µg/mL

[a]Varies depending on the specific indication for treatment.

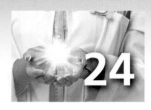

24 Odds and Ends

ROUTINE HEALTH MAINTENANCE

There is no compelling evidence that regular checkups of asymptomatic, healthy patients reduce morbidity or mortality. They do increase the cost to our health care system and can lead to false positives, overdiagnosis, and unnecessary treatment. So why do we bother? Although for most healthy adults there are no clear-cut reasons to insist on an annual evaluation, periodic checkups may nevertheless offer some benefits:

- Strengthen the bond between the patient and the health care provider

- Increase compliance with current screening recommendations and vaccinations

- Mitigate cardiovascular (and other) risk factors

So the decision to undergo the occasional checkup is really a balancing act and should be driven largely by patient preference after a thorough discussion of the pluses and minuses.

What, then, is the role of the laboratory in the periodic "wellness" examination?

Routinely ordering a complete blood count (CBC) or comprehensive metabolic panel (CMP) is not recommended. However, there are a few lab tests that actually do make sense in the right clinical context. Ordering anything beyond the following recommendations should, in most instances, be driven by a focused history and physical examination.

 Diabetes Screening

Guidelines here vary. Some recommend screening all patients of any age who are overweight (body mass index [BMI] ≥25) or have any other risk factors for diabetes mellitus, such as a positive family history. Others suggest that screening should start at age 45 even if there are no risk factors, and that additional screening should be carried out every 3 years. The suggested tests can be either a fasting glucose or hemoglobin A1c (see Chapter 19).

For patients with impaired glucose tolerance who do not meet the criteria for full-blown diabetes, annual screening should be considered.

Lipid Screening

Screening for hyperlipidemia should be part of a patient's overall cardiovascular risk assessment. Regular screening often starts around age 40. One-time screening in late adolescence/early adulthood is also a common practice. In particular, it is reasonable to start at a younger age in patients with a family history of early cardiovascular disease or in those who have multiple cardiovascular risk factors such as hypertension, diabetes, or a smoking history. Although the most commonly ordered test is a complete lipid panel, it is adequate to start with just a non-HDL cholesterol. If the results of lipid screening do not mandate any significant clinical intervention (see Chapter 6), then repeat screening can be carried out every few years.

 ## *Screening for Infectious Diseases*

All individuals 15 to 65 years should be screened at least once for HIV; the CDC recommends starting at age 13. For anyone with ongoing risk factors for HIV, regular screening is recommended and can be done annually or even more often if deemed advisable.

Everyone should be screened one time for hepatitis C infection between the ages of 18 and 79. Patients at high risk should be rescreened as appropriate. The initial test should be for hepatitis C antibodies. If this is positive, then a polymerase chain reaction (PCR) test should be run to assess the viral load. The CDC also recommends one-time screening for hepatitis B for all adults; the recommended tests are a hepatitis B surface antigen and antibody (see Chapter 14).

Screening for other sexually transmitted diseases is discussed in Chapter 14.

 ## *Cancer Screening*

We discussed this topic in Chapter 20, so we will spare you the details here. As far as laboratory testing is concerned, you should become familiar with the recommendations regarding prostate-specific antigen (PSA) testing, cervical cancer, and colon cancer screening.

 ## *Tests That Should Not Be Ordered*

In healthy, asymptomatic individuals without significant risk factors for particular diseases, only the tests mentioned earlier should be considered a routine part of laboratory screening. In particular, tests that are frequently ordered but that are not supported by existing data include a thyroid-stimulating hormone (TSH) and serum iron level. Vitamin D should also not be routinely tested, although it may be appropriate in persons who are exposed to very little sunlight or who have intestinal malabsorption. Despite initial claims to the contrary, vitamin D levels in otherwise healthy individuals do not appear to correlate with meaningful clinical outcomes; it is also unclear what constitutes a "normal" vitamin D level.

The Medicare Wellness Exam

In the United States, as of this writing, Medicare covers the following tests as part of an annual wellness examination:

- Lipid panel

- Diabetes testing, up to two screenings per year for persons at risk

- Hepatitis C, if at risk or if born between 1945 and 1965 (In the latter case, if the patient is not at risk, then the test is approved for one time only.)

- HIV, annually for anyone aged 15 to 65, or anyone below 15 or above 65 if at risk; repeat testing up to 3 times is approved for patients who are pregnant.

- PSA, annually for men over 50

- Sexually transmitted infection (STI) screening—chlamydia, gonorrhea, syphilis, and hepatitis B—for those who are pregnant or who are at risk

PREOPERATIVE EVALUATION

The primary reasons for performing a preoperative evaluation are to identify any acute disorders, chronic illnesses, or significant risk factors that would affect management before, during, or after an invasive procedure and to lower the risk of perioperative complications. Patients requiring emergency surgery should go right to the operating room without waiting for further evaluation. At the other end of the spectrum, patients undergoing low-risk procedures (eg, most ambulatory procedures, cataract surgery, and endoscopic procedures) or who have no significant cardiovascular or other risk factors can also proceed directly to surgery.

The major take-home point here is that routine laboratory testing should be discouraged. It simply hasn't been shown to meaningfully alter outcomes. Only in specific situations is laboratory testing indicated, and even in many of these circumstances, the benefits are unclear. It is safe to say that in the vast majority of cases, the patient's functional status at the time of the planned procedure is far more important than any lab result.

Lab tests that are often considered are listed next, along with the circumstances where they may be helpful. The likelihood of finding something important that had previously gone unrecognized is low. A careful history and targeted physical examination will usually point you in the right direction.

Table 24.1 Targeted Preoperative Laboratory Testing

Lab Test	When It May Prove Useful
Electrolytes	Use of medications that can impact electrolyte balance (most commonly diuretics), underlying renal disease, hypertension
Creatinine	Renal disease, the older adult
Liver function tests	Liver disease of any kind
Glucose and hemoglobin A1c	Diabetes, patients on glucocorticoids
Hemoglobin	Fatigue or dyspnea, history of anemia, renal disease, bone marrow disease (eg, myelodysplasia), patients in whom you anticipate extensive loss of blood during the procedure
White blood cell count	Active infection, myeloproliferative disease, use of medications that suppress the bone marrow
Platelet count and coagulation studies	History of bleeding, liver disease, use of anticoagulant therapy, history of thrombocytopenia
Urinalysis	Signs or symptoms of urinary tract infection, planned urologic procedure
Pregnancy test	Consider in women of childbearing age

THE PATIENT WITH MULTIPLE UNEXPLAINED SYMPTOMS

Many patients are seen for a constellation of nonspecific symptoms persisting for months to years that do not point to a specific diagnosis and therefore challenge the diagnostician. Fatigue is often foremost among these, sometimes accompanied by concerns about diffuse aches and pains, headache, abdominal discomfort, diarrhea, constipation, dizziness, or exertional dyspnea. Provided the patient is up to date on age-appropriate cancer screening— and there is nothing in the history of physical that points to a malignancy (eg, profound weight loss)—the initial laboratory evaluation should typically include the following:

- CBC with differential

- Fasting glucose or hemoglobin A1c

- CMP

- TSH

- Erythrocyte sedimentation rate (ESR) and C-reactive protein (CRP) for those patients above 50 years old in whom you suspect polymyalgia rheumatica

Beyond these tests, which often come back within normal, random shotgunning of various lab tests is likely to prove fruitless and expensive. Rather, further testing should be guided by any signs, symptoms, risk factors, or abnormal initial results that suggest the possibility of one or more specific diseases.

Repetitive testing rarely turns anything up and often encourages patients to continue to seek answers that we, unfortunately, cannot give them with any degree of certainty. However—and we cannot stress this point too much—these patients are truly suffering, and any failure to pin down a precise diagnosis or establish a definitive cause is not their failing, but rather a reflection of the limitations of modern medicine. Even with all the tests at our disposal, we do not have all the answers. A strong and supportive health care provider-patient relationship is critical to achieving a good outcome and limiting unnecessary lab testing and imaging.

Section 4
Wrapping Things Up

So this book has turned out to be a bit longer than we had anticipated. It's just that there are so many lab tests out there, and we didn't want to leave out any of the important ones. You almost certainly won't remember everything you've read and that's ok—you can always look up the details later. But we hope that you've internalized the essential principles of laboratory diagnosis that we've harped on with such annoying persistence:

- A single test result rarely means much in isolation; it is just one part of a bigger picture.

- Know what you want to know, and order only those labs that will get you there. Do not order tests just because they are there and you can.

- Always ask: Will this lab test affect the management of my patient? What will I do with a positive result? With a negative one?

- Involve your patients in the decision-making process because who has more at stake than they do?

Thank you for spending some time with us. We hope you found the journey a useful and enjoyable one. We have been honored to have you join us!

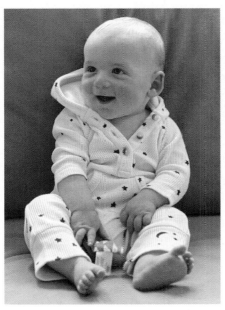

Figure S4.1 Miles Eli Thaler, ready to learn!

INDEX

Note: Page numbers followed by *f* indicate figures; those followed by *t* indicate tables.